Tolliver

Early
Childhood
Stuttering

FOR CLINICIANS BY CLINICIANS

Deanie Vogel and Michael P. Cannito, Series Editors

This book, *Early Childhood Stuttering*, is the 14th book in the For Clinicians by Clinicians series of texts on the diagnosis and clinical management of speech, language, and voice disorders. Each text provides a contemporary perspective on one major disorder or clinical area and is designed for use in clinical methodology courses and continuing education programs. Authors have been selected who represent a broad spectrum of clinical interests and theoretical positions and who hold the common belief that their viewpoints, experiences, and successes should be shared in order to provide a forum for clinicians by clinicians.

The idea for this series came from Dr. Harris Winitz, who served as editor of the series until 1997. During Winitz's tenure as series editor, many important titles were added to the series, including the following volumes: *Treating Language Disorders, Treating Articulation Disorders, Case Studies in Aphasia Rehabilitation, Treating Cerebral Palsy, Alaryngeal Speech Rehabilitation, Treating Disordered Speech Motor Control, Cleft Palate,* and *Language Intervention: Beyond the Primary Grades.*

The last six additions to the series, *Aging and Communication, Alaryngeal Speech Rehabilitation, Evaluation of Dysphagia in Adults, Treating Disordered Motor Speech Control, Vocal Rehabilitation for Medical Speech Language Pathology,* and this book, have been guided by the new series co-editors, Deanie Vogel and Michael P. Cannito. Their intent is to continue the rich tradition of this important series that was established many years ago by Dr. Winitz.

Early Childhood Stuttering

For Clinicians by Clinicians

Ehud Yairi
Nicoline Grinager Ambrose

With chapters by
Elaine Pagel Paden
and Ruth V. Watkins

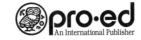

8700 Shoal Creek Boulevard
Austin, Texas 78757-6897
800/897-3202   Fax 800/397-7633
www.proedinc.com

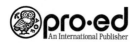

© 2005 by PRO-ED, Inc.
8700 Shoal Creek Boulevard
Austin, Texas 78757-6897
800/897-3202 Fax 800/397-7633
www.proedinc.com

Library of Congress Cataloging-in-Publication Data
Yairi, Ehud.
    Early childhood stuttering for clinicians by clinicians / Ehud Yairi, Nicoline Grinager
    Ambrose ; with chapters by Elaine Pagel Paden and Ruth V. Watkins.
        p. ; cm.—(For clinicians by clinicians)
    Includes bibliographical references and index.
    ISBN 0-89079-985-7 (hardcover : alk. paper)
    1. Stuttering in children.   2. Stuttering in children—Treatment.   I. Ambrose,
Nicoline Grinager.   II. Title.   III. Series.
[DNLM: 1. Stuttering—Child. 2. Stuttering—Infant. WM 475 Y14e 2004]
RJ496.S8Y357 2004
618.92′8554—dc22

                                                                            2004044333

Art Director: Jason Crosier
Designer: Nancy McKinney-Point
This book is designed in Minion and Eras.

Printed in the United States of America

1 2 3 4 5 6 7 8 9 10   08 07 06 05 04

Dedication

To Wendell Johnson—
His theory, research, clinical work, thoughtful writing, and sincere human interest in people who stutter and their families altered the course of the profession and have influenced generations of scholars and clinicians devoted to the advancement of knowledge of stuttering.

Dedication

To Dean Williams—
His broad perspectives, dynamic teaching, research, clinical work, and insight into the minds of people who stutter inspired us to develop our own "point of view about stuttering." Above all, his boundless optimisim and enthusiasm have been contagious.

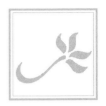

Contents

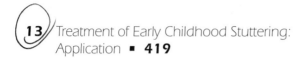

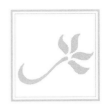

Contributors

Ehud Yairi, PhD, CCC-SLP
University of Illinois
Speech and Hearing Science
901 South Sixth Street
Champaign, IL 61801

Nicoline Grinager Ambrose, PhD, CCC-SLP
University of Illinois
Speech and Hearing Science
901 South Sixth Street
Champaign, IL 61801

Elaine Pagel Paden, PhD, CCC-SLP
Professor Emerita
University of Illinois
Speech and Hearing Science
901 South Sixth Street
Champaign, IL 61801

Ruth V. Watkins, PhD, CCC-SLP
University of Illinois
Speech and Hearing Science
901 South Sixth Street
Champaign, IL 61801

Preface

The idea of writing this book began in the 1990s, during the early years of the University of Illinois Stuttering Research Program. What began as an in-depth 4-year longitudinal study of about 40 children grew into a 14-year study with over 200 children, and we are now embarking upon variations on a theme in a multicenter, 5-year longitudinal study to identify subtypes of stuttering.

Our original agenda was to document the onset and development of early childhood stuttering. As the years went by, we were struck by how clearly the picture we obtained represented ideas at odds with dominant traditional views while reinforcing some old observations that had been either dismissed or rejected. The concept of the book then took on the role of disseminating information, directly observed and carefully documented, on the intricacies of early childhood stuttering. Our agenda, however, has been expanded by presenting new information within the context of past research findings and theoretical ideas pertinent to each topic, and by applying the findings to clinical issues of diagnosis, prognosis, and counseling. Finally, with practicing clinicians and graduate students in mind, we further expanded to include presentation and analysis of past and current approaches to therapy of early childhood stuttering. We hope that readers can share in our discoveries.

Acknowledgments

Foremost we wish to acknowledge the many children and their families who so graciously cooperated in long-term participation in the research project reported herein. Hopefully, their dedication will benefit future children and parents.

We are grateful to the United States National Institutes of Health, National Institute on Deafness and Other Communication Disorders, for its continuous generous financial funding of our research.

We wish to acknowledge the excellent technical support rendered to us by Mark Joseph throughout the many years of this research project.

We also extend our thanks to our colleagues who contributed excellent advice concerning the manuscript for this book. Carol Seery read and made insightful comments on the entire manuscript, Richard Curlee made editorial comments on Chapters 1 through 3, Nancy Cox commented on Chapter 9, and Charles Healey commented on Chapters 12 and 13. Our doctoral student, Jean Sawyer, spent many hours rereading, correcting, proofing, and formatting the entire manuscript. Two other doctoral students, Brent Gregg and Aishah Patterson, helped in many other ways.

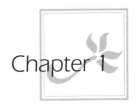

Chapter 1

Early Childhood Stuttering

An Introduction

In this chapter, we establish the general perspective for our book. Although the chapter focuses on research concerning early childhood stuttering conducted at the University of Illinois, the findings are presented within the context of past ideas and research, with special reference to their clinical relevance. The critical significance of information about the early stage of stuttering to the overall epidemiology of the disorder is discussed, and the multiple meaning, dimensionality, and heterogeneity of stuttering are recognized. A guiding theoretical frame of reference is established, stuttering is defined, and the importance and far-reaching influences of definitions of stuttering are explained.

Study Questions

1. *What epidemiological factors can best be investigated during the early stage of stuttering? Explain why.*

2. *What other factors related to stuttering are particularly useful to consider during the early stage of the disorder? List and discuss them.*

3. *What is the critical role of definitions of stuttering in the research and clinical arena?*

Objectives

Casual observers are likely to be impressed by the severe impact that stuttering can have on an individual's ability to communicate verbally. More sophisticated observers, including clinicians, know that stuttering eventually may have devastating consequences in emotional and social domains of the individual's life, and may affect career choice and overall success. Nevertheless, one should not exaggerate or unduly generalize the presence of such consequences from some members to the entire stuttering population. The fact is that individuals who stutter differ markedly not only in the ways they stutter, but also in the scope and degree to which they are affected by and cope with the disorder.

Preschool-age children also vary greatly in their stuttering and their reactions to it. Although they may exhibit very complex stuttering and be seriously affected by it, on the whole they constitute a significant portion of those individuals for whom the effects of the disorder appear to be limited in several respects. Nevertheless, the majority of all cases of stuttering begin in preschool years, and the prevalence of the disorder in very young children is higher than in any other age group in the population at large. Critical developments in stuttering occur in childhood, and several major factors, such as growth of language and phonology skills, have their greatest impact during that period. It is remarkable, therefore, that very few professional books devoted to early childhood stuttering have been published. Those few have focused on important clinical issues but have not included comprehensive presentations and discussions of basic scientific data concerning various domains of the disorder. This book seeks to correct the deficit and is written at a level that speaks to scientists but in a style that should also appeal to students and professional clinicians. It was initially motivated by a desire to consolidate in a single publication the various research activities and publications of the University of Illinois Stuttering Research Program from the 1980s through the present. This research has addressed a wide array of issues concerning the disorder of stuttering and its symptomatology throughout the age range, but undoubtedly its uniqueness can be attributed to the focus on early childhood. In this respect, the book is not limited to a presentation of the Illinois program. Rather, one of its goals is to project our work against a backdrop of the research and theoretical notions of those who preceded us, as well as the work of contemporaries. Thus, we have endeavored to provide a historical perspective and an appreciation of the progress that has been made in the field.

A mere presentation of a series of studies and their findings, however, is incomplete. Consequently, we present an exposition of our views on various aspects of early childhood stuttering related to this research. This is, after all, the fun and more intriguing part of scientific work that has consisted of long hours, over many years, of laborious data collection and analysis for each child and family. One must admit, however, that as long as a number of competing interpretations of stuttering research continue to circulate, the need remains for more and better data to enable scientists to arrive at more definitive answers. We, therefore, view our contributions only as a link in a chain that will probably be broken by future investigators, perhaps ourselves, and replaced with a stronger one that is followed by additional links.

This text was not intended to be a prime source of clinical direction, yet our objective is to emphasize the clinical significance of the findings, as can be seen throughout the chapters and at the conclusion of each chapter. This goal is of great importance. Although natural curiosity is a legitimate motivation in science, the acute needs of substantial segments of the population with communicative disorders provide the strongest justification for pursuing research endeavors motivated by practical considerations. Thus, one of our key aims has been to help fill the void in knowledge about stuttering in young children. Given the generous support from the U.S. government through its National Institutes of Health, National Institute on Deafness and Other Communication Disorders, which has sustained our research, the ultimate aim of shedding light on the clinical concerns of young children who stutter and their families has been paramount.

The University of Illinois Stuttering Research Program has operated with an overarching philosophy that the eventual purpose of much of the research in normal and pathological structures and processes of human communication, even the seemingly "basic science" research, is to generate information that can be used to improve the effectiveness of clinical services provided to those whose communication is impeded, and thus improve their quality of life. The phrase "improve quality of life" has been used so frequently that it has almost become a meaningless cliché. Unfortunately, however, many good people take so much for granted and are simply unable to appreciate what improvement of quality of life may mean to the child or adult who stutters. As a child growing up with severe stuttering, one of us (Yairi) used to cry in school whenever strangers visited the classroom and it was his turn to read aloud. The quality of his life for quite a few years could have been vastly improved if only there had been a way to ameliorate his overt stuttering and reduce the tension of constant anxiety and fear of being called upon to recite in class. Just imagine how the quality of your life would be changed if such fear blocked you from making or answering telephone calls. For example, instead of calling, you would ride the bus to and from the speech clinic just to inform the office that you must cancel your next appointment. Such behaviors are not uncommon among people who stutter. With these thoughts in mind, we stress throughout this text the clinical implications of research findings to diagnosis, prognosis, treatment, and counseling. Additionally, we dedicate four chapters to the evaluation and treatment of early childhood stuttering.

As many investigators, students, and clinicians quickly become aware, even the simplest phenomenon turns out to be increasingly complicated the closer one looks. Thus, as speech–language clinicians will attest, there is no "simple articulation disorder" or "simple language delay," to use once-popular terms. Likewise, there is no "simple, easy stuttering." The more one investigates an individual's stuttering, the deeper is the realization of its tremendous complexity. The multifaceted nature and character of stuttering are apparent from the first attempts to conduct a disfluency count, or from the initial clinical contacts with a child who stutters or a family member of that child. As scholars and clinicians, we understand that stuttering is not merely a disorder of speech. In complex and multidimensional ways, stuttering is interwoven with language and phonological development, cognitive skills, socioemotional competence, and other domains of development. This book recognizes the multidimensionality of stuttering by addressing the association between fluency and other relevant domains.

This book has several additional objectives. First, much stuttering research has yielded conflicting or inconsistent findings, which, for a long time, have been attributed to imprecise measurement techniques and observer disagreement. We have reason to conclude, however, that these varied findings are not the result of the observation techniques but rather the failure to recognize and account for the heterogeneity of those observed—that is, the people who stutter. Thus, we seek to highlight heterogeneity. Second, findings of the Illinois studies, primarily those related to epidemiology and etiology, have important implications for future research in childhood stuttering. In this book we want to emphasise these implications, which must be taken into consideration in order to build a stronger scientific basis of knowledge and clinical practice. Finally, we intend to place all of the findings, conclusions, and interpretations within a unifying theoretical framework that provides direction for future research.

Early Childhood Stuttering

Our focus on early childhood stems from a number of critical observations about stuttering and relevant research. First, there is overwhelming evidence that stuttering typically begins during the preschool years. Second, its onset occurs during a critical period of speech and language development, and strong evidence indicates that stuttering is associated with language functions. Third, stuttering occurs during a period of rapid neuromotor development and appears to involve problems in motor control. Fourth, stuttering begins and evolves during a period when the home environment has enormous influences on the child and on shaping of the disorder. Fifth, even though stuttering has been viewed as a single disorder, for the most part, present evidence points toward the diversity of subtypes that emerge during formative stages of the disorder. In support of our reasoning, it is interesting to note that approximately 5% of preschool-age children experience episodes of stuttering, but less than 1% of adults stutter. Nevertheless, until 20 years ago, more than 80% of basic and clinical research focused on issues and characteristics of adults who stutter (M. R. Adams, 1986). The result was a knowledge base that is incomplete and fragmented, with many key questions remaining unaddressed and unanswered. We believe that scientific information about early childhood stuttering is essential to establishing a sound theoretical grounding of the disorder, to planning a coherent line of scholarly inquiry, and to evaluating and interpreting research findings in a meaningful manner.

Epidemiological Factors

One of the most important domains of study of any disorder is its epidemiology—the relationship of various factors determining the frequency and distribution of the disorder. How many persons are affected? Where do they live? When does the disorder strike, and how long does it last? What are its signs and symptoms? What segments of the population (e.g., age, gender, race, socioeconomic class) are affected? Is it a familial disorder? Are there different subtypes? What are the personal characteristics of those affected? Although a considerable amount of sophisticated research employing the most advanced techniques has examined various aspects of stuttering, some of these basic questions have not been adequately researched. The absence of reasonably accurate epidemiological data has impeded progress in formulating credible theories of stuttering, designing research studies that adequately represent the stuttering population, applying genetic models to stuttering, planning clinical services, selecting appropriate clinical intervention strategies, and addressing many other critical issues.

Epidemiology reveals a great deal about the nature of a disorder, a fact that stuttering illustrates very well. Although stuttering affects a substantial number of people across a wide age range, including late adulthood, epidemiology indicates that it is, in several important respects, a disorder that triumphs in early childhood. The overriding basis for such a statement is that early childhood is *the* period when the representation of the stuttering population (i.e., those who ever stutter) is substantially superior to that of any later period in life. The following sections discuss various epidemiological factors that give weight to the view of stuttering as a disorder of early childhood.

Onset

Early childhood is the period when stuttering most often begins. According to data from our large sample, a great majority of stuttering onsets occur from 20 to 48 months of age, with a mean of 34 months. Undoubtedly, the biggest risk is in the lower half of this limited age range. Although Gavin Andrews (1984) concluded that 75% of the risk for stuttering is over by age 6, we suspect that a higher percentage (approximately 90%) of the risk is already over 2 years earlier, by 4 years of age. The Danish investigator Mansson (2000), who surveyed a whole population on the island of Bornholm, seems to agree that relatively few new onsets occur after age 3 or 4.

Natural Recovery

The early years of life are also the period when stuttering ends of its own accord without formal treatment (i.e., natural recovery) for a large majority of cases (Yairi & Ambrose, 1999a). Although natural recoveries can occur at any age, data reported by others, as well as our own, show that most natural recoveries occur from a few months to 3 years after stuttering began during the preschool years. Considerably more often than not, the entire cycle of a stuttering disorder, from beginning to end, is completed in early childhood.

Gender Distribution

Gender distribution is another key issue that underscores the special significance of early childhood stuttering to understanding the disorder. A common concept about stuttering has been that it is characterized by a substantial gender difference, in which males outnumber females at ratios that are usually estimated to vary from 3:1 to 6:1 in school-age children (Bloodstein, 1995). However, stuttering is much more evenly distributed between the genders during its earlier stages, with male-to-female ratios as low as 1:1 (Yairi, 1983) and 1.6:1 (Kloth, Janssen, Kraaimaat, & Brutten, 1995) reported near the time of onset. Because the ratio of males to females does increase with age, eventually reaching or surpassing a 6:1 ratio, it is reasonable to hypothesize that more girls recover from stuttering than boys, or more boys begin stuttering at later ages, or some combination of both. There is strong evidence to support the first option. First, data gathered from direct observations throughout our longitudinal studies (Yairi & Ambrose, 1999a) indicate a greater tendency for girls to recover. Second, our data and those of others show that much of the risk for children to begin stuttering is over after age 4, and certainly after age 6. Thus, the decreasing number of stuttering onsets cannot account for the large increase in ratio of males to females who stutter, and Bloodstein's (1995) contention that a substantial number of new stuttering cases continue to appear during school years is not well founded. In our opinion, stuttering must be studied in early childhood to fully appreciate the gender, especially the female, factor in this disorder.

Parents and Other Relatives

Regardless of one's view about stuttering, its roots in early childhood make it impossible to disregard the potentially important role of parents, either as contributors to its etiology or in shaping stuttering during its critical formative period—the early years of life (Yairi, 1997a). This is the time when parents and other family members (e.g., siblings, grandparents) have their prime influence on shaping the child. Keeping in mind unquestionable evidence concerning strong genetic components to stuttering, in many cases the role of parents is very direct in transmitting the disorder to their children. For example, up to 40% of children who stutter have parents, mainly fathers, or siblings who have stuttered, and up to 70% are raised in families with histories of stuttering in the extended circle of relatives. Although all parents are major sources of influence on children, those who have stuttered are likely to contribute special effects, not only in terms of their genes, but in terms of feelings, attitudes, and behaviors that reflect their personal experiences with the disorder. Yairi (1997a) concluded that, although the weight of the evidence does *not* support the view that parents of stutterers have abnormal personalities or suffer obvious emotional or adjustment problems, there have been repeated reports that these parents tend to experience heightened levels of anxiety and to be overprotective and anxious about their children compared to parents of normally fluent children. Other reports indicate that parents of children who stutter tend to hold negative evaluations of their children's personalities, which are also perceived by the children. Finally, there have been consistent reports of overt, sometimes negative, parental reactions to a child's stuttering.

As stuttering children become older, however, studies of their parents and other relatives become increasingly less important. As time passes, the value of parents' reports concerning the time when stuttering began, as well as of studies of their personalities, child-rearing practices, and responses to the child's stuttering, is greatly diminished. Thus, if parents are important in regard to stuttering, their primacy also supports the importance of studying the disorder in early childhood.

Epidemiologic Factors Combined

As children who stutter grow older, their stuttering follows one of its two most obvious developmental tracks—natural recovery and persistence—and the demography of the stuttering population undergoes substantial change. Not only does the incidence of new cases fall to low levels, but large numbers of this population exhibit natural recoveries. Many boys and increasingly higher percentages of girls who once stuttered are no longer members of the stuttering population, and the nature of their special characteristics and those of their parents are lost to further studies of the disorder. Undoubtedly, when investigators of stuttering examine adults, older children, or even young children 2 years or more after onset, they are looking at a biased, nonrepresentative sample of the people who ever stuttered. Those remaining in the sample are primarily males who have persisted in stuttering and represent a minority of the original population. The evidence strongly suggests that persons who recover from stuttering differ genetically from those who do not, which indicates that the validity of many findings and conclusions of past research has been diminished by the use of grossly biased samples of older stutterers.

Other Factors

Personality

There are additional reasons for placing high value on the study of stuttering in early childhood; however, these reasons do not involve factors that are classically epidemiological in nature. Personality is one of them. Although related to the issue of parental influences, it warrants separate discussion.

Theories suggesting that stuttering results from difficulties in personality development during early childhood were quite popular during the first two thirds of the 20th century. Psychoanalytic perspectives, in particular, exerted a major influence. Brill in 1923 and Glauber as late as 1958, as well as others during this period, expressed the view that stuttering is a symptom of a psychosexual fixation that originates from a child's unconscious conflicts over unsatisfied needs. It was also suggested that these conflicts could be traced to neurotic parental personalities and their conflict-motivated behaviors. Extensive research of the personality and emotional adjustments of persons who stutter, however, yielded inconsistent findings, with the majority of the better designed studies providing negative results. Consequently, the prevailing view for the past 35 years or so has been that people who stutter, as a group, do not exhibit significant emotional maladjustment or specific personality traits. Currently, however, there seems to be a renewal of interest in this domain.

Recent models of stuttering (e.g., Conture, 2001; G. D. Riley & Riley, 2000; A. Smith & Kelly, 1997) propose that personality factors, such as children's temperaments as expressed in sensitivity and self-perceptions, in addition to parents' temperaments and attitudes (Yairi, 1997a), influence the developmental course of stuttering. For the most part, these views have emphasized manifestations of personality in adults and school-age children who stutter. For example, school-age children who stutter are perceived by their mothers as having more sensitive temperaments and being more behaviorally inhibited than nonstuttering peers (Glasner, 1949; Oyler, 1996; Oyler & Ramig, 1995). Preliminary evidence is beginning to accumulate with regard to stuttering preschoolers' specific temperament traits, such as sensitivity, inhibition, reactivity, and others. This research suggests that preschoolers who stutter tend to have more negative attitudes about speaking (Ezrati-Vinacour, Platzky, & Yairi, 2001; Vanryckeghem & Brutten, 1997) and temperaments that are more sensitive and inhibited (Anderson, Pellowski, & Conture, 2001; Embrechts, Ebben, Franke, & van de Poel, 2000; Wakaba, 1998) than their nonstuttering peers. Insofar as it is believed that such traits are present at birth, are relatively stable over time, and operate during infancy and early childhood to form the foundation for later personality characteristics (Caspi, 1998), childhood stuttering should also be viewed from this perspective.

The Linguistic Connection

Linguistic factors have been considered as relevant to stuttering since the early investigation of S. Brown (1945) demonstrated their strong influence on the loci of stutters (i.e., the location in utterances where stuttering events occur). Later investigators became interested in the possible interplay of stuttering with such linguistic variables as phonology, language skills, and language complexity. Several investigators reported that children who stutter fall below norms in acquiring phonological skills (e.g., Louko, Edwards, & Conture, 1990), and Ryan (1992) reported that they tend to be delayed in their acquisition of language skills. Still other researchers reported that language complexity is a factor in stuttering (Au-Yeung, Howell, & Pilgrim, 1998), and some went so far as to suggest that stuttering is basically a disorder of language development (e.g., Chevekeva, 1967). On the other hand, our research over the past 13 years has found that children who stutter fall well within the normal range for language skills, and some, in fact, exceed normal limits. As a group, however, their phonological development tends to be a bit delayed.

In spite of a rich research history, there is no consensus on the precise role or contributions of linguistic variables to the onset of stuttering, its persistence, or natural recovery. Nevertheless, the fact that most cases of stuttering begin between ages 2 and 4, especially at ages 2 and 3 — precisely during the period when complex language, articulatory, and phonological skills are acquired and expanded (Yairi, 1983; Yairi & Ambrose, 1999a) — appears to be more than an interesting coincidence. Although conflicting findings have been reported in the past 15 years, particularly those indicating a slower pace of language development, interest in linguistic variables has shifted to other directions of inquiry, specifically imbalances or asynchronies in various aspects of verbal proficiency that are essential for the formulation and production of language, imbalances or asynchronies that might result in stuttering. In any event, the possible interactions between (a) the onset and progress of stuttering and (b) children's emerging speech and language skills further support the view of stuttering as a disorder rooted in early childhood and developmental processes.

Neuromotor Aspects

Kent (1999) stated that "ultimately it should be possible to frame speech development within a timetable of typical neural development" (p. 46).

Stuttering is a disorder that involves both motor speech control and language functions. Consequently, persons interested in understanding stuttering should also be interested in the development of neurological structures and processes that underlie language and speech functions. Because such information on these structures and processes is somewhat limited at present, we await further research advances regarding the development of, for example, neurotransmitters, neuronal interconnections, myelination, and hemispheric control, *in utero* and after birth. A closely related concept to such biological development is brain plasticity (i.e., the adaptive structural and functional changes that occur during development and in response to pathological conditions). We are intrigued by Dennis's (2000) ideas (a) that challenge the belief that there is greater brain plasticity in children compared to adolescents and adults, (b) that developmental plasticity cannot be understood solely by the age factor, and (c) that some impairments in young children increase in severity over time, some do not disappear with age, and new deficits may emerge later after injury. This perspective is compatible with our focus on the formative stages of stuttering during the early childhood period. Clearly, understanding of childhood speech disorders is closely tied to understanding the development of normal speech.

The Critical Period

A central, key point of the previous discussion is that much information concerning stuttering can be obtained only in early childhood, near its onset. Because of time-related changes that take place in stuttering and in a growing child, it is not possible to understand and generalize information about childhood stuttering from observations of the disorder in older groups. For example, many adults who stutter have strong fears about speaking and avoid speaking, or even being present, in situations likely to involve speaking. Such reactions have led to theories about the role of anxiety in the etiology of stuttering (Brutten & Shoemaker, 1967; Sheehan, 1958); however, clinicians and researchers who have frequent contact with young children who have just begun stuttering are usually impressed that a majority show no clear indications of even being aware of their speaking irregularities. Although some children show signs of frustration with their speech, rarely do they evidence anxiety reactions to their stuttering or speech in general.

Nevertheless, many years passed before the simple facts discussed above made an impact on the scientific activities of experts in the field. Until the mid-1980s, there was a dearth of physiologic data for childhood stuttering, only one large study of stuttering onset (Johnson et al., 1959), a single developmental study of reasonable size (Andrews & Harris, 1964), and no appropriately controlled treatment study of preschool children. As recently as 1986, Adams reported that most published research and clinical studies in this area have focused on adults who stutter. As late as 2002, at the time of this writing, in spite of commendable progress to achieving better balance, only three of the currently funded National Institutes of Health grants that support stuttering research are focused on young children who stutter. Because advanced stuttering often, but not always, differs from its incipient form, tending to be more complex, and because the population of adults who stutter appears to comprise a minority of 25% or less of all people who ever stutter, individuals who attempt to draw inferences about the etiology, nature, and treatment of stuttering based on data derived from adults, should recognize the limitations of their conclusions.

During the past 25 years, however, a few investigators, including our research group, began making dedicated efforts to bring research closer in time to the event of stuttering onset than ever before. Several studies (Yairi, 1983; Yairi & Ambrose, 1992b) reported unexpectedly large proportions of sudden onsets, many cases evidencing early struggled speech and concomitant physical or emotional stress. Many severe cases near stuttering onset were also reported (Yairi, Ambrose, & Niermann, 1993), as were marked differences in frequency, type, and duration of disfluencies near stuttering onset (Ambrose & Yairi, 1995, 1999; Zebrowski, 1991). Associated facial or head movements, long regarded as a later development, were found in beginning stutterers (Conture & Kelly, 1991; H. D. Schwartz & Conture, 1988), as was awareness of stuttering (Ambrose & Yairi, 1994). Physiologic aspects of laryngeal function were examined (Conture, Rothenberg, & Molitor, 1986), as well as acoustic characteristics (K. D. Hall & Yairi, 1992; Subramanian, Yairi, & Amir, 2003; Yaruss & Conture, 1993), phonological processes (Louko et al., 1990), language development (Bernstein Ratner, 1997; Bernstein Ratner & Sih, 1987; Logan & Conture, 1995; Ryan, 1992), and genetic aspects (Ambrose, Cox, & Yairi, 1997). Consequently, views of the early stage of stuttering as involving complex, diverse phenomena have been replacing long-held views of its onset and development as a simple, uniform, linear phenomenon. We do not believe, however, that early stuttering is fundamentally different from advanced stuttering.

A Theoretical Framework

A significant barrier to effective research, diagnosis, and treatment of stuttering has been the tendency of most investigators and clinicians to view stuttering as a single disorder—a pathognomonic monolith (St. Onge, 1963)—in spite of its readily apparent diversity. Although theoretical issues will be addressed in more detail later in this book, at this juncture we point out that, in contrast to this historical tradition, our general view of stuttering emphasizes its variability. Although we believe that only a few genes may be necessary for the behavior to develop, and that these genes may result in a relatively straightforward anatomical–physiological abnormality, our model involves the interaction of the effects of these genes with other genes and with multiple environmental factors, resulting in subtype diversity.

We assume that subtype differentiation is grounded in genetics and shaped by environment (Ambrose et al., 1997). Furthermore, the disorder of stuttering emerges and advances in young children due to a multilevel complex of genetic and environmental factors related to dynamic systems involving speech, language, motor, and psychosocial aspects. By dynamic, we mean that the timing and degree of influence of these domains or factors vary considerably, so that the disorder is nonlinear and does not progress or change systematically from simple to more complex forms along a steadily escalating path. Thus, differences in genetic loading and environment affecting speech and language processes, motor function, and psychosocial behaviors are reflected in different subtypes, as seen in varied symptom patterns and developmental courses. Nevertheless, certain characteristics are shared by all subtypes. Additionally, there is considerable fluidity (change of balance) within domains. Guided by this premise, we did not limit ourselves to a search for any predetermined subtypes, but we carefully documented stuttering and developmental characteristics across several domains of interest in children from close to onset to well into the school years. The data speak for themselves. The patterns that have emerged are presented in the remainder of the book.

Definitions: What Is Stuttering and Who Is Stuttering?

The importance of a workable definition of stuttering appears to be unappreciated. Indeed, researchers and clinicians alike have worked for years without a formal, widely accepted definition of stuttering. Many of the definitions used seem to be confounded with explanations. This state of affairs is exemplified by the tongue-in-cheek observation that everyone knows what stuttering is except the expert. However, the failure to define what stuttering is and clarify who is a person who stutters (i.e., a "stutterer") has had a significant impact in several fundamental ways that may not be fully appreciated by many academicians, speech–language clinicians, other professionals, students in the field, and the general public.

The Role of the Definition of Who Is Stuttering: A Point of View

A definition provides a powerful reference and general orientation to the disorder of stuttering. Definitions of "who is stuttering" that focus primarily on speech characteristics or personality dynamics would have direct influence on theory, understanding what phenomena are important, determining how the disorder is researched, and seeking approaches to its treatment. Clinicians educated in academic institutions where stuttering is defined or explained as an outward expression of inner emotional conflicts would likely emphasize counseling or perhaps other psychotherapeutic methods in treatment. Clinicians educated in academic centers where stuttering is defined by the presence of excessive numbers of certain types of disfluencies would likely administer speech modification techniques. Those from academic centers where stuttering is viewed as learned behavior might apply operant conditioning techniques in treatment. Thus, the road from abstract definitions to the practicality of treatment is short.

Points of Entry and Exit

One critical point for the role of definition is when parents need to decide whether their child has begun to stutter, which is the *point of entry*.[1] One of the most influential theories of stuttering (Johnson et al., 1959) proposed that the onset of stuttering involves a remarkable case of definitional confusion in which parents fail to distinguish between what falls under stuttering and what falls under normally disfluent speech. Such definitional confusion, revealed in mistakenly labeling certain normal speech

---

[1]We believe that the terms *point of entry* and *point of exit* in this context were used by Wendell Johnson but have been unable to identify the source.

phenomena as "stuttering," constitutes the very heart of the etiology of stuttering in young children. According to this theory, there would be no disorder of stuttering if parents would only define stuttering properly. The theory has had far-reaching consequences with long-lasting implications for clinical management philosophies and strategies for treating childhood stuttering. One specific consequence was guilt-instilling counseling provided to millions of innocent parents for several decades. This illustrates the enormous potential effects that a definition of stuttering may have, and not only in the theoretical sphere.

Once parents decide that their child is stuttering, clinicians face the challenge of having to make a professional diagnostic determination of the presence or absence of what they believe to be stuttering and to decide whether or not treatment is warranted. At a later point in time, they and the parents will have to determine whether the child is still stuttering and decide whether to continue or terminate treatment. That is the *point of exit*. In all of these decisions—when one enters the class of people who stutter and when one gets out of it, and when to initiate and when to terminate treatment—the role of definition is critical. Its consequences extend beyond the professional judgments and have ethical and financial implications, as well. Speech therapy can be expensive regardless of who is paying, parents or insurance companies. In our experience as investigators and clinicians, there has been very close agreement between us and the parents on the point of entry (i.e., that a child is doing a sufficient amount of stuttering to exhibit the disorder). There has been more discrepancy, however, between us and the parents on the exit point (i.e., when the child no longer belongs to the population of children who stutter). Surprisingly, in the majority of cases with differences of opinion, it is the parents who feel that the child has stopped stuttering, or at least does not exhibit a stuttering disorder, while we continue to perceive stuttering events in the child's speech and consider the child as still exhibiting the disorder. Although the point of entry is based on a decision of "what is stuttering," when it comes time for the point-of-exit decision, it is possible that the parents are shifting the frame of reference to applying the "who is a stutterer" question and are not considering any remnants of stuttering to be a problem any longer.

In practical terms, then, should termination of treatment be based on parents' or clinicians' definitions? Should it consider only what the World Health Organization considers functioning factors (body function and structure) or also consider disability (activity/participation) and contextual (environment and personal) factors (see Curlee, 1993a; Yaruss &

Quesal, 2004)? How long should parents or health insurance companies continue to pay for treatment of a disorder that they believe has ceased to exist? On whose definition should they base the decision, theirs or ours? As can be seen, what appears to be an abstract issue may have serious personal, financial, and moral implications.

Research: Who To Include?

Similarly, definitional issues have had a substantial impact on stuttering research, beginning with the basic task in the study of any disorder: determining its incidence and prevalence. The question of who should be counted is straightforward but not simple. To identify and count people who stutter, investigators are immediately confronted with questions about what are the characteristics of stuttering (i.e., its signs and symptoms) and how much of these characteristics is sufficient to identify a given person as "a stutterer" or, as some prefer, "a person who stutters." Few probably realize that incidence data can have a direct impact on other types of stuttering research, such as genetics. Various genetic models of stuttering are tested by comparing familial distribution of stuttering cases against the distribution assumed for the population. Thus, genetic knowledge depends on incidence data, which, in turn, depend heavily on definitions of who stutters. Genetics is not an isolated example; the quality and meaningfulness of all stuttering research rest on definitions. Such research begins with selecting participants for the stuttering (experimental) and nonstuttering (control) groups. In the latter case, the challenge is to decide what are *not* characteristics of stuttering and who is *not* a stutterer. Frequently, participants in past research were included in the experimental group on the basis of the simplistic argument that they were "regarded" to exhibit stuttering or because they were enrolled in stuttering treatment programs, and no other criteria were given. Likewise, participants were included as control subjects because they were "not regarded" to exhibit stuttering, even though stuttering was never defined.

Research: What To Measure?

The importance of definition extends into more advanced forms of stuttering research in which investigators study the effects of various independent variables on the dependent variable (i.e., stuttering events). For example, the effects of such independent variables as noise, time pressure, electrical shock, therapy, and the passage of time on various aspects of stuttering events have been studied. A fundamental question for all of these types of studies is, What has to be measured in order to document any "changes in stuttering" that may result from the numerous experimental conditions employed?

Complications

Defining the disorder of stuttering has proved to be such a difficult task that it is yet to be successfully accomplished in spite of numerous attempts over the years. Aside from the fact that many proposed definitions have been expressions of various points of view regarding the etiology or "nature" of the disorder or descriptions of selected characteristics rather than a definition, they also differ so greatly that one must wonder if all of them refer to the same disorder. For example, stuttering has been conceived by Coriat (1943) to be a psychoneurosis; by Eisenson (1958) to be a transient disturbance in communicative propositional language usage; by Van Riper (1971) to be a temporal disruption of the simultaneous and successive programming of muscular movement in the production of speech; and by Brutten and Shoemaker (1967) to be a form of fluency failure that results from conditioned negative emotion. According to just these four definitions, stuttering is described as a psychiatric disorder, a language disorder, a motor disorder, and a learned disorder, but more could be added. Perkins (1990), for instance, explained stuttering as an involuntary disruption of the continuing attempt to produce a spoken utterance whose key symptom is the speaker's feeling of loss of control of his or her speech. Thus, stuttering events are whatever the person who stutters feels them to be regardless of what listeners perceive.

Several reasons may account for these definitional difficulties. First is the multidimensionality of the disorder of stuttering. Clinical experience with persons who stutter soon leads to the realization that the disorder cuts across several domains of human characteristics and functions. Clinicians are well aware that stuttering disorders are not limited to disfluent speech, especially in older children and adults, and are frequently associated with physical tension, emotional reactions, and changes in cognitive processes. Furthermore, those familiar with stuttering through laboratory research also know that a host of other factors, including motoric, neurological, and linguistic features, also are associated with the disorder. Such complexity does not easily lend itself to a cohesive, all-inclusive definition but seems to invite observers to focus on just one or two domains or aspects of stuttering to the neglect, or insufficient consideration, of the entire disorder.

A second reason stems from confusion in the conceptualization of stuttering as a disorder in relation to stuttering events and, therefore, to what needs to be defined. For instance, is the disorder merely a surface phenomenon, comprising observable speaking difficulties and physical tensions, or is it a more general disorder, whose overt speech characteristics are but one symptom? Is it limited to verbal expression, or is it a disorder that involves the entire motor system? Or, is it a complex disorder that involves several systems and is expressed in functions other than just speech? Many discussions of stuttering fail to distinguish between the disorder of stuttering and stuttering events.

A third reason is the conceptual dichotomy between what listeners perceive as "stuttering" and a speaker's perceptions of "stuttering" (Perkins, 1990). In the latter case, stuttering might constitute a variety of different behaviors, processes, and experiences, such as loss of control, for different people who perceive themselves to stutter.

Clarifications

It is important to reduce some of the confusion about stuttering by recognizing the difference between defining stuttering in terms of speech events and defining it as a disorder afflicting persons who stutter or are perceived by listeners as being stutterers. Although these are related concepts, they are certainly not identical. Consider, for example, the following four possibilities:

1. A speech event that occurs in isolation may be perceived by listeners as normal, but when the frequency of such "normal" events exceeds certain limits in a person's speech, listeners are likely to perceive him or her as a stutterer.
2. A speech event that is perceived as normal in isolation or in the speech of a person considered to be a normal speaker, may be perceived as stuttering, even in isolation, when produced by a person believed to be a stutterer.
3. A speaker may produce one or more speech events, each of which is perceived in isolation as stuttering if listeners are asked to make yes–no judgments. Yet, if the events are produced infrequently enough, the speaker may still be perceived as normally disfluent.

4. A speaker may rarely, if ever, produce speech events that listeners perceive as stuttering but still may regard himself or herself as a stutterer.

Thus, some speech events may be perceived as stuttering not on their own merit but by virtue of who the speaker is, even though the same speech events coming out of a different mouth are perceived as perfectly normal. Such perceptual relativity is not uncommon for disorders of communication. Those who work with voice disorders realize that a high-pitched voice, which is normal for a 12-year-old boy, is likely to be perceived as grossly abnormal for a 25-year-old man. These examples simply illustrate that, even when confined to the most obvious surface phenomena (e.g., speech disfluency), definitions of *stuttering* or *stutterer* cannot be limited to absolute terms that describe overt speech characteristics. A specific speech feature, in itself, is not always sufficient. Its length, frequency of appearance, and distribution in a person's speech are extremely important influences on listeners' perceptions of what is normal or abnormal. Other factors, including the identity of the speaker, the speaker's beliefs about his or her speech, and, of course, the listener's perceptual set, all bear influence.

An Index of Stuttering

The World Health Organization's (1977) definition of stuttering—"disorders of rhythm of speech in which the individual knows precisely what he wishes to say, but at times is unable to say it because of involuntary, repetitive prolongation or cessation of a sound" (p. 202)—gives considerable weight to the inner experiences of the person while also including the basic symptomatology. It is our position that, whatever else the clinical disorder of stuttering entails, there seems to be relatively little disagreement that the term *stuttering* refers to the domain of motor speech production and its disruption by speech disfluencies. Physical, physiological, cognitive, and emotional components, regardless of how frequent or intense they might be, would not be labeled as "stuttering" if they did not accompany a speaker's disfluent speech. In light of the difficulties just discussed, we decided to employ a statistical approach to operationally defining, identifying, determining, and quantifying stuttering as events and, in turn, children who stutter.

As Bloodstein (1970) suggested for many years, we conceptualize stuttering in terms of *probability* based on both speech production and perception. That is, we consider those speech characteristics that young children who stutter tend to produce, and those that are likely to be judged by listeners as stuttering. Thus, children considered to stutter are inclined to exhibit interruptions in the flow of speech in the form of repetition of parts of words (e.g., sounds and syllables) and monosyllabic words, as well as by disrhythmic phonations—that is, prolongations of sounds and arrests of speech (blocks). We have referred to these overt speech phenomena as *stuttering-like disfluencies* (SLD). These are the most common disfluencies produced by children who stutter, as well as the speech events most likely to be perceived as stuttering (e.g., Yairi, 1996). These three elements also were listed in the definition suggested by the American Speech-Language-Hearing Association (1999).

Stuttering-like disfluency does not identify or precisely isolate whatever we believe stuttering to be. We simply count those types of disfluencies that have a high statistical probability of occurring in the speech of children who are perceived to be stuttering. Even though SLD are the most common speech disfluencies observed in children who stutter and are also readily identified by listeners as stuttering, we recognize that just about any type of speech disfluency, including interjections of "um" or repetitions of short phrases, may be perceived as stuttering under certain circumstances. Thus, we acknowledge the possibility of a two-way error: A relatively small percentage of the SLD counted may not be perceived by many listeners as stuttering, and other disfluency types present in a child's speech but not counted may be perceived as stuttering. We believe, however, that in the absence of a measure that assures the consistent and exact quantification of stuttering on all occasions for all people, an index that reflects the most relevant features of stuttering, most of the time for most people, is appropriate (Yairi, Watkins, Ambrose, & Paden, 2001), and we are willing to accept, as Conture (2001) suggested, a certain amount of error. SLD provide such an index, which we have used in our research program for a number of years to quantify stuttering in young children. Furthermore, the term *stuttering-like disfluency* is appropriate (a) in that by "like" we mean "characteristic of" and (b) given the fact that judgments of overt speech behavior as "stuttering" are made in the ear of the listener, and these judgments can be rather fluid (e.g., Curlee, 1981; Curran & Hood, 1977; Williams & Kent, 1958). *Stuttering-like disfluency* is also an appropriate term because what the listener hears as stuttering might be but the surface aspect of the disorder.

Admittedly, our use of this index has irked several investigators for a variety of reasons. Wingate (2001) objected to the inclusion of monosyllabic-word repetition as stuttering, whereas R. J. Ingham and Bothe (2001) argued that stuttering events can be determined only by direct listener judgments. As long as most scholars are uncertain about what stuttering really is, we believe that the link between disfluent behaviors and stuttering should be made in terms of what is *statistically* most probable to reflect both frequency of occurrence in persons who stutter and what listeners perceive as stuttering, rather than preconceived theoretical notions of what stuttering is or ought to be.

Chapter 2

The Illinois Longitudinal Studies

This chapter sets the stage for discussion of the main research project that is in the center of this book. Following a brief historical account of the University of Illinois Stuttering Research Program, we provide general information concerning the longitudinal investigation of the development of stuttering, such as descriptions of the general population from which children were drawn, the epidemiological principles for the study, and criteria for subject selection. We summarize descriptive information for the participating children, such as age, gender, racial and ethnic background, and stuttering severity scores. The methods of the study—parent interview, recording, testing, and follow-up—are described in details that provide guidance and practical hints for clinicians.

Study Questions

1. Why are comparative normative developmental disfluency data for children who stutter and normally speaking children important for theoretical and clinical purposes?

2. What considerations are important in selecting samples of children for research concerning the development of stuttering?

3. What methods were used to assess stuttering severity by the experimenters and by parents? Discuss.

Background

The University of Illinois Stuttering Research Program as currently known was established in 1977 when Ehud Yairi joined the faculty of the university's Department of Speech and Hearing Science. Historically, however, its roots can be traced to a series of studies of early childhood stuttering conducted or directed by Yairi during the early 1970s at Texas Tech University: Yairi and Clifton (1972) compared the disfluent speech of preschool children, high school students, and geriatric persons; Yairi and Jennings (1974) examined the relationship between disfluency of preschool children and that of their parents; and Yairi's student, Gail Roman (1972), wrote a master's thesis that compared the disfluent speech characteristics of parents of children who stutter with a group of control parents. These investigations indicated a turn in the direction of Yairi's first scientific activities related to stuttering, which had focused on the school-age population (e.g., Yairi, 1972; Yairi & Williams, 1970, 1971), although research with other groups, including those with Down syndrome (Otto & Yairi, 1976) and brain damage (Yairi, Gintautas, & Avent, 1981), and conditions, such as noise (Yairi, 1976), continued for a while. From the early 1970s, the primary focus of Yairi's research has been on the early stages of stuttering and specifically on preschool-age children.

After moving to the University of Illinois in 1977, Yairi used small university research grants to carry out investigations of speech disfluency in normally speaking 2- and 3-year-old children (Yairi, 1981, 1982a), stuttering onset (Yairi, 1983), disfluent speech near onset (Yairi & Lewis, 1984), and other topics. During the early 1980s, Yairi initiated a small, longitudinal study of preschool-age children who stutter. Influenced by widely accepted developmental systems or models that depicted stuttering as progressively increasing in frequency and complexity (Bloodstein, 1961; Bluemel, 1932; Van Riper, 1954), Yairi began to record speech samples of a small group of 30 stuttering children at periodic intervals to quantify and document the natural evolution of stuttering. This preliminary investigation, the results of which were published by Yairi and Ambrose (1992a), led to the development of a protocol that has formed the foundation for the main research endeavor at the University of Illinois Stuttering Research Program during the last 15 years. The program has received the generous and continuous support of the National Institute on Deafness and Other Communication Disorders (NIDOCD), part of the National Institutes of Health, since 1989. Nicoline Ambrose, now the codirector of the program, first joined as a graduate assistant while working on her master's degree. She became research associate and project coordinator when National Institutes of Health funding was initially awarded, while also working toward her doctoral degree. Kelly Hall, the first doctoral student in the program, helped establish the laboratory and set the pace for other doctoral students, including Nicoline Ambrose, Rebecca Throneburg, Ofer Amir, Anu Subramanian, Shu Lan Yang, Brent Gregg, and Jean Sawyer. There were also many graduate assistants working on master's degrees who performed the tedious, exacting, and crucial job of transcribing speech samples that provided the basic data for many of our studies. Additionally, several faculty members, particularly Elaine Paden, Ruth Watkins, and Adele Proctor from the University of Illinois and Nancy Cox from the University of Chicago, made critical contributions to this research program. Together, all involved formed a research team dedicated to the long-term, intensive study of childhood stuttering.

Over the years, the Illinois stuttering program has expanded considerably. At the time of this publication, the program is composed of five major components: development of stuttering, stuttering in African American children, genetics of stuttering, subtypes of stuttering, and imaging studies. The first four have been supported with different grants from the NIDOCD. This book is based primarily on the project pertaining to the development of stuttering.

Objectives

Despite all of the published descriptions of early stuttering, how it changes over time, and theoretical accounts of its onset and progression, basic normative data about such characteristics of stuttering as the amount and type of disfluency that occurs at different age levels were not available toward the latter part of the 20th century. This contrasts noticeably with the knowledge available about disorders of language and phonology; clinicians treating children with these disorders have a pretty good idea of developmental norms and the kinds of errors expected of children at different ages. Therefore, the initial primary objective of the University of Illinois Stuttering Research Program was to document the onset and evolution of symptoms of early childhood stuttering. We were especially interested in how its defining characteristic—disfluent speech—varies over time. As the largest data-based, longitudinal investigation of the pathognomonic development of childhood stuttering to date progressed, however, it also provided us with unique opportunities to test hypotheses pertaining to genetic liabilities and the domains of motor speech, language, phonology, and cognition, as they relate to the onset and evolution of childhood stuttering.

We had additional goals. Both theoretical and clinical considerations resulted in our gathering of comparative data from normally fluent children. Although such comparisons are important in the study of other communicative disorders, this is particularly true for childhood stuttering because of several influential theories (e.g., Brutten & Shoemaker, 1967; Johnson et al., 1959) that link it to normal disfluencies. Wendell Johnson, for example, believed that parents are responding to normal disfluencies when they first think that their child is stuttering, and his ideas have continued to cause many speech–language clinicians to be concerned about distinguishing between incipient stuttering and normal disfluency. Thus, what disfluencies and associated characteristics are normal, and what is to be considered stuttering, becomes a very significant question. This led to the second major objective of the program: the differentiation between normally fluent speech and early stuttering.

The study had progressed for some time before we noticed that a substantial number of stuttering children apparently exhibited natural recovery. Documenting the magnitude and timing of this phenomenon became our third major objective. Then, as children continued to be monitored by the program for several years and reached the point at which they could be classified as either having recovered or having persistent (i.e., chronic) stuttering, it became apparent that data obtained soon after stuttering onset (i.e., the point of entry to the study) provided information that was potentially a powerful means for early identification of which of these two developmental tracks a child was following. As a result, the differentiation of subgroups of children who stutter, in general, and the early prediction of children with high risks for developing chronic (i.e., persistent) stuttering, and those with high chances of recovery, became the program's fourth objective.

To track the children who stutter over time, and to compare them with each other and with normally fluent control children, we used counts of disfluencies and associated behaviors obtained from audio and video recordings; acoustic analyses of temporal and frequency dimensions of speech samples; tests of phonologic, linguistic, and motoric skills; and assessments of nonverbal cognitive functions and other areas. By applying various statistical methods to the data obtained from the children at frequent intervals, we were able to discern subgroups that emerged along diverging trends and to identify factors that may influence these trends. We are hopeful that this information will provide the scientific basis necessary for developing theoretical models of the natural evolution of stuttering, predicting eventual outcomes and responses to treatment, and determining clinical intervention strategies, such as recommending intervention, timing of intervention, and rationales for intervention methods.

The Children

Recruitment of Participants

From the outset, three important principles guided recruitment and selection of the program's participants. First, we sought a reasonably accurate representation of the population's social and ethnic factors within the geographic constraints of the program's location. Second, we wanted the sample to represent the population of all young children who *ever* stutter, rather than a typical clinical caseload in which a large percentage are families or clients who actively sought professional advice or treatment for stuttering. Third, and most important, the pool of subjects had to be epidemiologically sound, which meant that we wanted children from the earliest possible stages of stuttering to participate in the investigation so that the entire range of each developmental path of early childhood stuttering could be fully traced across time. Thus, any child identified by parents as stuttering and confirmed by the investigators using a set of established criteria was considered important to include. We strongly disagree with the frequently expressed notion that a child must stutter for at least 6 months to be considered to stutter. The exclusion of short-term patients from research of any disorder would result in misleading scientific and clinical information about the nature of the disorder. For our research, requiring children to be at least 6 months past the onset of stuttering would have introduced major errors, as have been committed in past studies. Such a sample would have bypassed important developmental changes in stuttering, and therefore missed a significant number of recovered cases while being heavily biased in favor of persistent cases. To illustrate and amplify the point, if surveys of infant mortality exclude children under 1 year of age, they would miss a large percentage of babies who die. Accordingly, children who were within 12 months of stuttering onset were targeted regardless of the duration of their stuttering, as long as they were properly identified and classified.

The program participants were preschool-age children and their parents recruited from Champaign-Urbana, a community of approximately 100,000 residents surrounded by small towns, family farms, and several industrialized communities in east central Illinois. Families were drawn from all of these sources, within approximately a 90-mile radius of the university, and parents represented a wide range of backgrounds, including academics, professionals, blue-collar workers, farmers, and welfare recipients. A key factor in the success of this longitudinal investigation was the relatively large number of families who contacted us initially and chose to cooperate and stay with the program for several years. Parents' sincere interest in the well-being of their children and in the outcome of this research motivated them to keep returning for periodic reevaluations. Their patience with our many calls for setting up appointments, reminders, and various other requests as the need arose was truly amazing.

The active participation and broad socioeconomic representation of this sample was due, in large measure, to the program's recruitment and publicity efforts. We met with individuals and groups of area pediatricians and speech–language pathologists, appeared on radio programs, solicited articles about the program, and placed ads in the area's newspapers. One of our more fruitful methods for recruiting participants was to mail letters to approximately 350 speech–language clinicians, pediatricians, nurses, and day care centers at the beginning of every school year. The letters described the purposes of the program and emphasized the importance of early referrals to ensure the scientific integrity of the research. Considering the wide referral network and selection criteria used, we believe that the program's sample satisfies all of our three principles: It is geographically and ethnically representative, not restricted to clinical cases, and inclusive of all who fall under the rubric "ever stuttered." The program's nonstuttering control children were recruited primarily from day care centers located in the same areas.

Criteria for Participation

In view of the multidimensionality of stuttering, the difficulties encountered in defining it, and the various measures employed to tap it, one of the program's most critical tasks was operationally specifying what stuttering is and who a child who stutters is. Clinicians are faced with similar challenges in their routine practice. When Johnson and his associates (1959) studied the onset of stuttering during the 1950s, they adopted a unidimensional criterion. A parental diagnosis of stuttering was the only requirement for a child to be included in the experimental group. Conversely, children whose parents indicated that their child neither stuttered nor had a history of stuttering were placed in a nonstuttering control group. In our view, this criterion was too simple.

The University of Illinois Stuttering Research Program took a more conservative approach and employed multiple criteria, which included the subjective perception of parents, clinically experienced investigators' judgments, and speech data documenting each child's stuttering. Subsequently, when parents or other relatives of a potential study participant contacted us, an elaborate protocol was followed that included detailed interviews, direct observations of the child and parents, a battery of tests for child and parents, and extensive recordings of speech.

The following criteria were used to verify that a child was stuttering and qualified to participate in the study:

1. The child was 6 years of age or younger, so that only those children with stuttering onsets in early childhood were included. Andrews (1984) estimated that 90% of all stuttering onsets occurred prior to age 6.

2. Parents believed the child had a stuttering problem. Parental diagnosis of stuttering was required as an independent verification of the disorder, because parents' reports about onset and further changes in stuttering were essential to the study. Parent ratings of early stuttering severity reached a level of at least 2 on an 8-point scale (0 = *normal*, 7 = *very severe*).

3. Both investigators (i.e., Yairi and Ambrose) believed the child had a stuttering problem, to reduce any doubts that stuttering had existed in a child who was later reported to have recovered.

4. Stuttering severity was rated by experimenters as greater than 1 on an 8-point severity scale (0 = *normal*, 1 = *borderline*, 7 = *very severe*), a criterion that allows maximal inclusion of the population of preschool-age children who stutter, while excluding those at borderline levels.

5. The child exhibited at least three stuttering-like disfluencies (SLD) per 100 syllables of spontaneous speech. This criterion reflects the opinion of many speech–language pathologists that young children whose speech includes these types of disfluencies this frequently are stuttering (e.g., Conture, 2001) and is consistent with the disfluency

data reported by Johnson et al. (1959) for a large number of children who stutter.

6. The child had no reported history of neurological disorders or abnormalities. We wanted to avoid including children with a major organic condition that might overshadow the dynamics of stuttering that we wished to study, but thought it unwise to eliminate children with other communication disorders that might possibly be related to stuttering. We believed also that it was important to be as inclusive as possible in sampling the population of early childhood stuttering.

The use of these multiple objective and subjective criteria ensured that every child admitted into the study exhibited stuttering of clinical significance.

As we had hoped, these criteria were effective in screening out children who did not meet the program's objectives, but there were good reasons to obtain as much data as possible from them even though they were not included in the main longitudinal study. A small group of children met the above criteria but were already more than 12 months postonset. They were, therefore, studied as a separate group, who could provide data comparable to those of the children seen closer to onset, as they progressed over the years in the program. Members of this group have been excluded from studies that focused on specific questions but were included in others when justified. For example, because their postonset period was not relevant to the genetically oriented research of the program, they were included in these studies.

Children participating in the normally fluent, control group had to meet the following criteria:

1. The child had to be 6 years of age or younger.
2. Parents reported no history of stuttering.
3. Both investigators agreed the child did not stutter.
4. The parent severity rating had to be less than 1 on the 8-point scale.
5. Both investigators' severity ratings had to be less than 1 on the 8-point scale.
6. The child had to exhibit fewer than three SLD per 100 syllables.
7. Parents reported no history of neurological disorders or abnormalities.

Several admission criteria need further explanation, particularly the rating scales and the disfluency measures. The Parent Severity Scale requests a rating of overall recent stuttering severity that ranges from 0 to 7, and allows parents to choose points halfway between the numbered intervals. Zero is defined as *normally fluent,* 1 as *borderline,* and 2 as *mild* stuttering. The interval between 1 and 2 is designated as *definite but very mild to mild* stuttering. Point 3 is defined as *mild to moderate,* 4 as *moderate,* 5 as *moderate to severe,* 6 as *severe,* and 7 as *very severe* stuttering.

Clinicians' severity ratings involve several elements and are based on overall impressions of the child's speech throughout the evaluation. The scale we devised drew from scales developed by Darley and Spriestersbach (1978) and Riley (1981) and included four components of stuttering that were rated: frequency, duration, tension of disfluency, and accessory characteristics. The first three were rated from 0 to 6, and their mean was calculated. For these components, 0 represented levels typical of normally fluent speech and 6 indicated characteristics of severe stuttering. Accessory characteristics were rated from 0 to 1, and this rating was added to the mean of the first three components. Thus, a maximum score of 7 (*very severe stuttering*) could be obtained if frequency, duration, and tension were rated 6 and accessory characteristics rated 1. The Illinois Clinician Stuttering Severity Scale, shown in Figure 2.1, was found to be highly reliable. Ten videotapes of participants' speech samples were randomly selected and rerated by Yairi and Ambrose independently. The mean difference in their ratings was 0.17 of a scale interval. When the ratings of the two investigators differed as much as 0.50, the rating was set at the higher of the two estimates. In those rare cases in which a greater difference occurred or there was uncertainty, the sample was reviewed until a mutually agreed upon rating was achieved.

Initial Evaluation Procedures

Many of the program's data-gathering procedures resembled clinical routines of a diagnostic workup but were more extensive and more uniform. Each child received a comprehensive initial evaluation over two sessions, approximately a week apart, which usually required 3 to 4 hours to complete. Research with young preschoolers often requires patience and the flexible use and adjustment of data-gathering procedures if precious, rare data from very early stuttering are to be obtained. Sometimes 2-year-olds do not produce speech samples of sufficient length or quality to analyze, or do not cooperate with testing during their appointment, and can present creative challenges to obtaining worthwhile speech samples and reliable

ILLINOIS CLINICIAN STUTTERING SEVERITY SCALE

Name _____ Date _____

Session # _____ Rater _____

Instructions

1. On the scale from 0 to 6 as indicated, circle the number of Stuttering-Like Disfluencies (SLD) (part-word repetitions, single-syllable word repetitions, and blocks or prolongations) per 100 syllables.
2. Rate the length of the average of the 5 longest disfluencies in repetition units (bu-bu-but = 2 units, and-and-and-and = 3 units) or average length of prolongations, whichever is more predominant and severe.
3. Rate the tension of disfluencies.
4. Assign points for secondary characteristics.

SLD	Score	Duration or Repetition Units	Score	Tension	Score
0–3	0	none	1	0	none	0
3–5	1	none/fleeting	1+	1	none to slight	1
5–7	2	<.5 sec	1.5	2	slight	2
7–10	3	<1 sec	2	3	slight to moderate	3
10–15	4	<1.5 sec	3	4	moderate	4
15–20	5	<2 sec	4	5	moderate to excessive	5
>20	6	>2 sec	>4	6	excessive	6

Secondary Characteristics

.25 ___ mild, very few, infrequent, minimal; not noticeable unless looking for it

.33 ___ mild, few and occasional; barely noticeable

.50 ___ moderate, few and sometimes; noticeable

.66 ___ moderate, some and/or often; obvious

.75 ___ severe, many and/or frequent; distracting

1.00 ___ severe, many and frequent; severe and painful looking

(SLD points + Duration points + Tension points) divided by 3 = _____

(_____ + _____ + _____) = _____ /3 =   _____

Additional points for secondary characteristics   _____

Total Severity Score

Comments:

Figure 2.1. Illinois Clinician Stuttering Severity Scale.

test findings. As many clinicians have experienced, we encountered a few children who initially refused to talk, said only "Okay" or "I don't know," seemed angry or upset, or appeared simply tired and cranky. Some whispered or talked purposely in a "funny" voice. Consequently, we had to improvise. Several such participants were recorded on the floor in an office instead of in the recording room, required us to change the order of their tasks or to modify their assessment in several other ways, or were seen for additional sessions. We have encountered similar reactions with children who were being evaluated for other speech disorders, as well as with normally speaking control children. Therefore, there is no reason to suspect that such reactions reflect the social impact of stuttering problems.

Parent Interview

Parents were the main source of information about the child's background and the family's history of stuttering and were informed at the beginning of the interview about the program's objectives and that regular clinical services were not included. Mothers were usually the primary informants, and supplementary information was solicited from fathers and grandparents as needed. Interviews followed a standard format that elicited information pertaining to family background, the child's health and developmental history, and the circumstances and characteristics at onset and of early stuttering. Typically, parent interviews lasted 1 to 1½ hours over two visits and were supplemented by additional sessions if needed.

The first section of the interview focused on the onset and early characteristics of stuttering and began by documenting the onset as well as possible. Special care was taken to narrow down the date, manner, and circumstances at onset. To help identify the time and situation of onset, parents were encouraged to consult their child's baby book and to recall concurrent events or the proximity to other dates. We found it particularly helpful to use a systematic bracketing pattern of questioning that narrowed the time range for identifying the time of onset. In a number of cases, stuttering onset was pinned down to a specific date with apparent confidence that was confirmed independently by both parents. The following example was typical of such bracketing:

EXAMINER: When did the child begin stuttering?
PARENT: Last winter.

EXAMINER: When during winter?

PARENT: Around Christmas.

EXAMINER: Before or after Christmas?

PARENT: I am sure it was after.

EXAMINER: Before or after New Year's Day?

PARENT: After. He did not stutter on New Year's Day.

EXAMINER: Was it a few days or weeks later?

PARENT: It was a day or two after we returned from vacation and just before I went back to my job at school. I remember this very clearly.

EXAMINER: When did you go back to work?

PARENT: January 5th.

EXAMINER: So, we are pretty close to pinning it down.

PARENT: It must have been between January 3rd and 5th.

We also sought details about "how" stuttering began to help us identify how sudden or gradual onset was. We asked for specific information about the situation, how the child spoke, and the time period in which the disfluency developed into what the parents decided was stuttering. Using a system similar to the previous example, we asked the general question, "How did stuttering begin?" If a parent reported either a definite, quick change in the child's speech or a slow change, follow-up questions attempted to determine how gradual or sudden the change was, as in the following example:

PARENT: He just started stuttering.

EXAMINER: What do you mean? Did he go to bed speaking normally and wake up the next morning stuttering?

PARENT: Not quite, but it was very fast.

EXAMINER: So, you say that it was very fast but not a matter of one day to the next?

PARENT: Almost, but not quite.

EXAMINER: Did it take several days for you to realize that he started stuttering?

PARENT: It was a matter of one or two days.

In a few cases, parents could immediately provide the exact day, time, and place when stuttering was first noticed. Here is one example.

PARENT: It happened last Thursday, about 11:30 in the ice cream parlor. She asked for cho-cho-cho-cho-cho-chocolate chip ice cream and I was shocked to hear her stuttering.

EXAMINER: Did it ever happen before?

PARENT: No. It was the first time.

We treated responses indicating a gradual onset similarly, presenting parents with gradually increasing periods (e.g., from "several days" to "more than 5 weeks") during which stuttering evolved, from which they could choose.

Parents also described or imitated the child's stuttering at onset and rated its severity using the 8-point scale that we describe in Chapter 3. We probed circumstances surrounding onset, focusing on the presence or absence of any significant events or changes occurring around that time. After obtaining information regarding onset, we asked a series of questions concerning the changes in stuttering that had occurred from the time of onset to the present. We asked parents to describe how stuttering had changed, as well as any reactions they or the child had to stuttering, and to rate the current severity of the child's stuttering.

The second portion of the interview gathered information on the child's birth, health, and physical, motor, and speech development, as well as the mother's health during pregnancy and the circumstances of labor and delivery. Any history of speech, language, or hearing disorders or therapy was noted. Basic information was also sought concerning the child's family, which included the parents' education, occupation(s), income, residence, other children, languages spoken at home, and so on. Finally, to obtain data concerning possible genetic influences in stuttering, we requested a detailed pedigree of the child's family, which included grandparents, uncles, aunts, cousins, and siblings, to identify any relatives who ever stuttered, as well as any possible hereditary or other significant disorders that should be noted.

Parent Counseling

Following the child's examination and the parents' interview, we met with the parents to provide feedback about the child's stuttering, its nature and severity, and related factors. We explained and discussed findings from the various tests that were administered, and mailed a formal written report to their home.

We also gave parents general information about stuttering, such as its incidence and characteristics, persistence or remission, and common explanations about causation and the scientific evidence that supports or refutes these views, and we addressed any questions or concerns they raised. We then provided a brief review of several frequently cited conditions or behaviors that might help children who stutter, such as providing a relaxed environment, encouraging slow speech, and avoiding negative corrections of the child's speech. We then reminded parents that, even though the program did not provide treatment for stuttering, the child's welfare was our most important consideration, and we encouraged them to jot down any notable events or changes in the child's stuttering and to call us at any time if there was a marked change in stuttering, or if they had questions or concerns about the child's speech or any reactions to it. Parents always had the choice of whether their child received treatment for stuttering, and referrals for treatment, either in the family's community or at the University of Illinois Speech and Hearing Clinic, were available and offered whenever requested by parents or believed to be in the child's best interest by program staff.

Speech Samples

Recording

The most important information obtained by the program was derived from tape-recorded samples of each child's speech. These tapes provided the "hard evidence" about the evolution of stuttering. Conversational speech samples lasting about 40 minutes were audio- and video-taped in a sound-treated recording suite during somewhat structured and controlled interactions between the child and parent and between the child and one investigator in two sessions approximately 1 week apart. The samples consisted of conversations while the child played with clay and included several standard, open-ended questions about the child's favorite toys, TV shows, movies, siblings, and school or day care experiences, as well as talk about ongoing play. Most samples ranged from 1,000 to 2,000 syllables, but a few were shorter or longer. When the samples were analyzed, those that were longer than 1,500 syllables were shortened by excluding portions from the beginning or end of the recording. Although obtaining speech samples in such an organized fashion is efficient most of the time, clinicians should know that excellent data can often be obtained in less formal situations and conditions that stimulate children's spontaneous speech. Therefore, in addition, we made sure to exploit each opportunity to note the child's stuttering in several locations in the clinic during the two sessions, including such conditions as running along the hallways, playing in the waiting room, or playing on the floor in the experimenter's office, using small handheld portable recorders.

Many of the measures of interest to this investigation were derived from the spontaneous language samples of each subject, and several steps were taken to ensure collection of representative, high-quality samples. First, a portion of each sample was with a comfortable, familiar conversational partner, the child's parent. Second, adults interacting with the children during sampling were instructed to use open-ended comments and questions, such as "Tell me more about what you're making" or "What happened in that movie?" and to limit questions that invite yes–no or one-word answers, such as "Who are your friends?" or "Do you like to watch TV?" Third, in addition to the standard questions, the experimenters included topics that had been identified by parents as especially exciting to the child, such as recent minor mishaps, pets, and special toys. Fourth, the speech samples were significantly larger than those often reported (e.g., 300-syllable samples) in studies of childhood stuttering (Conture & Kelly, 1991; Meyers, 1986; Yaruss, 1997) or the 100-utterance lengths used in many studies involving language analyses. Some disfluency types that occur in low frequency cannot be adequately assessed in short speech samples, and several scholars have suggested that reliability and validity are significantly enhanced by the use of longer samples (Lahey, 1988; Lund & Duchan, 1993). Fifth, the samples were obtained on 2 different days to minimize the effects of moods, conversational topics, and fluctuations in stuttering frequency.

Analysis

Several program staff members, each having several hundred hours of experience analyzing disfluent speech, transcribed the tapes orthographically and identified disfluencies. Each disfluency was defined in plain linguistics terms (e.g., "word repetition") or with other descriptors (e.g., "disrhythmic phonation"), relying heavily on the work of Johnson and other investigators at the University of Iowa, which has been used in stuttering research for several decades. We, however, reduced their original eight specific disfluency categories (Johnson et al., 1959) to six. (More information about this system is provided in Chapter 4.) The three disfluency types most typical of stuttering in young children (part-word repetition, monosyllabic word repetition, disrhythmic phonation) were combined to form a global category that we labeled Stuttering-Like Disfluencies (SLD). The remaining three types (interjection, revision–incomplete phrase, multisyllabic word and phrase repetitions) were labeled Other Disfluencies. The latter disfluencies are more typical in the speech of normally fluent children. Every disfluency was tabulated in each taped sample and coded as to type. The *Systematic Analysis of Language Transcripts* (Miller & Chapman, 1996) was used for transcript and disfluency entries. Previous studies (Yairi, Ambrose, & Niermann, 1993) had found SLD measures to be the most sensitive index of variations in stuttering over time, whereas the number of Other Disfluencies remained relatively invariable. For example, variations in SLD closely parallel subjective severity ratings of clinicians and parents.

Because measures of repetition units (i.e., the number of times that a unit is repeated) have been shown to differentiate children who do and do not stutter (Ambrose & Yairi, 1995; Yairi & Lewis, 1984), there is a good reason to consider this measure, as well as other measures of length of disfluency, when studying changes in the classification of children as either stuttering or nonstuttering speakers. Therefore, another measure that we used was the mean number of extra iterations (i.e., repetition units) in each part-word and single-syllable word repetition. For example, if "but" were uttered as "but-but-but," it would contain two repetition units (i.e., two extra repetitions).

Inter- and Intrajudge Agreement

Ambrose relistened to approximately 70% of the speech samples in their entirety. Any difference found between her identification of disfluency and the identification made by the other staff members was resolved by repeated listening, and hers was the final judgment used in the counting. All transcripts were listened to by at least two trained transcribers. The interjudge agreement of Ambrose and the transcribers on 50 samples, representing both early and later visits, averaged 86% for SLD frequency counts, including both type and location. A recheck of the count of repetition units found 98% agreement on number of units. Interjudge agreement on syllable counts of 50 utterances that were randomly selected from each of 24 samples found a mean difference in syllable count of about 1.50 syllables per sample, ranging from 1.33 to 1.83 syllables across the 24 samples.

Additional Testing

After recording speech samples, we administered a battery of speech, language, hearing, motor, psychological, and other tests. Included were the *Assessment of Phonological Processes–Revised* (Hodson, 1986), the *Preschool Language Scale* (Zimmerman, Steiner, & Pond, 1979), and the *Arthur Adaptation of the Leiter International Performance Scale* (Arthur, 1952) to assess nonverbal cognitive skills. Additional important information, such as expressive language and acoustic measures, were later obtained from the recordings of spontaneous speech samples.

The function of such testing was twofold. First, we wanted to know if the children's phonological development, receptive and expressive language, cognitive skills, and hearing were within normal limits, information comparable to that obtained in a typical diagnostic evaluation. Second, this information would aid our search for possible subtypes of stuttering or subgroups of children who stutter. Other testing included structure and function of the speech mechanism, repetition of standard sentences, and a simple test of awareness of stuttering. Parents also completed the *Parenting Stress Index* (Abidin, 1986) and the *Walker Problem Behavior Identification Checklist* (Walker, 1983), indicating their child's behavior and their own stress levels in response to the child. Children were administered the *Child Anxiety Scale* (Gillis, 1980), the Communication Attitude Test (Brutten & Dunham, 1989), and the *Revised Children's Manifest Anxiety Scale* (Reynolds & Richmond, 1994) when they were at appropriate ages for these instruments, as described in Chaper 8.

Follow-Up Procedures

Telephone and mail follow-up reminders and flexible scheduling and rescheduling of visits, including weekends and holidays to suit a family's needs, were effective in maintaining families' participation in the study. A few children who moved before completing the study were recorded in their new locale by local speech pathologists or parents. Each family received $30 for each two-session follow-up visit. The overall rate of subject attrition (i.e., children who completed less than 1½ to 2 years of the study and whose data were not usable as longitudinal information) approximated 5%, which is low for longitudinal research conducted in a modern mobile society such as the United States.

Direct observations, recordings, and testing were conducted every 6 months for all participants for 2 years, then yearly for 2 additional years. A final follow-up visit 5 to 8 years later was also completed. Speech and language tests were readministered yearly. Similar to the procedures for the initial evaluation, the 6-month follow-up visits were conducted over two sessions, approximately 1 week apart. Again, the two experimenters had several opportunities during these visits to observe the child in various speaking situations, both in and outside the clinic, and in the recording–testing room. The investigators noted whether the child stuttered, any changes observed in stuttering, and the child's overall severity of stuttering using the Illinois Clinician Stuttering Severity Scale. They also noted any indications of the child's awareness of stuttering and any behavioral problems. Speech samples containing at least 1,000 syllables, approximately 40 minutes long, were audio- and video-recorded over the 2 days.

Parents were asked to keep notes about their child's stuttering between visits and to call us at any time if a significant change in stuttering occurred. At each follow-up visit, parents provided standard progress reports, which included information on general trends in stuttering during the prior 6-month period. They were asked about the presence and overall frequency of each of several types of disfluencies in the child's speech, associated physical characteristics, situational variations in stuttering, the child's awareness of stuttering, indications of such emotional reactions as avoidance or word substitutions, and any comments by relatives, friends, or neighbors about the child's stuttering. Additionally, they were asked to rate the severity of the child's stuttering on the parent stuttering severity rating scale mentioned above. Information was also obtained regarding parents' reactions to and handling of the child's stuttering, including whether any speech therapy had been provided. The child's health status during the preceding 6-month period and any behavioral concerns that had arisen were discussed, as well.

The Children at Initial Evaluation

A total of 183 children, referred because of suspected stuttering, were originally evaluated; 158 were European American, 10 African American, 13 multiracial, and 2 Asian. Of this initial pool, 169 children were diagnosed as stuttering; 14 no longer stuttered and were excluded from the study. There were 146 children whom we first examined within 12 months of stuttering onset (Early Experimental, or EE, group). Parents of 11 of these children chose not to continue in the program after the first or second appointment; the remaining 135 children who were seen during their first year of stuttering were followed over a period of years. Twenty-three children were seen initially more than 1 year following onset; of these, 6 were seen for only one or two appointments. These 6 were excluded from the study, leaving 17 children in the Later Experimental (LTE) group.

Seventy-five control children were initially evaluated; 68 were European American, 2 African American, 2 Hispanic, and 3 multiracial. Of these, 46 were followed longitudinally, 16 were seen once or twice, and 13 chose not to participate or were excluded because of possible histories of stuttering.

Thus, we were able to gather data over the years on 163 children who were brought to us for evaluation of suspected stuttering. Their ages at the time of their initial examination and their parents' interview ranged from 23 to 75 months. Included were 2 children under age two years (23 months), 59 two-year-olds, 67 three-year-olds, 33 four-year-olds, 1 five-year-old, and 1 six-year-old who was included because he had begun to stutter only 6 months earlier. The ages of the control children were similar, ranging from 27 to 63 months, including 20 two-year-olds, 26 three-year-olds, 13 four-year-olds, and 3 five-year-olds. The average ages for these three groups are presented in Table 2.1. An interesting trend is that the boys' and girls' mean ages were relatively close in each group.

Socioeconomic status was determined by parents' education, profession, and income, which extended over a substantial range. Only a few parents did not complete high school; the remainder ranged from high school graduates to those with higher degrees. Parental occupation and income also ranged widely, from those on public assistance, to unskilled and skilled workers, and to higher income professionals. Although the socioeconomic status of the families varied substantially, middle-income households dominated, with only a few that could be defined as very low or very high income. Eighty percent of the children lived with both parents; the rest lived with one parent or grandparents. The health and developmental histories of most children were unremarkable. A few children were diagnosed with attention-deficit/hyperactivity disorder or had asthma.

Upon entrance to the study, the participants exhibited a range of stuttering severity, reflecting the admission criteria. As explained earlier, severity of stuttering can be determined in several ways, such as the number of disfluencies; their length; a weighted measure that includes frequency,

Table 2.1
Children's Mean Age (in Months)
and Standard Deviation (*SD*) at Initial Evaluation

Group	N	Mean Age	(SD)
Early Experimental			
Male	101	38.87	(8.83)
Female	45	39.02	(9.55)
Total	146	38.92	(9.02)
Later Experimental			
Male	10	48.10	(6.21)
Female	7	47.14	(4.60)
Total	17	47.71	(5.46)
Control			
Male	40	41.35	(9.62)
Female	19	40.32	(10.89)
Total	59	41.02	(9.96)

length, and type of disfluency; and subjective ratings of severity by parents and clinicians. Because the means of the EE and LTE groups on these measures were nearly identical, we present the means for the entire group of 163 children. During the initial evaluation, these children's mean frequency of SLD was 10.95 per 100 syllables (*SD* = 6.65), which is considered to be moderate or moderate–severe stuttering on several scales (e.g., Darley & Spriestersbach, 1978; Van Riper, 1971). Length, as measured by the mean number of repetition units (i.e., the number of extra iterations in each repetition) was 1.53 per repetition (*SD* = .50), well within the range reported for young stuttering children (Ambrose & Yairi, 1995). The weighted SLD measure was 19.25 (*SD* = 16.31), which would also be considered moderate stuttering. The mean stuttering severity rating by parents at the initial evaluation was 3.74 (*SD* = 1.36), and that by clinicians was 3.90 (*SD* = 1.40). Both of these mean ratings are above the midpoint of 3.50 on the 8-point scale (0–7) that was employed. Based on these five measures, the group's stuttering severity resembles a normal distribution. Mild stuttering was exhibited by about 25% of the children, moderate by close to 50%, and severe by around 25%.

The results of the various standardized tests administered indicated a wide range of skill levels among the children. As mentioned previously, tests used were the *Assessment of Phonological Processes–Revised* (APP–R) for phonology, *Preschool Language Scale* (PLS) for language, and *Arthur Adaptation of the Leiter* for nonverbal cognitive skills. Scores for the EE and LTE groups are reported separately because of the two groups' performance differences. Table 2.2 presents the mean scores at initial testing. For the APP–R, higher scores reflect poorer phonology skills and are expected to be higher among younger children. Interestingly, the EE group had higher (i.e., poorer) scores than did the control group, even though their ages were matched. Within each group, a few children showed no impairment and a few showed severe impairments. The LTE group showed the lower (better) scores, as expected due to their age.

Table 2.2

Children's Test Scores (and Standard Deviations) at Entry to the Study

	Test			
Group	APP–R	PLS–AC	PLS–VA	Leiter
Early Experimental				
Male	23.32 (13.39)	122.63 (19.96)	117.13 (19.43)	121.14 (18.91)
Female	20.62 (12.00)	122.29 (17.95)	117.01 (17.90)	120.84 (21.62)
Total	22.49 (13.00)	122.53 (19.33)	117.10 (18.92)	121.06 (19.60)
Later Experimental				
Male	11.88 (7.05)	118.67 (17.21)	111.98 (15.61)	116.61 (18.35)
Female	13.14 (12.96)	115.64 (25.71)	114.38 (25.17)	128.09 (26.07)
Total	12.44 (9.70)	117.61 (19.95)	112.82 (18.85)	121.20 (21.66)
Control				
Male	18.65 (13.61)	127.06 (16.09)	125.20 (16.37)	124.64 (15.28)
Female	18.04 (16.53)	127.39 (18.86)	125.40 (18.97)	131.20 (16.46)
Total	18.45 (14.50)	127.17 (16.87)	125.26 (17.09)	126.69 (15.81)

Note. APP–R = *Assessment of Phonological Processes–Revised* (Hodson, 1986); PLS–AC = *Preschool Language Scale* Auditory Comprehension subtest (Zimmerman et al., 1979); PLS–VA = *Preschool Language Scale* Verbal Ability subtest; Leiter = *Arthur Adaptation of the Leiter International Performance Scale* (Arthur, 1952).

For the language comprehension test (PLS–Auditory Comprehension), the control group scored highest, and the LTE group scored slightly lower than the EE group, but the means of all groups were above normal limits. For the expression portion of the test (PLS–Verbal Ability), the control group again performed better than either experimental group. The same pattern of scores was present for the Leiter, although to a lesser degree. A few children scored slightly below the normal range on the language test (5 experimental, 1 control) or cognition test (4 experimental), but none was seriously impaired.

Thus, we believe that the rigorous entry criteria and broad array of assessment procedures provided us with a good chance of documenting stuttering from onset through its early development and of discovering the characteristics and paths that different subgroups might follow. The following seven chapters describe our journey of discovery. Those chapters are followed by several others concerned with clinical management of early childhood stuttering and one chapter concerning theoretical perspectives.

Chapter 3

The Onset of Stuttering

The onset of stuttering represents a definite event marked by a loss of an already established normal domain of speech. Although ideas and information about onset have had important implications to theory and clinical aspects of stuttering, onset is very difficult to study. Our data indicate an earlier age at onset than has been previously reported, with the greatest concentration during the third year of life—the period when significant speech and language development take place. Contrary to past ideas that emphasized uniformity in stuttering onset, new data indicate substantial variability in the manner of onset, speech characteristics, awareness, emotional reactions, and so on. Also contrary to past ideas, new data indicate a wide range of stuttering severity at onset. Overall, our data negate the classical diagnosogenic theory of stuttering.

Study Questions

1. What is the theoretical and clinical significance of information concerning the onset of stuttering? State and discuss the significance.

2. What diversities have been reported regarding the characteristics of the manner of onset?

3. What diversities have been reported in speech, emotional, and physical symptomatology at the onset of stuttering? Discuss them.

The Event of Onset: Theoretical and Clinical Significance

To appreciate the potential impact of stuttering on very young children and their families, the reader should keep in mind that, in the vast majority of reported new cases of stuttering, the disorder seems to begin after a period when the child's speech was regarded as normally fluent. As we have stated on several occasions (e.g., Yairi, 2001; Yairi & Ambrose, 1992b), in this respect, stuttering differs from the more common language and phonological or articulation disorders in early childhood. Typically, these disorders do not have an identifiable onset. That is, children with normal phonology do not simply wake up one morning speaking unintelligibly. Instead, parents come to a gradual realization that something—normal acquisition of speech and language skills—has *failed* to happen rather than a sudden realization that something unusual *has* happened. Nothing new or unusual happens. In phonological and language disorders, no dramatic changes mark the beginning of a new condition; affected children do not lose an already established normal function. It is unlikely that those children feel a difference, such as a sudden inability to communicate as effectively as they used to. In contrast, the onset of stuttering is marked with definite changes: a loss of an existing function (fluency) that was regarded as normal, and the appearance of new, unusual speech characteristics to which both child and parents may react quite strongly.

It has been suggested that even prior to observable stuttering, the child's speech contained various imperceptible speech aberrations, such as abnormal timing of movement. A group of Dutch investigators found that children who later began stuttering spoke faster than other children a full year before they were diagnosed as exhibiting stuttering (Kloth, Janssen, Kraaimaat, & Brutten, 1999). Nevertheless, the speaking rate of these children was still within the normal range. Thus, the presence of clear speech aberrations long before stuttering begins has yet to be convincingly demonstrated. Even if minute aberrations exist, perceptible changes that are considerably larger in magnitude or substantially different take place and are recognized by most people as the beginning of the disorder.

Inasmuch as the onset of stuttering is an identifiable event, among the first questions to be asked are, When does it happen? How does it happen? What happens? To whom does it happen? What and who else is involved? and Why does it happen? Theoretically, the nature and timing of the onset may have far-reaching implications. Rapid neurological maturation and corresponding cognitive and motor developmental changes occur during the preschool years. For example, several authors have commented that when stuttering begins under age 3 (true for a large proportion of cases), it may coincide with qualitative and quantitative advancements in the child's articulation, phonology, morphology, and syntax (Bernstein Ratner, 1997; Chevekeva, 1967; R. V. Watkins & Yairi, 1997; Yairi & Ambrose, 1992b). Therefore, the potential association between stuttering onset and language skills becomes intriguing.

Other theories of stuttering could also be evaluated against information about the onset of the disorder. Environmental circumstances and behavioral responses have been implicated in the development of early stuttering. A learning point of view (e.g., Wischner, 1950) would seem to imply that stuttering should begin and develop in a relatively gradual manner, a process of forming and changing behavioral patterns as a consequence of environmental responses. On the other hand, notions of traumatic causation, whether organic or psychological, would be commensurate with more sudden onset (e.g., Mowrer, 1998). According to a second learning theory (Brutten & Shoemaker, 1967), authentic early stuttering is a motor disintegration expressed only in sound or syllable repetitions and sound prolongations that occur following strong emotional anxiety, generalized via classical conditioning, and secondary characteristics are acquired later. Information about the presence or absence of physical concomitants at the time of onset could shed light on this theory. The demand and capacity model (M. R. Adams, 1990) would predict that the presence of excessive pressure of various kinds prompts the onset of stuttering. Again, valid data on the background, circumstance, and symptomatology of very early stuttering would provide important means to evaluate this view.

For readers more interested in treatment and counseling, the clinical implications of information pertaining to stuttering onset also abound. For example, if onset is shown to be associated with physical or psychological traumas, orientation to treatment would be influenced accordingly. Or, if there are several types of onset, there might also be different etiologies and subtypes of stuttering. Indeed, Van Riper (1971) suggested that the manner of onset is predictive of eventual persistent or recovered stuttering pathways. According to him, a persistent course tends to follow sudden onset, whereas a course of natural recovery is more likely to follow gradual onset. It might be that detailed information on the nature of the onset of stuttering could be an important element in efforts to identify subgroups within the population of people who stutter, or to discern diverse developmental patterns and to make early prognoses for children at risk of becoming chronic stutterers and those who are likely to recover. At the very least, accurate knowledge of the time of onset is necessary to determine the length of the history of the disorder in a given case. Indeed, recent findings from the Illinois studies (Yairi & Ambrose, 1992a, 1999b; Yairi, Ambrose, Paden, & Throneburg, 1996) strongly suggest that a key factor in determining risk for persistent stuttering and for making a decision regarding initiating treatment is the length of time following onset.

Research Approaches and Concepts of Onset

In spite of the theoretical and clinical importance of the nature and timing of stuttering onset, the amount of relevant scientific research focusing on this issue has been surprisingly small. It was not until the late 1930s that systematic dedicated research on the onset of stuttering was begun at the University of Iowa with the work of G. Taylor (1937) and continued later with the much better known studies of Wendell Johnson and his associates (Johnson, 1942; Johnson et al., 1959). With a few exceptions, however, these research efforts have remained limited, primarily due to the inherent difficulties in making direct observations of authentic "first stuttering."

Four research approaches can be used to study the onset of stuttering:

▶ 1. *Direct observations of authentic first stuttering in a sample of the general population.* This is a difficult approach to follow because it would require close monitoring for several years of a huge number of children beginning at about 18 months of age (the age that a few children begin stuttering). About 1,000 children would be required in order to identify and observe 50 cases of stuttering onsets. Under the best circumstances, the chance for an experienced investigator to observe and record a child's first stuttering is not very realistic. It is too difficult to predict when a child will begin stuttering.

▶ 2. *Direct observations of newly born children in families with high risk for stuttering.* Although this method also requires close monitoring of a good number of children, the number is considerably smaller than in the first method, especially if the population is selected based only on parents who have stuttered. The problems with this method are that selected high-risk families having a child close to the age at which stuttering begins are difficult to find in one geographic area, the number needed is still not small, and the potential sample of children is very biased to a particular segment of the stuttering population. Also, even in families with high risk for stuttering, it is impossible to predict when, or if, a child will begin stuttering.

▶ **3.** *Intentionally inducing stuttering.* Although this is theoretically a potential experimental avenue, clearly such an attempt would be viewed as unethical. To our knowledge, there has been only one study (Tudor, 1939) in which inducing stuttering in children was possibly considered. The stated objectives of that study, however, were to increase the level of disfluency in normally speaking children, not to induce stuttering.

▶ **4.** *Retrospective reports.* These are typically obtained from parents of children who have stuttered. The main advantages of the approach are the relative low costs and the relatively large number of children who can be included because the identification of stuttering was already performed outside the realm of the study. The obvious disadvantage is the real risk of low accuracy in reporting past events, particularly the details required for scientific research. A very different disadvantage is that of underrepresentation. Important data are lost about onsets in children who have already recovered from stuttering, especially those who recovered within a short period after onset. Parents of these children typically do not participate in such studies.

The retrospective approach has been by far the most commonly used. In general, for a long period, only a small number of qualified speech therapists had the interest or capability to observe and record early stuttering. In the past, lack of professional personnel and appropriate equipment did not facilitate direct recording even if it were possible to do so. As late as 1965, the total membership of the American Speech-Language-Hearing Association was approximately 8,000. Even if parents were actively seeking professional help and advice, they might have had difficulties locating an experienced therapist or researcher to observe the case of early stuttering.

Also, electrical recording equipment to store and analyze speech samples was not readily available or sufficiently sophisticated and mobile during the first two-thirds of the last century. Another obstacle was that many parents of beginning stutterers adopted a wait-and-see strategy. In our experiences, passivity is encouraged by the family's experiences with naturally recovered stuttering, as well as the notion circulating in many segments of the population that calling attention to stuttering is more dangerous than helpful. A national survey that yielded responses from more than 500 pediatricians (Yairi & Carrico, 1992) indicated that such an attitude is encouraged by the child's pediatrician.

The kinds of methodological obstacles to directly observing authentic first stuttering have had their influence on the type and quality of information that has been gathered about the onset of stuttering. Reviewing the scientific literature of the early part of the 20th century reveals two types of sources. The first consists of casual commentary and anecdotal single-case studies that lacked detailed data (e.g., Fogerty, 1930; Green, 1924; Hoepfner, 1911–1912). Second, several well-known clinicians (e.g., Bluemel, 1932; Froeschels, 1921) provided information in the form of general impressions from their extensive experience over the years, although these were lacking in verifiable quantified data. Given the obstacles inherent in direct observations, later investigators who were intent on obtaining scientific data were forced to rely primarily on the fourth source listed above: retrospective parent reports (Andrews & Harris, 1964; Glasner & Rosenthal, 1957; Johnson et al., 1959; Yairi, 1983; Yairi & Ambrose, 1992a). Such second-hand sources continue as the main providers of information in the research on very early stuttering, although awareness of the desirability of more authentic data and the widespread availability nowadays of recording equipment at home have improved the research conditions.[1]

Unfortunately, as indicated above, much of the retrospective data reported by several investigators, supposedly about the very early pathognomonic characteristics of stuttering onset, were obtained from informants long after the disorder had erupted. For example, when Milisen and Johnson (1936) sought information about the age at onset of stuttering, they questioned the parents of individuals then between ages 3 and 22 years. To answer, those parents had to search their memories as far as 20 years into the past. Such a demanding task is one of the main weak-

---

[1] A recent case history reported by Mowrer (1998) provided rare video recordings of early stuttering.

nesses of the Iowa studies, the most well-known research concerning the onset of stuttering, carried out by Johnson and his associates (1959), who interviewed parents of children then up to 8 years of age, and of the British study by Andrews and Harris (1964), whose subjects were between 9 and 11 years old. Knowing, as we explain later, that stuttering typically begins between ages 2 and 4, it is clear that parents of many, though not all, participants in these studies had to try to remember events that took place at least several years in the past. The accuracy of data that depend on such long-term memory is naturally called into question. Can parents be taken at their word in saying that the child repeated syllables such as "bu-bu-but" rather than whole words such as "but-but-but"? Can they be expected to recall the child repeating only two or three times in each instance and with only "some" or "without any" tension? Yet, far-reaching conclusions and sweeping ideas, such as Johnson's diagnosogenic theory of stuttering, have been based on such data of questionable accuracy and reliability.

As we indicated earlier, we made a major effort in our study to identify children whose reported onset of stuttering was within 1 year before the initial examination. Our goal of increasing the accuracy of the information obtained from parents required a fair amount of constant public education and maintaining awareness of various professionals who were in a position to make referrals. Luckily, we were quite successful. The range of post-onset interval for the major group, the Early Experimental, was 0 to 12 months, with a mean of 5 months, which is less than one third as long as the mean postonset interval of 18 months in the Iowa studies conducted by Johnson and associates (1959).

Age at Onset

Surveys of different sample sizes and varied scientific quality reported from around the world (see Van Riper, 1971) indicate that stuttering begins within a wide age range, but most commonly during early childhood. Although many studies show no onset after ages 7 or 8, others have reported a few cases that began during the teens (e.g., Daskalov, 1962; Preus, 1981). Onset in adulthood is quite rare, and a good number of those few cases seem to be associated with either emotional (Mahr & Leith, 1992; Roth, Aronson, & Davis, 1989) or physical trauma such as brain damage (Canter, 1971; Rosenbek, Messert, Collins, & Wertz, 1978; Yairi, Gintautas, & Avent, 1981). We had the experience of working with a woman, however, who began to stutter in her 40s without *any* apparent reason. Another woman in her 30s related that she began stuttering at age 30, when she was under emotional stress during the completion of her doctoral dissertation. In both cases, early emotional reactions to the speaking difficulties, not a frequent characteristic of developmental stuttering, was obvious. More important, however, both clinical observations over many years and research studies have pointed out convincingly that stuttering is primarily a disorder that begins in early childhood. The question, then, is when do most children begin to stutter?

As is always the case, there are some variations in what investigators have reported. Those who attempted to answer the question found that the youngest age for onset among the individuals being surveyed was 18 months (Milisen & Johnson, 1936; Yairi, 1983) and the oldest was 13 years (Meltzer, 1934). As mentioned previously, clinical experiences have revealed adulthood stuttering onset in isolated cases. Most studies did not report onset past age 9, not even studies in which some of the surveyed stutterers were as old as 22 years (Milisen & Johnson, 1936). The mean age at onset was reported as low as 28 months (Yairi, 1983) and as high as approximately 62 months (Seider, Gladstien, & Kidd, 1983). Such differences reflect expected sample randomness, variations in sample size, and, to some extent, the influence of the age range of the children. Although it is possible to assume that studies in which the age range of the population under study was extended to include older children would yield older, more valid, mean age at onset, such a conclusion is rather risky for two reasons. First, the older the sample being surveyed, the longer is the stuttering history and the greater is the risk that parents' memories are inaccurate. Second, when samples do not include young enough ages, children who had very early onset and who have already recovered are missed, and their influence on the mean age is thus lost. Keeping in mind all these considerations, when we averaged data from 11 past studies (Yairi, 1997a), the overall mean age at onset was approximately 3½ years.

Our own data on this subject are based on the information obtained during initial interviews of parents of 163 children whom we evaluated for stuttering. Because of the improved research methods, including the use of many children of younger ages than in most previous studies, interviewing parents considerably closer to onset, and taking extreme care in establishing the time stuttering first occurred, there is ample reason to believe that these data are more accurate than those reported in past studies.

Table 3.1

Means (and Standard Deviations)
for Age at Onset (in Months) and Months Postonset

Group	N	Mean Age at Onset		Mean Months Postonset	
Early Experimental					
Male	101	34.02	(7.66)	4.89	(3.50)
Female	45	34.24	(8.76)	4.73	(3.46)
Total	146	34.09	(7.98)	4.84	(3.48)
Later Experimental					
Male	10	29.20	(7.42)	18.90	(6.24)
Female	7	24.57	(6.48)	22.57	(6.55)
Total	17	27.29	(7.23)	20.41	(6.44)
Total Experimental					
Male	111	33.59	(7.23)	6.15	(5.53)
Female	52	32.94	(9.07)	7.13	(7.29)
Total	163	33.38	(8.16)	6.47	(6.14)

Our records show that stuttering was first observed in these 163 children from 16 to 69 months of age, with a median and a mean of 33 months. In view of our concern that information on children obtained longer than 1 year after they began stuttering might be inaccurate, the data for the two experimental groups were analyzed separately and are presented in Table 3.1. On average, the children first seen within 12 months of stuttering onset (i.e., Early Experimental group) began stuttering just prior to 3 years of age and showed only minimal gender difference. In contrast, the children first seen more than 12 months postonset (i.e., Later Experimental group) were reported to have begun stuttering at ages that were 7 months younger, on average, than that of the children in the Early Experimental group. This finding might be of special significance because the Later Experimental group included proportionately more children whose stuttering later persisted, and the few girls in this group were 5 months younger, on average, than were the boys at the onset of stuttering. Although parents' memories of onset may be less accurate a year or more later, many of the parents of this group gave very specific, detailed information about onset, as described in Chapter 2. Nevertheless, it seems unlikely that chronic stuttering is associated with very early onsets. In fact, Yairi and Ambrose (1999a) reported that mean age at onset was 32.55 months for 62 children who recovered from stuttering, but 33.13 months for a group of 22 children whose stuttering persisted, a statistically insignificant difference. We will return to this issue in Chapter 5.

The mean age at onset of the University of Illinois Stuttering Research Program's 163 children was 33 months, which is about 9 months younger than the mean calculated from the data published in 11 prior reports (Yairi, 1997a). It is also more than ½ year lower than the 41.2 months reported by Johnson et al. (1959) and more than 2 years lower than the 5 years reported by Andrews and Harris (1964). More revealing than overall mean ages, however, is a detailed analysis of the relationship between onset and age presented in Figure 3.1, which displays the percentage of onsets occurring at 6-month intervals. The patterns for males and females are similar. Over half (59%) of stuttering onsets occurred during the third year of life (24–35 months). By 42 months of age, over 85% of onsets had occurred, increasing to 95% by age 4 years. Thus, only 5% of the children

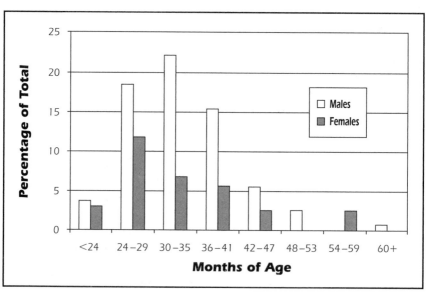

Figure 3.1. Age at onset of stuttering for males and females.

in this study began to stutter after age 4. We wonder about the possibility that the trend toward earlier age at onset is changing in society. If so, what could be responsible for this trend? If true, is this trend a reflection of earlier language acquisition?

The data in Figure 3.1 indicate that, even within the narrow age range spanned by these 163 children, stuttering onsets are concentrated between 24 and 42 months of age, in the lower half of the age range spanned, a period when complex language and articulatory skills are acquired. We focused on recruiting children close to the onset of stuttering but accepted children up to 6 years of age. Even so, substantially fewer onsets were reported in the upper half of the 18- to 72-month age range, especially after 48 months of age. These findings suggest that onsets of stuttering occur predominantly during the third year of life. Furthermore, we suspect that, had we been able to contact every new case of stuttering within our recruitment area during the program's existence, the percentage of onsets among children under age 3 years would have been even higher. This would be consistent with the information provided us by parents and others about unreported cases of children who began and stopped their stuttering before they were seen by any professional, as well as the findings reported by Yairi (1983), who found a mean age at onset of 27.8 months in a much smaller and younger sample of 23 children. Although the intriguing question of whether age at stuttering onset has gradually declined over the last 50 to 70 years is yet to be answered, it is apparent that a majority of onsets occur from 2 to 3½ years of age at the present time.

Uniformity and Diversity in Onset

Information on manner of onset is important to any epidemiological study, and variations in the onset of some disorders are clinically significant to speech–language pathologists. For example, an aphonia with sudden onset is much more likely to have a psychogenic etiology than is an aphonia that has developed gradually. For a long period, concepts of stuttering onset and its characteristics emphasized simplicity and uniformity. Early writers, such as Froeschels (1921, 1943), Hoepfner (1911–1912), and Bluemel (1932), characterized stuttering onsets as having uniformity in terms of (a) gradual appearance, (b) effortless repetitions of syllables or words, (c) lack of physical tension, and (d) lack of awareness and affective reactions related to the stuttering. Such a rigid view was clearly expressed by Froeschels (1943), a prominent pioneer in the study of early stuttering, who said that only in rare cases did stuttering onset deviate from this pattern. To underscore the distinct simplicity of early stuttering, Bluemel (1932) referred to it as "primary stuttering," which he viewed as a "pure" speech disorder that differed from the later emergence of what he called "secondary stuttering," a disorder complicated by emotional and physical components. Perhaps the most important feature of these traditional views, however, was the assumption that the early signs and symptoms of stuttering are essentially normal and later turn into "real" stuttering through parent–child interactions or other environmental influences. Such models reflect an inherent assumption that there is a transitional phase between normal and abnormal disfluency. Thus, views of stuttering onset as gradual were likely influenced by the belief that a passage of time was needed for this transition to take place.

The influence of these ideas persisted for several decades. Although Johnson and his associates (Johnson, 1942; Johnson et al., 1959) did report some variability in the characteristics and severity of stuttering at onset some years after Froeschels and Bluemel's early work, they continued to pointedly emphasize the commonplace circumstances of stuttering onset, the absence of any unusual happenings at the time, and the gradual appearance of the first stuttering. These researchers' tendency to overlook important differences in their own data remains a puzzle to us. Perhaps there was a theoretical motivation to highlight the similarities between stuttering and normally fluent children, which supported the view that the onset of stuttering is a misdiagnosed variation of normal speech. Investigators who believe that there are no differences between early stuttering and normal disfluencies may also be apt to overlook variations in "typical" onset within the stuttering group. A few years later, Andrews and Harris (1964) reported variations in the disfluent speech characteristics at onset but still concluded, "The children had begun with a mild repetitive stutter" (p. 130). Similar stereotypic views of the onset of stuttering were expressed as late as 1995 by Bloodstein.

The field's recognition of the heterogeneity of stuttering onsets can be found in the writing of several authors, such as De Ajuriaguerra, De Gobineau, Narlian, and Stambak (1958), but it became more common in the early 1970s. A major influence was Van Riper's (1971) work on the development of stuttering and his conclusion that stuttering progresses along

one of four developmental tracks. Significantly, such onset-related variations as age at onset (early vs. late), manner of onset (sudden vs. gradual),
and severity of stuttering at onset were important parameters in differentiating his tracks.

Manner of Onset

The manner of onset drew particular attention as investigators became
increasingly aware that, in a substantial percentage of children, parents
perceived the onset as sudden. Three such studies supported these parental
reports. Van Riper (1971) found sudden onset in 10% of 114 children,
Yairi (1983) in 31% of 23 children, and Yairi and Ambrose (1992b) in 31%
of 87 children when sudden onset was defined as "within 1 day" and in
44% when defined as "within 1 week." Other sources—for example,
Morley (1957) in England, Preus (1981) in Norway, and Mowrer (1998) in
the United States—also mentioned the occurrence of sudden onsets in
either group samples or individual case studies. Of course, an important
point to keep in mind is that parents' decisions that (a) stuttering has occurred and (b) onset was either sudden or gradual, are strongly influenced
by how they perceive or define stuttering. Indeed, it is quite possible that
onset is always sudden and that parents' reports of gradual or sudden onsets reflect whether early symptoms are mild or severe.

In our current study, we asked parents how stuttering began, and then
followed with requests for specific details and clarifications. Their responses were placed into one of six categories that were later organized as
three general onset types: Sudden onset consisted of responses reporting
onsets of 1 day or 2 to 3 days; intermediate onset included reports of 1 or 2
weeks; and gradual onset consisted of reports of 3 to 5 and 6 or more
weeks. It is not clear what is happening during the 3 or more weeks of
gradual stuttering onsets. Presumably, parents are aware that their child is
talking differently at times and they may be looking for greater consistency
or severity in his or her disfluencies before deciding that the child is stuttering. The percentage of children in each of the six categories and three
general types is shown in Table 3.2. Nearly 30% (48 children) were reported to exhibit onset over one *day*, and such onsets were distinctly remembered as discrete events for many children. Together with onsets over

Table 3.2

Percentage of Children in Each Onset Category

Occurrence of Onset	Percentage
Sudden	
One day	29.6
2 to 3 days	11.1
Total	40.7
Intermediate	
1 week	8.0
2 weeks	24.1
Total	32.1
Gradual	
3 to 5 weeks	11.1
6 or more weeks	16.0
Total	27.1

2 to 3 days, the total percentage of children with sudden onsets was over 40%. Intermediate onsets, still representing a relatively brief window, comprised almost 33% of the cases reported. Gradual onsets, which traditional views believed were the most common onset, were in fact the least frequent type among these 163 children, including a bit more than 25% of the sample. One might wonder if the children who were initially seen longer after onset, when parents' memories were perhaps cloudy, received fewer discrete reports of onset; however, the data indicate such was not the case. For example, 1-day onsets were reported by parents 0 to 26 months after their child's onset of stuttering; 2-week onsets were reported 0 to 19 months postonset; and gradual onsets of 6 or more weeks were reported 3 to 32 months postonset.

Males and females were distributed similarly across the three types of onset ($\chi^2 = .50$, $p = .78$), as shown in Figure 3.2. Thus, the difference in percentage between genders in each onset category remained relatively close to the 2:1 male-to-female ratio of the entire sample.

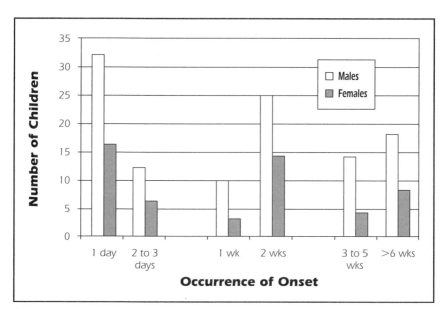

Figure 3.2. *Manner of onset of stuttering for males and females.*

As mentioned earlier, more than a few parents provided specific details of sudden onsets that had occurred only a few weeks or days prior to their interview. The following are excerpts from transcripts of the initial interviews of mothers of two boys (E: examiner; P: parent).

Case 1

E: I would like you to tell me how the stuttering of your son began. What happened? When did it happen? Do you have specific recollections of that time?

P: Okay, we first noticed it the morning that we were leaving on vacation. It was February 10th.

E: Today is April 20th, so it was about 10 weeks ago?

P: Yes.

E: Okay.

P: We got up, got ready to go, and at first that morning I thought it was because he was excited. He would start saying, "When when when when are we leaving?" Like that. But as the day progressed, and later in the day in the back seat of the car, he had word blocks also. He couldn't get any words out.

E: You said it was on February 10th. Are you sure it was not before that day?

P: I would say 99% sure, because I'm a very overprotective mother so I notice anything that happens with him, and that is the very first time we noticed it—me and his father and grandmother.

E: So you were not the only one at the time?

Case 2

E: Let's talk about when he first began stuttering. Just tell me in your own words what you remember about his stuttering—when he began stuttering and what happened? Today is November 12, I believe. Okay?

P: It was on Sunday. I know it was the 8th because it was my birthday and it was immediate onset.

E: You mean the very last Sunday?

P: Right, Sunday prior to this Thursday. It was immediate. My husband and I thought that he was doing it as an attention-getting trick.

E: What do you mean when you say "immediate"?

P: He was having a hard time getting words out, and we had never noticed that before. It was just something that he just seemed to just start doing. And we originally thought he was doing that to try to [get attention]. He's in competition with his brother a lot, so we thought that maybe he was trying to get our attention by doing this. He was having problems with multiple words in a sentence. He would repeat the first sounds.

E: Like what? Show me.

P: He would say like "g g g g g ga come here," and most times he would repeat the sound 8 to 10 times.

E: Eight to 10 times?

P: Sometimes it got as bad as 12 to 15 times. There were some times we had difficulty understanding anything he was saying in a sentence. We could pick out one or two words throughout a sentence.

E: Let me just make sure. Today is Thursday, and you say that he began stuttering 5 days ago, since Sunday, and you are sure because it was your birthday?

P: Right.

E: Now let me ask you this. Are you sure that there was no stuttering a day or a week before this, or 2 weeks before this?

P: I feel fairly certain that there wasn't. If there had been, it was very, very insignificant and very minor.

E: Okay.

P: When we first noticed it, it was pretty severe, and he goes to a pre-school day care 3 days a week, and they had noticed it on Monday when I picked him up. His teachers had noticed it as well.

E: They had not noticed it before? So you also have confirmation from the preschool?

P: Right.

E: Now what about the father? Did he notice it before?

P: He noticed it initially. He noticed it before I did on that Sunday. In fact, he actually scolded Troy [a fictitious name] after the first couple of times, and Troy started crying because he didn't know why he was being scolded. He didn't know why he was in trouble. So, my husband had not noticed the stuttering prior to that either.

E: Okay, go on. What happened then?

P: Okay, so it was in school. I asked his teachers if any other children stuttered or stammered, and they weren't aware of any other child that had a stuttering problem. And Tuesday it continued, Wednesday it continued, and then we came here Thursday. There was one particular time when he was speaking to my mother Wednesday night where I could only pick out two words of the entire conversation. It seems to get worse at night. He does wake up stuttering, but I don't know if maybe being tired or fatigued increases it.

E: Did you say that he wakes up during the night and he stutters?

P: No, not in the middle of the night. When he wakes up first thing in the morning, he is stuttering somewhat, but then it seems to progress and get worse the later it gets.

E: So we are now saying that he began stuttering on Sunday. On Monday you heard from the school and then through today (Thursday) he was waking up in the morning mostly stuttering and then it gets worse during the day?

P: I think, yeah. By night time, by bedtime it's considerably more pronounced.

Environmental Characteristics

Environmental Events

Literature sources from past centuries, including a number from the first half of the 20th century, attributed stuttering onsets to physical events, such as illness, or events that caused emotional turmoil. Although some sources were based on authors' experiences with a single case, others summarized impressions based on rather large personal caseloads or surveys. Makuen (1914) reported that onset of stuttering occurred after shock or fright in 28% of his caseload of 1,000 persons who stuttered. West, Nelson, and Berry (1939) estimated that 16% to 20% of their caseloads began stuttering after illnesses. As late as 1962, Katsovaskaia reported that stuttering onset was preceded by illness in 35% and emotional shocks in 27% of 200 children examined.

As mentioned earlier, specific physical injuries or mental stresses have been reported to precipitate or to be associated with the onset of stuttering in adults for several decades. Although such views are widely accepted with regard to adult onsets of stuttering, that is not the case with regard to the onset of developmental stuttering in young children, primarily as the result of two major modern investigations. The Iowa studies on the onset of stuttering by Johnson and his associates (1959), in which parents of 246 children who stuttered and their matched controls participated in individual interviews, yielded two pertinent conclusions. First, seldom did onset of stuttering occur under dramatic circumstances, and only in very few cases was there a temporal association of onset with illness, injury, shock, or fright. Second, the health histories of children who stutter did not reveal more childhood diseases than those of control children. Five years later, Andrews and Harris (1964) compared the health histories of 80 stuttering and 80 control children in England and found no significant difference in the incidence of diseases between the two groups.

In spite of the impact of these studies, the notion that stuttering onset appears to be associated with specific physical or emotional stress in a number of cases has remained and gained ground in recent years. One of the more dramatic and convincing examples is a case study of a 2½-year-old boy described by Mowrer (1998). In this exceptionally well-documented study of sudden onset, the author provides rather compelling grounds to suspect that strong emotional reactions triggered the child's stuttering. Poulos and Webster (1991) reported that individuals who stuttered but had no family history of stuttering tended to have experienced earlier events such as anoxia, head injury, and anesthesia, and that could have resulted in early brain damage. This exciting lead, however, has yet to be substantiated. In one of our earlier studies of stuttering onset (Yairi & Ambrose, 1992b), we found that the histories of 43% of the children contained reports of either physical or emotional stress; however, a breakdown between the two types of stress was not specified, unfortunately. Consequently, we decided to revisit the onset–stress relationship in an analysis of our present data.

Physical and emotional stresses were included in several questionnaire items pertaining to the child's health history and current health status and were covered during the initial evaluation and parent interview. These items probed the occurrence of stress in close proximity to onset and elicited a variety of parental responses. Examples of emotional stress included such events as divorce of parents, moving, death of a beloved pet, birthdays, excessive sibling rivalry, family vacations, or difficult day care situations. Physical stresses occurring just prior to onset included such conditions as respiratory problems, surgery or illness requiring hospitalization, asthma requiring medical treatment, and acute illness. Data from parents of the Early Experimental group seem to agree with opinions more typical of the early part of the 20th century. We found that 14% of the children were reported to experience illness or excessive fatigue just prior to onset, and over 40% experienced emotionally upsetting events in close proximity to onset. In addition, behavioral or developmental stress or change, such as toilet training, giving up "blankies" or bottles, family rivalry, and so on, were described as occurring around the time of onset for 36% of the children. Taken together, such events, which could be termed sources of "general stress," were reported for almost half of the children. There was not a significant difference, however, between the genders in any of the three stress categories, which is incompatible with Schuell's (1946, 1947) suggestion that more males than females stutter because of the extra stress put upon males.

Although we agree with Van Riper's (1971) analysis that many early reports on stuttering onset are open to question due to the lack of, or weak, scientific controls, we do not believe they should be dismissed altogether. Our data indicate that physical or emotional stresses might play an active role in stuttering onset. If a child possesses predisposing (i.e., genetic) factors to stutter, aggravating physical or emotional stresses might very well trigger the onset.

Developmental Changes

During the third year of life, a period when stuttering onsets are very common, children's speech and language undergo rapid growth. As a child's vocabulary becomes richer and sentences grow longer and more grammatically complex, verbal communication evolves into a more adultlike form (R. Brown, 1973; Golinkoff & Hirsh-Pasek, 2000). The stuttering–language connection, accompanied by pertinent data, is covered in Chapter 7. Briefly, parents' observations and speculations about the relationship between stuttering onset and their child's rapidly developing speech and language skills are illuminating. We asked parents if their children were undergoing such changes during or close to the time of stuttering onset. Over 40% described their children as rapidly developing in language skills, and 43% commented that they seemed to be having difficulty finding the right words to express themselves. Taken together, over 50% of the children were reportedly undergoing such language "stress." Such reports occurred similarly often for boys and girls. When one mother was asked what was the cause of her son's stuttering, she responded,

> I really don't know; he has always been very verbal. He has always spoken earlier than my other son. He has a much broader vocabulary than my other son, and he's extremely articulate for his age, much more so than his peers at school [be]cause his teachers have told me this.

Another one said, "We noticed every time that she had an episode of stuttering was in correlation of a growth spurt, either physical, or emotional, or with her vocabulary. When she began stuttering, she was having a vocabulary spurt." Such reports were common, as were parents' comments that their child stutters because his or her mind works faster than his or her speech. Their expressed opinions provide an impressive indication of their conjecture that some connection exists between the onset of stuttering and their child's speech and language development.

Overt and Covert Characteristics

Having shed some light on how stuttering begins and under what circumstances, the next question is, What is actually happening? How do young preschoolers talk, sound, and look when they first begin to stutter? What is it that begins either gradually or suddenly? What other behaviors are associated with the speech that we call "stuttering"?

Speech Characteristics

Many early writers (e.g., Bluemel, 1932; Gutzmann, 1894; Hoepfner, 1911–1912) relied primarily on their clinical impressions and typically limited their descriptions to a simplistic pattern of repetition of syllables and words, which were free of any so-called secondary characteristics, such as head and neck movements or other signs of physical tension. It appears, however, that these were descriptions of stuttering during the initial months or first year after onset of the disorder, which may not be the speech patterns that were present *at onset*. Somewhat later, in a better documented clinical source, Froeschels (1952) relied solely on the spontaneous comments of parents about onset. He reported that parents specified repetitions of syllables or words as the first, and *exclusive*, sign of stuttering in *all* 800 cases of childhood stuttering that he had seen. Froeschels appreciated the importance of speaking rate and physical tension in stuttering and opined that the early repetitions of stuttering children were of normal tempo and without tension.

The belief that repetitions are the primary, if not the only, speech characteristic of stuttering at onset and throughout its incipient stage prevailed, with few exceptions, during the first half of the 20th century. An early departure from this simplistic view of stuttering symptomatology at onset can be found in a study of the parents of 47 stuttering children ages 3 to 7 years that was conducted at the University of Iowa by G. Taylor (1937). Although 85% of these parents reported repetitions, especially of whole words, as the most frequent sign, 12% of the children were reported to evidence sound stoppages, and 11% to exhibit such secondary characteristics as head movements and gasping. Taylor's study, which has been largely ignored in the literature, appears to have set the stage for the series of Iowa studies directed by Wendell Johnson. In 1942, Johnson initiated the largest investigation dedicated specifically to the onset of stuttering. In three studies extending over a 20-year period, Johnson and his associates (1959) interviewed the parents of 250 children who stuttered and reported that the majority of parents said that the speech first labeled as "stuttering" consisted of effortless, brief repetitions of syllables, whole words, or phrases, usually at the beginning of utterances. However, other patterns of more complex and severe onsets of stuttering were also found. For example, approximately 33% of the children were described as exhibiting some force that accompanied their first stuttering, and 12% to 15% had sound prolongations and complete blocks. Such findings were deemphasized in writings of Johnson and his associates.

In spite of the obvious variability in parents' descriptions of stuttering onset, Froeschels and Johnson went on to pronounce that the disfluencies of first stuttering do not differ from the "normal" repetitions observed in the speech of all young children. The idea that early stutterings are essentially normal disfluencies or emerge from them, and become "real" stuttering through parent–child interactions or other environmental influences is a distinctive, and perhaps the most important, feature of the traditional model of early childhood stuttering. As we have already mentioned, such a model requires an assumption that there is a transitional phase in stuttering onset between normal and abnormal disfluent speech, a view with which we strongly disagree.

Other investigators, such as McDearmon (1968), examined and reanalyzed Johnson's data and concluded that the speech features most parents described at the time of stuttering onset consisted of disfluencies that characterize stuttering, not normal speech disfluencies. It also appears that the Iowa research team overlooked the importance of the length of stuttering children's disfluencies, another important oversight in our opinion. Another study mentioned that parents had described initial stuttering as repetitions of syllables and words "averaging about three repetitions per stutter" (Darley, 1955, p. 138); however, Johnson (1959) referred to such repetition as "brief." The failure of the Iowa investigators to realize that 3 to 4 iterations per instance of repetition is *much* above the normal, which is 1.1 iterations (Ambrose & Yairi, 1995), was a major reason, in our opinion, for their making a fundamental error in interpreting their data as showing that stuttering children's disfluencies at onset were normal, an error that had far-reaching theoretical and clinical management consequences.

The realization that symptomatology of stuttering onset is diverse and does not always differ categorically from advanced forms of the disorder was advanced in Van Riper's (1971) work on the developmental heterogeneity of stuttering. He proposed that there were four different developmental subgroups or tracks and that unhurried multiple- and single-syllable word repetitions were the onset characteristics of the largest subgroup (the children who followed Track I). However, such onset characteristics as fast-rate repetitions, silent gaps, prolongations, complete blocks, vocal fry, breathing abnormalities, pauses associated with grunting, tongue protrusions, wide-open jaw, and lip tremors were listed for children in the other subgroups (those who followed other tracks). In a later study of 61 stuttering children, whom he had personally examined within 3 weeks of onset, Van Riper (1982) reported that 80% of the children repeated syllables or words at least three times per instance, 28% had prolongations longer than 2 seconds, and 15% had indicated their awareness of stuttering.

More recent research by Yairi (1983), who interviewed the parents of 22 very young children who were seen less than 6 months from the time of onset, on average, provided similar results. A large majority of these children were reported to exhibit syllable and word repetitions at onset, but 85% of the parents also reported that syllables and words were repeated three to five times per instance. In addition, 36% reported sound prolongations at onset, 23% conspicuous silent intervals in speech, 14% blocks, 18% facial contortions, and 18% respiratory irregularities. Only 32% of these parents described the onset of stuttering as characterized by easy, simple repetitions that were devoid of any sign of tension or force. Indeed, most perceived early stuttering to be associated with some degree of force, with 36% reporting moderate to severe tension. Contemporary case study reports (e.g., Mowrer, 1998) also support this impression, as did Yairi's (1974) observations of the severe, complex symptomatology of his son's stuttering, which included as many as 15 consecutive repetition units of words or syllables, within days of onset.

Parental reports of the onset of stuttering in the Early Experimental group of 146 children indicate that almost 50% exhibited only repetitions at onset, higher than the 33% reported in Yairi's (1983) study. Six children (>4%) were recalled as having *only* blocks and prolongations when they began stuttering. Slightly less than 50% evidenced repetitions and disrhythmic phonations (primarily sound prolongations) at onset. Taking into consideration that parents' memories may not be totally accurate, it is still abundantly clear that stuttering begins, about half the time, with more than just easy repetitions. The following exchange with one mother is an example (E: examiner; P: parent):

E: You mentioned that in the afternoon [of the day of onset] he had these kinds of blocks. What do you mean by blocks? Can you show me?

P: Okay, it was when he was really tired and he would go "aaaaa ...," tried to get [a] word out or "wheeee," like that, he couldn't speak the word at all.

E: So this was still on the very first day?
P: Yeah.

Not only do many parents describe early stuttering as being markedly different from typical childhood disfluency, but the project's recorded speech data of 23 children who were seen within 1 month of stuttering on-set provide direct empirical support. Analyses of their speech samples showed that the frequency of just word and sound repetitions was over 9 per 100 syllables, on average, and that disrhythmic phonations occurred more than 3 times per 100 syllables, together totaling 12.63% Stuttering-Like Disfluencies (SLD). This is well above the 1.33% SLD expected for normally fluent 2- and 3-year olds (Ambrose & Yairi, 1999).

Two other features may be even more distinctive of early childhood stuttering onset. First, in terms of length, the mean number of times a seg-ment was repeated during each repetition was just under 1.75, which is sub-stantially above (more than 5 standard deviations) the mean number of it-erations per repetition (1.10) of normally fluent children (Ambrose & Yairi, 1999). The repetitions of some children did indeed involve only one extra segment most of the time. Of course, even short repetitions that occur at frequencies much higher than normal make them highly noticeable, even distracting, to parents and other listeners. Nevertheless, the number of ex-tra iterations was substantially higher for other children in the group, rang-ing as high as 17 for a single instance of disfluency, and one child averaged more than five extra iterations per repetition. We are convinced, therefore, that a large number of long disfluencies (e.g., repetitions containing two or more iterations) plays a major role in parents' decisions that their child has begun stuttering.

Second, the presence, even dominance in some cases, of blocks and sound prolongations indicates that these features can be core elements of very early stuttering, just as some parents described them. In contrast, the frequency of what can be considered as more typical of normal disfluency, such as interjections, revisions, and phrase repetitions, was comparable to what is expected for normally fluent young children.

Physical Concomitants

Nonspeech behaviors that accompany stuttering are referred to by several terms: physical concomitants, accessory behaviors, and, more commonly, secondary characteristics. The latter term, secondary characteristics, reflects the view that such behaviors emerge later in the development of stuttering, as reactions to it, not as core characteristics of real stuttering that are present at onset. In the 1980s and 1990s, the findings of several studies corroborated each other by documenting the presence of such concomitant behaviors close to stuttering onset (H. D. Schwartz, Zebrowski, & Conture, 1990; Yairi, Ambrose, et al., 1996). Most parents (53%) of the 146 children we saw within 1 year of onset reported that their children exhibited at least one specific physical component at stuttering onset, including abnormal, visible tension or movement of the face, eyes, lips, tongue, jaw, and neck; respiratory irregularities; and tense movements of the head or limbs. These reports provided additional evidence for the presence of so-called secondary characteristics right at the time of onset. Again, there was no difference in the percentages of boys and girls who exhibited such symptoms, as is true of all of the features of stuttering onset discussed so far.

Emotional–Cognitive Aspects

Judgments of preschool-age children's emotional or cognitive reactions to stuttering present a serious challenge to scientific investigation. Questionnaires and interviews are often too abstract, and the validity of parents' interpretations of what occurs in their child's mind can be difficult to assess. There are a number of ways to explore emotional or cognitive issues despite such difficulties. First, parents can be asked to report what children actually say about their stuttering. More than 20% of the parents we interviewed reported that their children were aware of the problem at onset. It is perhaps surprising to note how often parents report their children's specific comments regarding their stuttering, such as "My words are stuck," "I can't talk," or other similar, unsolicited comments. One mother of a child whom we interviewed less than 2 months after onset related,

> I think he had noticed, you know, over the last 2 months because he [had] been able to speak easily and clearly. Before, but more in the past 10 days, he has told me, he'd say, "I can't talk." He would be stuttering, couldn't get it out, and just stopped and said, "I can't talk."

The mother insisted that her son had said this more than once. Another mother, talking about the day of onset, reported, then he would just, er, that is, he started getting really frustrated. He would get mad, I mean because the words wouldn't come out, his face start[ed to] turn red. And then, that day, and that's the only day I've heard him say it, he said, "I just can't talk."

Second, observations of children during stuttering can reveal their emotional or cognitive reactions. During evaluations, we often heard similar statements and were able to observe and document facial expressions, vocalizations, and body language clearly indicating sudden discomfort during a severe moment of stuttering. For example, a 2½-year-old boy, who was seen less than 2 weeks after onset, repeated "unh" 17 times before he could finally say, "Mom," whereupon he put his head in his mother's lap, with a very unhappy expression on his face. Such behavior during the evaluation occurred only in association with his stuttering.

Third, we developed a testing procedure in which the children viewed brief videotape segments displaying one fluent and one disfluent puppet and were then asked, "Which one talks the way you talk?" Ambrose and Yairi (1994) reported that this procedure indicated that some 3-year-olds who stutter are aware of their stuttering. Our current data on 64 children within 12 months of onset reveal that almost 10% of the children showed indications of awareness based on puppet identification.

Overall Severity or Complexity

Notwithstanding our discussion of how stuttering begins, it is apparent that most investigators and clinicians are inclined to associate gradual onsets with a mild disorder and sudden onsets with a more severe, noticeable disorder. It is not surprising that early writers, such as Bluemel (1913), who conceptualized stuttering onsets as uniformly gradual, were strongly inclined to describe stuttering at onset as being easy, effortless repetitions, always mild in severity. This view seems to have influenced many researchers and clinicians in the field, including Wendell Johnson (1959), Gavin Andrews and Harris (1964), and Charles Van Riper (1954), thereby forming the stereotypical view that all cases of stuttering at onset are low or mild in severity. More than 50 years after the publication of Bluemel's text, Andrews and Harris (1964) expressed a similar idea in writing that "the children had begun with a mild repetitive stutter" (p. 130). It is not surprising, therefore, that when clinicians obtain a different report from parents, they tend to suspect that the parents' descriptions of a child's early stuttering are exaggerated, motivated by anxiety.

Another reason for our interest in the severity of stuttering at onset is that satisfactory data on severity and its distribution among children and adults who stutter at various ages and phases of the disorder, are not available. Soderberg's (1962) finding that the majority of his 105 subjects ranked their stuttering as "mild" was based on the reports of college students. Perceptions of stuttering severity are influenced by the complex interaction of such factors as frequency, type and duration of disfluency, observable tension, associated physical movements, listeners' tolerance and experiences, and so forth. We do not discuss these issues here but believe that it would be inappropriate to generalize Soderberg's conclusions to other age groups. Yet, information concerning perceived severity at onset is important for understanding not only the nature of onset, but also the further developmental course of stuttering. For example, is there a relationship between natural recovery and the severity of stuttering?

As is true with other parameters of early stuttering, it appears that its heterogeneity at onset extends also to perception of severity. Deviations from traditional descriptions of mild stuttering at onset are present in the writings of several investigators and clinicians. Yairi (1983), for example, found that only 63.6% of the parents of the 22 very young children in his sample described them as having had mild or easy stuttering at onset, whereas 13.6% felt that stuttering at onset was severe, with the rest, 22.7%, rating it as moderate. Likewise, Mansson (2000), an investigator working in Denmark, found that a significant number of children in his sample had severe stuttering at onset. Mowrer's (1998) exceptionally detailed case history described a boy who exhibited severe stuttering when it began, including repetitions of 3 to 4 iterations, blocks, and numerous secondary behaviors such as body rocking and breath holding.

To determine what clinicians should expect to hear from parents about the overall severity of their child's stuttering when it began, we asked parents to rate the severity of the child's earliest stuttering that they could recall using an 8-point scale, with 0 being *normal speech* and 7 being *most severe* stuttering. When the data of 146 children were grouped into three severity levels, the following results were obtained: Onsets were rated as *mild* (ratings 1–3) for 63% of the children, as *moderate* (ratings 3–5) for 31%, and as *severe* (ratings 5–7) for 6%. The distribution of severity levels was virtually identical for boys and girls, and these findings are similar to those reported by Yairi in 1983 for a different sample of children. The following excerpt is from an interview with a mother who was absolutely confident about the exact date of onset, approximately 10 weeks prior to this interview.

> E: Tell me what you think about the way that he talked that afternoon, when he had all those blocks that you mentioned. If I asked you to rate the severity of stuttering during that particular time—like 0 being normal speech; 1 being kind of borderline; 2, mild stuttering; 3, mild plus; 4, moderate; 5, moderate plus; 6, severe; and 7, very severe— where would you place him?
>
> P: In that afternoon?
>
> E: That afternoon.
>
> P: Seven.
>
> E: Seven?
>
> P: I mean, it scared me to death. Because I have never been around it or it had never happened to him, I didn't know if he was having a stroke or something.

Relationships Among Factors

One of the more intriguing questions arising from our data is whether the variables we investigated in relation to stuttering onset are interrelated in ways that may shed more light on onset or contribute to the identification of subgroups. We explored such relationships in several ways, prior to which we had to consider the issue of gender. Even though stuttering is gender biased in its incidence, the data that we have presented in several prior sections showed that boys and girls are similar in terms of the variables that we examined, at least at onset. We decided, therefore, to combine the data of the two genders for the following analyses.

The children were divided into two groups according to their age at onset: early (onset occurring by age 36 months) and late (onset at or after age 36 months). Also, for this particular analysis, they were divided into only two categories of manner of onset—sudden (1 day to 1 week) and gradual (2–6 or more weeks)—and into two stuttering severity levels— mild or moderate–severe.

In Table 3.3, the relation of these factors to the presence of some type of stress in language is depicted. The table shows the percentage of children whom parents reported as exhibiting or not exhibiting signs of language stress (e.g., a spurt of language growth, trouble finding the right

Table 3.3

Percentages of Children Reported With or Without Language Stress
at Onset, Early or Later Onsets, Sudden or Gradual Onsets, and Mild
or Moderate–Severe (Mod–Sev) Stuttering Severity at Onset

| | Onset | | | | |
| | Sudden (1 day to 1 week) | | Gradual (2–6 or more weeks) | | |
Onset Age	Mild (<3.0)	Mod–Sev (3.0–7.0)	Mild (<3.0)	Mod–Sev (3.0–7.0)	Totals
Early (<36 mos.)					
Stress present	7.6	7.0	20.8	5.1	40.5
Stress absent	9.5	8.2	5.1	2.5	25.3
Later (≥36 mos.)					
Stress present	3.2	4.4	7.6	3.2	18.4
Stress absent	4.4	4.4	4.5	2.5	15.8
Totals					
Stress present	10.8	11.4	28.5	8.3	58.9
Stress absent	13.9	12.6	9.6	5.0	41.1

words to express themselves, or having their minds ahead of their mouths)
immediately preceding stuttering onset. If all of these factors were randomly distributed, then we would expect 6.25% of the children to occupy
each box. The most notable deviation is the much higher percentage of
children with early, gradual onsets of mild severity (20.9%) who were reported as having language stress.

In Table 3.4, the same information is presented for children reported
to have experienced physical or emotional stress preceding stuttering onset. Although it may be tempting to speculate that if gradual onsets are associated with language growth stress, then sudden onset may be associated
with illness or emotional stress, these data reveal that such was not the case
for these children.

A more comprehensive examination of the various combinations of
factors was performed using the Spearman correlation shown in Table 3.5.
These included age at onset in months, manner of onset in the six categories

Table 3.4

Percentages of Children Reported With or Without Physical
or Emotional Stress, Early or Later Onsets, Sudden or Gradual Onsets,
and Mild or Moderate–Severe (Mod–Sev) Stuttering Severity at Onset

| | Onset | | | | |
| | Sudden (1 day to 1 week) | | Gradual (2–6 or more weeks) | | |
Onset Age	Mild (<3.0)	Mod–Sev (3.0–7.0)	Mild (<3.0)	Mod–Sev (3.0–7.0)	Totals
Early (<36 mos.)					
Stress present	7.5	8.8	10.6	5.0	31.9
Stress absent	10.0	6.3	15.0	2.5	33.8
Later (≥36 mos.)					
Stress present	3.1	3.1	4.4	3.1	13.7
Stress absent	4.4	5.6	7.5	3.1	20.6
Totals					
Stress present	10.6	11.9	15.0	8.1	45.6
Stress absent	14.4	11.9	22.5	5.6	54.4

specified previously (from 1 = 1 day to 6 = 6 weeks or more), stuttering severity (from 0 to 7), and presence or absence of rapid language changes or of illness and emotional upset. Only three significant associations were found. First, greater severity was significantly associated with sudden onsets ($r = -.297$, $p < .001$), which intuitively makes sense. It would be more difficult to have a sudden mild onset because it would be less noticeable than an abrupt change. A gradual severe onset would seem to be much less probable, perhaps impossible. If stuttering were severe initially, onset would not be gradual, and if it were mild initially and then became severe, it would not be severe at onset. Second, there was a significant association between the presence of physical or emotional stress and greater severity at onset ($r = .158$, $p = .047$). It would seem logical that, to associate a stuttering onset with a particular stress situation, stuttering would likely be more than mild; otherwise it would be much less likely to have caught parents' attention. Interestingly, there was not a significant association between sudden onset and

Table 3.5
Spearman Correlation Coefficients
and Significance Among Factors Related to Onset

Factor	Onset Age		Manner		Severity		Physical or Emotional Stress	
	r	p	r	p	r	p	r	p
Manner	−.040	.613						
Severity	.027	.730	−.297	<.001				
Physical or emotional stress	−.047	.551	−.087	.271	.158	.047		
Language stress	−.076	.337	.238	.002	−.012	.886	−.036	.653

physical or emotional stress. Third, and of greatest interest, there was also an association between gradual onsets and the presence of a recent spurt of language growth or children's difficulty finding words to express themselves, resulting in a significant correlation ($r = .238, p = .002$). This finding has implications for theories pertaining to the interaction of language skills and fluency. Rapidly emerging or precocious language skills may place excessive demands on the fluency-generating system, thereby gradually precipitating stuttering in children with predispositions to stutter. Synchrony of speech and language systems development may also be a factor in recovery from stuttering, and later chapters will discuss this issue in more detail.

The lack of relationship between age at onset and either manner, severity, or language factors, or between manner of onset and associated physical or emotional stress is surprising. It would not be illogical to hypothesize that a significant relation between gradual onset and language stress might occur more often when onset is early, or that sudden, more severe onsets might be more typical of later onsets, or that physical or emotional stress might be associated with sudden onset. However, no such patterns are evident in the data shown in Table 3.5.

Racial and Ethnic Factors

Because of the small number of children representing minority groups in our sample, our data have not been analyzed to study possible differences between European American children and other groups with regard to various characteristics of stuttering onset. Nevertheless, we were interested in finding out whether the groups vary in the occurrence of stuttering. Thus, we conducted a rather large-scale survey of 3,404 preschoolers, including 2,223 African Americans, 942 European Americans, and 239 others. To identify children who stutter, we went to day care centers and schools in many towns and cities in Illinois with high concentrations of African American children.

A child was identified as exhibiting stuttering based on individual speech screenings and teacher reports. For some children, it was also possible to obtain parental judgment. Our team (Proctor, Duff, Patterson, & Yairi, 2001) reported a prevalence of 2.46% for the entire sample, with no group differences for African Americans, European Americans, and other minorities. Although prevalence of stuttering in the population at large is known to be at approximately 1%, a higher figure should be expected for the preschool-age subpopulations where most stuttering onsets occur.

Conclusions

The Changing Nature of Research Concerning Stuttering Onset

The 20th century saw significant changes in the nature, quantity, and quality of information about early childhood stuttering, accompanied by a parallel evolution in conceptualizations of the early stages of the disorder. Anecdotal case studies and casual observations, as well as clinicians' general impressions of how stuttering begins based on their caseloads (e.g., Froeschels, 1921), were primary sources of knowledge during the first third of the century. The concept of onset as a uniform disfluency pattern limited solely to "simple" repetitions, perhaps slightly deviate from normal, prevailed throughout this period. During the middle of the century, however, a major effort was undertaken to introduce more sound scientific methods to the study of this domain through systematic collection of data from large groups of children and their parents (Andrews & Harris, 1964; Johnson et al., 1959). This research drew heavily on information obtained from parents. The seminal work of Johnson and his colleagues at the University of Iowa, which concluded that stuttering begins gradually, literally as normal repetitions and under ordinary, uneventful circumstances, gave rise to a revolutionary theory that blamed the onset of stuttering on parents' misjudgments of a child's normal speech as being pathological.

During the latter third of the century, as the focus of research on stuttering gradually shifted from adults to children, it became apparent that quantification and characterization of the onset of stuttering required additional research. A few investigators, who used relatively small groups initially, sought to improve the quality of research methods employed in studying onset. They began by studying younger children in narrower age ranges considerably closer to the time of onset (Buck & Lees, 2000; Yairi, 1983; Yairi & Ambrose, 1992a) and looking into subgroup differences as well (Van Riper, 1971). Initial attempts to study the speech and other characteristics of children *before* they began stuttering (Kloth et al., 1995) were also begun, and the availability of home video equipment allowed authentic recordings of very early stuttering to be made (Mowrer, 1998).

Many of these methodological improvements were incorporated in the University of Illinois Stuttering Research Program, which was expanded in scope to become the largest study of early childhood stuttering conducted during the latter third of the 20th century and into the beginning of the 21st century. This research, and that of studies completed during the latter third of the last century, has resulted in conclusions that differ significantly on a number of critical issues from those reached by Johnson and his associates years earlier at the University of Iowa.

The Fall of the Diagnosogenic Theory of Stuttering Onset

The widespread, international acceptance of Johnson's diagnosogenic theory over more than three decades has gradually crumbled as the scientific evidence in four areas has mounted.

▶ 1. *The nature of the speech disfluencies exhibited by children at the onset of stuttering compared to those of normally speaking children.* The contribution of our research in this area has been particularly notable. A substantial body of data gathered by several investigators has indicated that (a) disfluencies are present in the speech of all young children, but most produce only a few of them (e.g., Yairi, 1981); (b) the disfluencies of children at stuttering onset appear to be abnormal and differ substantially in several dimensions from those of nonstuttering children from the start (Ambrose & Yairi, 1999;

Throneburg & Yairi, 1994; Yairi & Lewis, 1984), and Johnson et al.'s (1959) own disfluency data do not support his assertions as shown by McDearmon (1968); and (c) many parents perceived abnormal speech in their child from the first day of stuttering (Yairi, 1983).

▶ **2.** *Experimental punishment of stuttering.* Evidence in a second area that directly negates the diagnosogenic theory's main assumptions comes from studies showing that aversive contingencies on stutter- ing, which have included negative verbal responses, mild electrical shock, bursts of loud sounds, and so forth, often result in substantial declines in stuttering, exactly the opposite effect than would be pre- dicted by Johnson's theory (Costello & Ingham, 1984). Even experi- ments with preschool children (e.g., Martin, Kuhl, & Haroldson, 1972) found that when attention was called to the children's stutter- ing, the stuttering dropped to near-zero levels, and there was clear evi- dence that the children were aware of the reactions to their stuttering.

▶ **3.** *Parental correction of stuttering.* Studies of parental reports that they had asked their children to "stop" or "slow down" when they stuttered, obviously calling attention to the stuttering, found that these parents' "negative reactions" did not adversely affect the chil- dren's recoveries from stuttering (see review by Wingate, 1976).

▶ **4.** *Nonenvironmental etiologies.* The evidence of a genetic compo- nent to stuttering accumulated over the past 30 years has become so strong that finding the specific genes that predispose children to having the disorder is all but certain. Recently, Cox et al. (2000) identified three chromosomes suspected as possible locations for such genes, and other scientists have found anatomical differences in the brain structure of adults who do and do not stutter (Foundas, Bollich, Corey, Hurley, & Heilman, 2001).

The Critical Period for the Risk for Stuttering

We have concluded that children under age 3 have the greatest risk for be- ginning to stutter. More than 60% of the children who stutter begin prior to that age and more than 85% by 3½ years of age. This conclusion varies from Andrews and Harris's (1964) estimate that 75% of children's risk for stuttering is over by age 6. Although the upper age limit of our sample may account for some of this discrepancy, our focus on including children as close as possible to onset resulted in the inclusion of younger children with earlier onsets, a group that was not well represented in previous studies. Locating stuttering children at very young ages and close to onset is a key factor in epidemiological research on stuttering. In addition, our large sample and its age distribution justify our conclusion that stuttering, on average, tends to begin at earlier ages and within a narrower range than has been assumed previously. There appears to be a critical period that rarely allows stuttering to occur prior to age 2, even though the child is talking, and relatively infrequently after age 4.

The maturational processes of the brain, neurological and functional, that occur during this period, especially during the third year of life, must be better understood for researchers to identify the factors that precipitate stuttering onset. Although many avenues of research undoubtedly need to be explored, the temporal proximity of stuttering onsets prior to age 3 to the acquisition of complex articulatory and syntactic skills (Yairi, 1983; Yairi & Ambrose, 1992b) invites particularly intriguing speculations that interferences in these maturational processes may involve stuttering–articulation–language relations. As advances continue in understanding the genetic and brain structures and functions associated with language–articulation disorders (K. Watkins, Gadian, & Vargha-Khadem, 1999) and their parallels in stuttering, a better understanding of such relations can be expected. Such overlap seems less likely to exist for onsets that occur after age 4, and different combinations or dynamics of factors are more likely to be involved beyond this somewhat arbitrary age. We suspect, therefore, that onsets of childhood stuttering that occur after this critical period should be investigated as a potential separate subtype.

Clinical Applications: The Nature of Onset

The evidence accumulated during our investigation, as well as from other studies over the past 30 years, supports the conclusion that stuttering on-sets are characterized by a wide range of circumstances and even more vari-ability in symptomatology. This conclusion is reflected in several findings:

• Stuttering may begin in many ways and is distributed similarly across sudden, intermediate, and gradual manners of onset, with a somewhat greater proportion of children in the sudden category, most of whom evidence an abrupt onset.

- Only about 20% of children begin to stutter under what appear to be fully unremarkable circumstances. The data show that the onsets of many of the children's stuttering are associated with at least some degree of various physical, emotional, and language stresses.
- The first signs of stuttering vary. Repetitions of initial syllables and short words are virtually universal, but initial symptomatology is rich and may also include sound prolongations and articulatory fixations (i.e., blockages), which may even be a primary early symptom. Although some children repeat easily, repetitions associated with tension are described in many cases, and, even more important, the number of repeated units is often reported to be twice or more per repetition than found in normally fluent children.
- Variations also occur with respect to the behaviors that accompany stuttering (i.e., secondary characteristics), such as tense movements of various parts of the body, especially the head, face, and neck. About 50% of children exhibit one or more movements early on, and the other half do not. Thus, such characteristics are not always signs of advanced stuttering.
- Quite a few children provide clear signs of being aware of or bothered by their stuttering, but the majority do not.
- There are large differences in parents' perceptions of the overall severity of stuttering onset, with approximately 65% reporting mild onsets and 35% moderate to severe.
- There may be an association between a gradual onset of stuttering and unusually rapid language growth.

These findings suggest that the diversity in age, manner, stress, and other factors at onset should be given greater recognition in published descriptions of childhood stuttering, as well as in standard clinical evaluations of young children who begin to stutter. Currently, however, there is still insufficient evidence that initial variations in onset provide useful diagnostic and prognostic differentiation of young stutterers, a possibility we raised a decade ago (Yairi & Ambrose, 1992b). Except for a few hints about the possible connection between gradual onsets and language development spurts, no reliable relationship has been found among the other factors we have investigated.

Based on our extensive parent interview data and direct observations of children, especially those whom we examined very soon after onset (whose speech samples are discussed in the next chapter), it is clear that parents and others who knew the child viewed the onset of stuttering as a definite change from the child's normally fluent speech to what was perceived as different or abnormal. In most cases, including those reported as gradual onsets, stuttering commences in a rather clear, definite manner and within a relatively brief period of time. Furthermore, there is evidence that the parents not only *perceived* a definite change, but were reacting to real changes in the child's speech and accompanying physical characteristics. In our opinion, the stuttering that is emerging in such situations does not reflect parental misdiagnosis or unrealistically high standards for a child's speech development. We posit that the changes parents perceive are legitimate causes for concern. In this respect, our conclusions are diametrically opposed to the beliefs fostered by the conclusions of Johnson and his associates (1959). In our view, stuttering does not arise from normal disfluency, but begins as abnormal disfluency. We cannot, therefore, prevent normal disfluency from becoming stuttering, a position that has important implications for intervention and counseling, as we discuss in Chapters 11 through 13.

Most of the data presented in this chapter reflect different parents' individual perceptions and standards for normal disfluency, stuttering, perceptions of severity, sudden or gradual onsets, stress, and so on. The data also reflect parents' ability to accurately recall and describe details of past events. In spite of the enormous methodological difficulties and financial costs involved in obtaining direct data on stuttering onset, such investigations are necessary if a scientifically credible understanding of the onset and natural course of this disorder are to be obtained. It is important, therefore, as a final caveat, to keep in mind the possibility of error or bias in the findings just presented, at least until other carefully conducted studies on stuttering onset replicate these findings and, thereby, establish their validity.

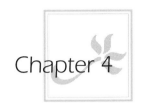

Chapter 4

Disfluency Characteristics of Early Stuttering

The various interferences in the progress of speech utterances, referred to as "disfluency," are the central feature of stuttering. Stuttering and disfluency, however, are not synonymous. Whereas stuttering reflects a perceptual judgment of quality, disfluency is used for descriptive purposes. Also, the latter may be used to describe the former, but not the other way around. Early research of disfluent speech began with a very limited disfluency system but has evolved into various disfluency schemes attempting to differentiate speech of children who stutter from that of normally fluent peers. It is important to be aware, however, of the many factors, including the metric used to quantify disfluency, that may influence the data. Although initial findings led researchers to believe that disfluencies of the two groups are very similar, we report normative data that establish marked differences in terms of the frequency–type distribution, length, and so forth. In this chapter, we illustrate and discuss a new measure that combines frequency, type, and length of disfluency into a single score, and we present data concerning other parameters, such as clustering of disfluency and associated physical movement.

Study Questions

1. *Discuss the difference between disfluency and stuttering. When does disfluency stop being normal and become stuttering?*

2. *In what ways is disfluency relevant to theory, research, and clinical aspects of stuttering?*

3. *What are the bases and the rationale for the index known as Stuttering-Like Disfluency?*

4. *What is the contribution of the length of disfluency (such as repetition units) in regard to quantifying disfluent speech?*

The Prominence of Disfluency

Disfluency and Stuttering

Stuttering traditionally has been described as a complex, multidimensional disorder that involves cognitive, physiological, physical, emotional, sociological, and other domains. Although the disorder can be characterized according to these dimensions, especially in persons with chronic stuttering, it is first and foremost a disorder of speech. As early as 1932, Bluemel suggested that, during its incipient stage, stuttering is a "pure" speech disturbance, and that physical tension and other reactions "have nothing to do with primary stammering" (p. 188). We question the totality of his statement but agree that, although other aspects of the disorder, such as awareness or affective reactions, may be present during early stages, they are less apparent than the disordered speech in a substantial number of children (Ambrose & Yairi, 1994). Furthermore, even the speech domain of stuttering can be narrowed. Whereas speech attributes, such as vocal quality, vocal pitch, articulatory rate, and formant structure, may be perturbed as part of the overall disorder, it is the observable interference in the continuous progress of utterances, commonly referred to as "disfluency," that constitutes the immediate, earliest, most common, and most obvious characteristic of stuttering.

The literature clearly reflects two major orientations to measuring interruptions in the speech of people who stutter. One is based on categorical yes–no responses that require the listener to judge each speech segment as either stuttering or normal. Such segments can be defined in terms of a specified time interval (e.g., 2 seconds of speech) or in terms of linguistic units (e.g., words or syllables). Thus, the number of "stutterings" in the speech sample is counted (R. J. Ingham, Cordes, & Gow, 1993). The second approach relies on counting instances of "disfluency" that include different types of interruptions. For this purpose, linguistic terminology such as "word repetition," as well as other descriptive references such as "revision," is used to define each of these interruptions or disfluencies (M. R. Adams, 1977). Although counting instances of stuttering is an acceptable method, we advocate disfluency counts. The implementation of a behavioral taxonomy of disfluency types, as opposed to listener judgment of stuttering, represents a more objective method that should, by its nature, be less biased (Yairi, Watkins, Ambrose, & Paden, 2001).

The term *disfluency* can be misleading in that it may refer to events that interrupt an utterance but are not themselves disfluent, such as interjections, or word and phrase repetitions. In these cases, the flow of speech is continuous, although progress through the utterance is hindered. To complicate matters further, the term also has been used at times as a synonym for *stuttering;* however, stuttering, as a phenomenon, and disfluency are *not* synonymous on at least two grounds. First, in terms of speech *production,* disfluency occurs in the speech of normally speaking persons as well as in those who stutter. Substantial data show certain overlap in disfluent speech of normal and stuttering populations, including comparable groups of young children (Johnson et al., 1959; Yairi & Lewis, 1984). The overlap is seen in both the types of disfluency produced and the amount of disfluency. Concerning type, all conventionally recognized and defined disfluencies found in children who stutter also occur in the speech of normally fluent children; however, as we explain later, there are apparent differences in features of the same disfluency type for normally fluent speakers and those who stutter. Although these differences are difficult to perceive, they can be observed with the aid of powerful technology, such as computer-based acoustic analyses. Regarding amount, occasionally normally speaking children are as disfluent as their stuttering peers, or even more so. Conversely, children who stutter may exhibit less disfluency than normally speaking children. As we discuss below, however, the overlap is small, and the proportional distribution of types is markedly different.

Second, stuttering and disfluency are not synonymous in terms of listener *perception.* The average listener may identify some events as unequivocally stuttering, and others as clearly normal. The differentiation, however, is not that simple. Sometimes, disfluencies uttered by people who stutter are perceived as normal, and vice versa. As we elaborated in Yairi and Ambrose (2001),

> the literature is replete with data that reflect great listeners' disagreement in perception of disfluent speech as "stuttering" ([M. A.] Young, 1984) as well as various conditions that change listener judgment of same disfluent events as being either "normal" or "stuttering" (e.g., Williams & Kent, 1958). It is quite likely that a listener who identifies several disfluencies as "stuttering" in a tape and was biased toward thinking that the speaker is a "stutterer," will tend to hear more subsequent disfluent events as stuttering. (p. 869)

This point is highlighted in Bloodstein's (1970) suggestion that "there is no test for determining the precise point at which speech repetitions stop being 'normal' and become 'stuttering'" (p. 31). Instead, he offered the continuity hypothesis, positing that stuttering and normal disfluencies are not categorically different. Disfluency indices, such as our Stuttering-Like Disfluencies (SLD) or Conture's (1990) "Within Word Disfluencies," were developed in part to diminish such bias by employing counts of defined, describable, and differentiated speech events.

In spite of some areas of overlap in production of disfluencies, potential perceptual confusion, and frank listener disagreement, disfluent speech events have remained what Yairi (1997, p. 49) termed "obligatory signs of stuttering," and have been the single most frequently used parameter to describe and define stuttering or stutterers in many practical domains. All the reservations that have been raised concerning the use of disfluency counts (e.g., Cordes & Ingham, 1996; Onslow, Gardner, Bryant, Stuckings, & Knight, 1992) cannot negate the reality that they have been *the* classic metric of the disorder. More important, such reservations have apparently overlooked the practical significance of disfluencies in research and clinical practices, as discussed in the next section. Other metrics that have been suggested, such as percentage of speech intervals judged as containing stuttering (Ingham et al., 1993), number of stutterings per minute (Ryan, 1974), or the length of fluent speech (Starkweather, 1990), have not been widely adopted by either clinicians or researchers.

Relevance to Research, Theory, and Clinical Matters

In the *research arena,* changes in the level of disfluency in response to different experimental conditions have been used as the dependent variable in various studies (e.g., Conture & Brayton, 1975; Yairi, Gintautas, & Avent, 1981). Transformations in disfluency patterns (e.g., easy repetitions to tense blocks) have been a cardinal feature in work that focused on developmental sequencing of stuttering (e.g., Bloodstein, 1960b; Van Riper, 1971). Describing changes in the characteristics of overt stuttering during the course of the disorder would have been difficult, if not impossible, if such changes were to be limited only to the number or length of instances of "stuttering" without reference to the vastly distinct features observed in whatever is meant by "stuttering." In another research area, investigators have shown the potential usefulness of different disfluency types in the subgrouping of young children who stutter (H. D. Schwartz & Conture,

1988). Our own research group has employed disfluency profiles in the study of differentiation of persistent from recovered subgroups (e.g., Throneburg & Yairi, 2001; Yairi, Ambrose, Paden, & Throneburg, 1996).

The critical importance of disfluency and its normal–abnormal contrast is also readily seen in the *theoretical arena*. Stuttering theory was profoundly influenced when Johnson (1942) concluded that whatever parents regard as the first stuttering is nothing else than normal disfluency commonly produced by young children. In other words, improper normal–abnormal disfluency distinction brought about the onset of stuttering. This was a sharp shift from physiological and psychological orientations to the semantic and learning spheres that dominated the thinking in the field for several decades and left deep marks on therapeutic approaches. Other theoretical notions, such as the covert-repair hypothesis (Kolk & Postma, 1997) and operant conditioning (Shames & Sherrick, 1963), also have disfluencies at their core. The former explains how disfluencies are formed; the latter describes how they develop from normal to abnormal.

The theoretical (and practical) significance of describable, specified disfluency is also reinforced by the simple fact that defining stuttering has leaned heavily on the use of descriptive disfluency types. The core of Wingate's (1964) classical definition of stuttering consists of specific disfluencies, primarily syllable repetition, single-syllable word repetition, and sound prolongation. Without the use of specific types of disfluency, definitions of stuttering would be restricted to vague statements that stuttering is what listeners perceive as stuttering.

Disfluency also serves significant functions in the *clinical arena*. For the practicing clinician, the question of what constitutes normal and abnormal disfluency may become a routine issue to consider on at least two occasions that were discussed in Chapter 1. First is the *point of entry*, when deciding whether the child's disfluency constitutes stuttering and whether it merits clinical intervention (Manning, 1996). As scientific advancements have brought better understanding of the distinction between disfluencies of normally speaking people and of those who stutter, the prominence of disfluency measures has risen. Disfluency information has been weighted heavily in formal and informal diagnostic instruments for early childhood stuttering, especially in the differentiation between normal disfluency and incipient stuttering (M. R. Adams, 1977; Campbell & Hill, 1987; Curlee, 1980; Gordon & Luper, 1992; Pindzola & White, 1986), and in those methods designed to predict stuttering chronicity (Conture, 1990; Cooper & Cooper, 1985; Curlee, 1999b; G. D. Riley, 1981). The second occasion is the *point of exit,* in determining whether the disfluency of a child receiving therapy has become normal, warranting dismissal from treatment. For the practitioner, however, the importance of disfluency extends to other issues. The child's progress between the entry and exit points is monitored by examining not only the total number of interruptions or "stutterings," but also the changes in the frequency–type pattern of disfluency. Additionally, the number of disfluencies, especially of certain types, has been regarded as the most important index of stuttering severity (Van Riper, 1971).

One reason for the wide adoption of disfluency counts and their relevance to theoretical, research, and clinical purposes has been a strong inclination to attach significance to the unique features of the diverse disfluencies and a desire to make the most of such diversity. The ability to express the specific characteristics of a stuttering event—for example, whether it is repetition of syllables or sound prolongation—is diminished when other metrics, such as percentage of words stuttered, are employed. A count of 20 "stutterings" in a speech sample tells us little about how the speaker talks when he or she stutters. On the other hand, information that the 20 instances of disfluency in the speech sample contain 12 repetitions of syllables, 2 repetitions of phrases, and 6 prolongations of the /m/ sound provides the clinician with a better picture of the unique characteristics of the client's stuttering. Furthermore, the implementation of disfluency systems and disfluency counts allows direct comparisons between people who stutter and normally fluent speakers in ways that would have been impossible if instances of "stuttering" or "not stuttering" were to be compared without specifying their characteristics. For example, comparisons of temporal properties, such as duration, of interruptions in speech of children who stutter and normally fluent controls (Throneburg & Yairi, 1994), necessitated specifications of the target segments as single or double units of syllable repetition.

Finally, analysis of children's disfluency data by trained investigators has yielded remarkably satisfying reliability estimates. Reviewing the literature, Yairi (1997a) showed that point-by-point (location and type) interjudge agreement on the occurrence of disfluent events in studies reported during the 1980s and 1990s is generally between .82 and .93. These data provide the backing for our disagreement with the position advocated by several investigators (e.g., Cordes & Ingham, 1994) that low agreement among observers regarding identification of disfluency threatens the validity of results from several decades of research on stuttering. Hubbard (1998) demonstrated that reliability of disfluency identification in speech of preschool-age children is as good as that of stuttering identification. A potentially important development in the reliable identification of disfluency has been reported by Howell, Sackin, and Glenn (1997), a group of investigators from Great Britain, who developed automatic computer recognition of specific types of disfluencies with up to 78% identical identification to that of human judges.

Given that absolute differentiation between disfluency found in speech of people who stutter and in normal speech is impossible at present, many investigators in the field have sought a distinction on the basis of statistical probability (e.g., Bloodstein, 1970; Yairi, 1996). That is, these researchers have attempted to isolate disfluent features that, with high probability, are different, or occur in an appreciably greater frequency, or occur in different patterns, in speech of people who are known to exhibit stuttering as compared with speech of normally fluent persons.

Historical Perspectives of Disfluency Research

The Retrospective and Impressionistic Era

As discussed in Chapter 3, practicality has dictated that almost all past data pertaining to early speech characteristics, especially disfluency at the onset of stuttering, were obtained from indirect sources, namely retrospective parental descriptions. Such descriptions are limited in capturing much of the detail under the best of circumstances, and are further weakened by the reporting parent's selective or failing memory. Secondhand sources, however, were unavoidable because investigators could not be present in an unpredictable place and time to record a child's first stutters. Unfortunately, unrecorded, unverified subjective data were used in the past even for the postonset stages of stuttering, after the disorder had been recognized and duly diagnosed and the children became available for close direct examination. Major work in the field, such as Froeschels's (1964) very detailed descriptions of the development of stuttering, Bloodstein's (1960a, 1960b) cross-sectional study that yielded four developmental stages, and Andrews and Harris's (1964) landmark longitudinal investigation concerning persistence and recovery, were all based on the clinician–investigator's impressions, not on systematically gathered, quantified speech characteristics. It is an interesting historical fact that such influential studies were based on either indirect or unquantified data that could be easily questioned as to the strength of their scientific grounds. Fortunately, a considerably more solid data bank derived from speech samples of children has been accumulated over the years.

Early Disfluency Studies

To date, much of the existing information about speech characteristics in young beginning stutterers has centered around the frequency of occurrence of several types of disfluency that were defined with linguistically related terms such as "syllable repetition" and "sound prolongation" or with other descriptive terms. That information appears to underscore the historic fact that systematic research of disfluent speech began with the study of language development in normal children. Brandenburg in 1915 and Nice in 1920 each studied a single child, but just a decade or two later, investigators moved on to observe groups of normally developing preschool children (S. Adams, 1932; Fisher, 1932; McCarthy, 1930; M. Smith, 1926). They all commented on the general presence of repetitions, but these were neither defined, nor differentiated, nor quantified.

Quantitative, large-scale research of disfluencies began at the University of Iowa in the late 1930s, probably as Wendell Johnson was mulling over the initial version of his diagnosogenic theory, which linked stuttering onset to parental overreactions to normal disfluencies. To defend the theory, he had to demonstrate that disfluencies were commonplace in young children. This was accomplished through a series of studies of normally speaking preschool children's speech conducted from the late 1930s to the mid-1940s by Johnson and his students, including Davis (1939), Branscom (1942), Hughes (1943), and Oxtoby (1943), who investigated several discrete age groups between ages 2 and 5. In those days, however, tape recorders were not readily available, and the investigator had to transcribe the children's speech by hand while simultaneously marking disfluencies on the transcripts. These technical disadvantages reduced accuracy in recording children's utterances and disfluencies, and restricted the range of disfluency types included in the research. Their initial repertoire included only three types: (a) syllable repetition, (b) word repetition, and (c) phrase repetition.

The serious limitations of these studies did not prevent the investigators from arriving at the crucial conclusion that repetitions were common and frequent in normally fluent children. The lasting influence of apparently erroneous interpretations of data is astounding. To this day, many laypersons as well as health and educational professionals, including speech–language pathologists, advise parents that excessive repetition is quite common in the speech of all young children. Not only do we strongly disagree with the conclusion that normal repetitions are frequent, but the way in which this conclusion has been transmitted to the public is a cause for concern. We have heard from many parents who were advised by physicians that some stuttering is a normal stage. A nationwide survey of pediatricians, members of a health profession that exerts an enormous influence on parents, showed that 70% of this group hold similar beliefs (Yairi & Carrico, 1992).

More critical, however, was Johnson's (1942) idea that not only was disfluency common but whatever the parent originally diagnosed as the beginning of stuttering was nothing but normal disfluency. This idea became one of the central tenets in his theory regarding the cause of the onset of stuttering: that the disorder begins when overanxious parents react negatively to normal disfluency, which only later progresses and transforms into real stuttering. Johnson's critical determination that parents were diagnosing normal disfluencies as stuttering was based on his interpretations of their verbal descriptions of what they remembered, not on speech-based evidence. Others proposed similar perspectives. For example, Shames and Sherrick (1963) thought that stuttering began with normal disfluency, which was transformed into stuttering through selective reinforcement, and Bloodstein (1970) claimed that there was continuity between normally fluent speech and stuttered speech.

Later Disfluency Studies

The Iowa Study
Since Davis (1939) began systematic studies of children's disfluency, much of subsequent research has attempted to delineate the number and types of disfluencies produced by normally speaking children. Advances in electronic recording of speech samples made it possible to capture the topography of disfluent speech in greater detail and allowed repeated listening, which improved data reliability. The next step was to expand research of disfluency to young children who stutter.

In 1959, Johnson and his associates reported a study in which they obtained recorded speech samples from 89 children, ages 2 to 8, regarded by their parents as exhibiting stuttering, and from matched normally fluent controls. In spite of significant shortcomings, this study served as the main source on the disfluent speech of young children who stutter, and its data were viewed as norms. In the most general terms, the findings showed a mean *total* disfluency of 18 per 100 words for the stuttering group, nearly 2½ times larger than the comparable mean of approximately 7 disfluencies per 100 words for the nonstuttering controls. In spite of the large difference, as well as even sharper group differences in several specific disfluency types, the investigators emphasized the extensive overlap between the two groups. Their two chief arguments were that (a) one third of the normally speaking children had more total disfluency than one third of their stuttering peers and (b) every type of disfluency was present in the speech of the two groups. Most important, they concluded that if extensive overlap existed long after the stuttering onset, when the speech samples were recorded for the study, greater overlap must have existed at the time of onset. In other words, Johnson and associates extrapolated from a data point at an average of 18 months postonset back to the time of onset, where, according to his theory, disfluencies had just transformed from being normal to being stuttering as a result of diagnosis by the parent. As illustrated in Figure 4.1, the researchers assumed that there was a gradually sloping line connecting these points; that is, stuttering was mild at onset, followed by an accelerated course.

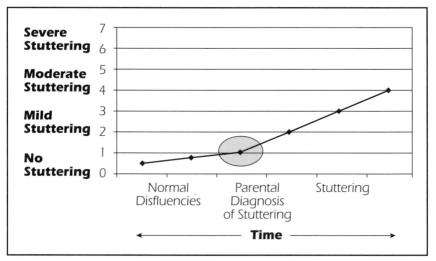

Figure 4.1. Wendell Johnson's model of onset and development of stuttering: Normal disfluencies are shaped into stuttering over time.

Other Studies

A new wave of studies reporting the frequency–type distribution of disfluency in preschool children rose during the 1970s and 1980s, throwing new light on the central question of what is normal and what is abnormal disfluency. A series of studies reported by Yairi and his students for discrete single-year preschool (Yairi, 1981, 1982a; Yairi & Clifton, 1972; Yairi & Jennings, 1974) and school-age (Yairi, 1972) groups provided new data for normally speaking children. These data helped dispel the myth that repetitions occur frequently in the speech of normally speaking young children.

Particularly relevant is Yairi's (1981) investigation of 33 two-year-old children, the largest modern-era disfluency study of this critical age group at that time. It clearly showed that a substantial number of these children produced disfluent speech rather infrequently. Nearly 30% of the children had only 2 or fewer total disfluencies per 100 words, and over 50% had 1 or fewer syllable or word repetitions per 100 words. Furthermore, the study demonstrated that a small number of the children accounted for most of the group's disfluency. This result should not have come as a surprise had data reported in previous studies been carefully examined. A close scrutiny of the data in all of the early Iowa studies of normally speaking children leads to similar conclusions. For example, the famous Davis (1939) report reveals that more than 25% of her 62 children ages 2 through 5 did not produce syllable repetitions, and nearly 50% had fewer than 0.5 repetitions per 100 words. These figures are not tantamount to being "very common" as many experts and laypeople have been led to believe. We suspect that Johnson's strong theoretical motives during that period to prove the normalcy of disfluency led those investigators, as well as those who came later, to misread their own data. Therefore, Yairi (1981) concluded from his findings that "the concept of 'normal disfluency' should not be mistaken to mean a frequently occurring or a predictable average behavior" (p. 484). Furthermore, a critical analysis of 16 studies of normally speaking children conducted by different investigators over a period of 55 years reveals an impressively similar general outcome (Yairi, 1997a). It appears, then, that the belief held by many speech–language pathologists that disfluency, especially repetition, is a pervasive normal phenomenon, and that all children go through a stage of heightened disfluency, is not supported by scientific data.

During this period of renewed research interest in disfluency of normally speaking children, Yairi and his students obtained additional disfluency data for young children in the early stage of stuttering. Particularly significant was a small study by Yairi and Lewis (1984). Unlike Johnson et al. (1959), these two investigators strove to obtain data that met two criteria: being recorded close to the onset of stuttering and representing a narrow age range of children. Their subjects, 10 stuttering and matched control children, were between 25 to 39 months of age and the children who stuttered were within 2 months after onset ($M = 6$ weeks). This compares with a postonset interval of up to 3 years, with a mean of 18 months, in Johnson et al.'s investigation. Yairi and Lewis found that large deviations from normal disfluency exist almost from the very beginning of stuttering, differences that were even larger than those reported by Johnson et al. These results provided direct evidence contradicting the assertion that the disfluent speech of the two groups of children is essentially the same when recorded closer to the time of stuttering onset, further undermining Johnson's diagnosogenic theory. These findings were recently confirmed in a large-scale study reported by Ambrose and Yairi (1999), which showed little overlap between the two groups.

Regardless of the specific findings, however, what constitutes normal and abnormal disfluency has been a significant issue with profound influence on theory, diagnosis, and treatment of the disorder for more than 50 years. In the clinical domain, the issue has created undue concern that it is difficult to decide whether a child's disfluency represents early stuttering that merits clinical intervention (Manning, 1996). Our brief review has highlighted the important role of disfluency metrics in all domains of stuttering research and has concluded that recent research has yielded powerful metrics for distinguishing children who stutter from their normally fluent peers.

A more detailed summary of the salient features that differentiate between early stuttering and normal disfluency is presented in Chapter 10. From a historical perspective, however, it should be noted that research concerning disfluency has taken several directions over the years. Researchers have focused either on normally fluent children, children who stutter, or the differences between these populations. Several investigators analyzed children's disfluencies in terms of the *proportion* of each disfluency type (e.g., Yairi, 1972; Yairi & Lewis, 1984; Zebrowski, 1991); their motivation was to investigate disfluency patterns for each group as reflected in the relative weight of each disfluency type instead of the absolute frequency. Information on the *spatial distribution* of disfluency events—that is, their tendency to occur in clusters—was reported by Hubbard and Yairi (1988) and LaSalle and Conture (1995). More recently, interest in the dimension of *length* of young children's disfluency has drawn increasing research activity (e.g., Ambrose & Yairi, 1995; Kelly & Conture, 1992; Throneburg & Yairi, 1994; Yairi & Hall, 1993; Zebrowski, 1991). Others have looked at the *variability* of disfluency in different situations (Silverman, 1972; Yaruss, 1997), with conversational demands (Weiss, 1995), and during interaction with parents (Bernstein Ratner, 1992; Kelly, 1994; Meyers, 1986). The association between disfluency and *secondary characteristics* was also studied (Conture & Kelly, 1991; H. D. Schwartz, Zebrowski, & Conture, 1990; Yairi, Ambrose, et al., 1996). Conture, McCall, and Brewer (1977) studied *physiological correlates* of disfluencies.

The Evolution of Disfluency Systems

Types of Disfluency

As just mentioned, considerable research on disfluent speech of children has been conducted since the period of the early studies. As investigators sought more and better data, methodological developments evolved from the original three-type repertoire of syllable repetition, word repetition, and phrase repetition. In 1959, Johnson and associates introduced an eight-type disfluency scheme that greatly influenced the work in this field. It was composed of (a) sound and syllable repetition, (b) revision, (c) word repetition, (d) incomplete phrase, (e) phrase repetition, (f) broken word, (g) interjection, and (h) prolonged sound. Further modifications by others followed. In 1968, Williams, Silverman, and Kools added a new type of disfluency, labeled tense pause, that was intended to account for unusual breaks associated with tense sounds between words. They also combined sound prolongations and broken words into a single category labeled disrhythmic phonation, and merged revision with incomplete phrase into a single type. These changes resulted in a seven-type system.

In 1981, Yairi separated word repetition into two different types: monosyllabic word repetition and multisyllabic word repetition, recognizing Wingate's (1964) conception that it is the short-element repetition that better characterizes stuttering. Other investigators have suggested additional specific disfluency types to create their working schemes. Meyers (1986) took the eight types of the Johnson et al. (1959) system, added tense pause from the Williams et al. (1968) system, and ended up with a nine-type scheme. Campbell and Hill (1987) used items found in the Johnson and the

Yairi schemes and added sound repetition, block, and hesitation to derive a total of 11 types. An interesting feature of their system is the use of the number of iterations as a factor in typing disfluency. For example, they regarded monosyllabic word repetition that contains three or fewer iterations as a different type from word repetition that contains four or more iterations.

More recently, our team (Ambrose & Yairi, 1999) opted to combine multisyllabic word repetition with phrase repetition because both involve more than one syllable and are typical normal disfluencies. This combination also acknowledges that multisyllabic word repetition is rather uncommon in the speech of young children. Additionally, we eliminated tense pause because it did not appear reliably identifiable.[1] We finally settled on a reduced system composed of only six disfluency types described below:

The Illinois Disfluency Classification System

▶ 1. *Part-Word Repetitions.* This type includes repetitions of sounds and syllables. No distinction is made between sound and syllable repetitions (e.g., "a-and," "f-five," "ba-baby," "mo-mo-mommy"). The part-word repetition type acknowledges the limitation of human ears with respect to the challenge of auditory discrimination between splintering of sounds versus syllables. There are times when a part-word repetition spans syllables (e.g., "ele-ele-elephant"). This speech disfluency cannot rightly be called any of these potential categories: sound repetition, syllable repetition, or monosyllabic word repetition. When more than one syllable is repeated (e.g., "becau-because," "anoth-another"), it is considered a multiple-syllable repetition.

▶ 2. *Single-Syllable Word Repetitions.* This category encompasses repetitions of whole, single-syllable words (e.g., "but-but," "and-and"). Words repeated for emphasis, as in "big, big," are not counted as disfluency. A repeated word with any intervening verbalization, such as an interjection, causes the repetition not to be counted as such. In-

---

[1] A type used in several of our early studies, tensions, or tense pause, refers to barely audible heavy breathing or tight vocal sounds. The disfluency is perceived to occur between words or nonwords (i.e., interjections). We have eliminated this type due to repeated indication of problems with reliability and confusion with extraneous noises.

stead, a revision is marked. For example, "I want um want to go now" is classified as "I want (revision) (interjection) want to go now." "I want mo- want some" is also a revision.

▶ **3.** *Disrhythmic Phonation.* This disfluency type includes sound prolongations or blocks (audible or inaudible sound prolongations), identified only within words. This kind of phonation disturbs the flow of speech and may be attributable to a block or prolonged sound, a stress or intonation pattern that is notably unusual, or a break in the word.

▶ **4.** *Interjections.* Interjections include extraneous sounds such as "um," "uh," "er," and "hmmm." An instance of interjection may include one or more units of repetition (e.g., "um" and "um-um"). Words grammatically considered interjections, such as "like" and "well," are *not* included in this category. Words and phrases such as "like," "well," or "you know" are not considered disfluencies but are counted simply as words.

▶ **5.** *Multiple-Syllable Word and Phrase Repetitions.* Repetitions of segments longer than one syllable or one word are included in this category. "Because-because," "Once up-once upon," and "I was-I was going," are examples of this type of disfluency.

▶ **6.** *Revision or Abandoned Utterance.* This disfluency type includes instances in which an utterance is modified or not completed. When the general content of the statement remains the same but a modification occurs, it is counted as a revision (e.g., "I was—I am going," "I want the ball—red ball," and "she gave him—he gave her"). An abandoned utterance occurs when a thought is not completed (e.g., "Yesterday I went—hey what's that over there?" or "I want another ...").

As explained, this taxonomy emerged gradually, and the various stages in which somewhat different disfluency types were incorporated in studies of the University of Illinois Stuttering Research Program are reflected in the publications of our group. The final version as described here has been in publications since 1999.

Classes of Disfluency

As researchers took a closer look at the diagnosogenic theory and its excessive emphasis on overlap in the disfluent speech characteristics of children who stutter and normally fluent children, it became quite apparent that disfluencies differ in the degree to which they are prevalent in the speech of the two groups. Although this idea was not entirely new, the growing realization resulted in at least five disfluency classifications that grouped several disfluency types to reflect this differentiation concept. All five classification systems are composed of two grand classes, each of which includes a number of disfluency types.

Several researchers have suggested that disfluencies can be organized into classes that may reveal their etiology. Manning and Shirkey (1981) offered two categories: formulative and motoric disfluency breaks. *Formulative disfluency* consists of (a) breaks in fluency between whole words, phrases, and larger syntactic units; (b) repetitions of these segments; and (c) interjections between the larger syntactic units. No tension is present during breaks. These breaks can be regarded as normal and are found in the speech of both stuttering and normally fluent children and adults. Although Manning and Shirkey did not explain their choice of the label "formulative" for these fluency breaks, it suggests a breakdown in the linguistic planning processes. A repetition such as "I want—I want to order out tonight" could have allowed the speaker extra time to plan, or formulate, the end of the utterance. *Motoric disfluency,* such as repetitions of short segments (parts of words), blocks, and prolongations, are characterized by (a) breaks in fluency between sounds or syllables, (b) obvious tension during the breaks, (c) pauses with possible cessation of airflow and voicing between small linguistic units, and (d) excessive prolongations of sounds and syllables. These are not considered normal and are more characteristic of the speech of people who stutter, although some are also present in the speech of nonstuttering individuals.

The first of Conture's (1982) two disfluency classes, *within-word disfluency,* is regarded as "stuttering." It includes sound repetition, syllable repetition, and prolongation. The second major class, labeled *between-word disfluency,* includes most other types and is depicted as "normal disfluency." One of the problems with this system is that it employs the term *stuttering* even when counting within-word disfluencies in the speech of normally speaking children. This terminology can be confusing. If children produce "stuttering," they should not be regarded as speaking normally. Another difficulty we encountered in the initial Conture classification is that it left monosyllabic word repetitions as an undefined category. According to our data, however, this is a very common element in the speech of young children who stutter and distinguishes them from normally fluent children. If single-syllable word repetitions are not included in research or clinical analyses of stuttered speech, it can be expected that approximately 25% of the disfluencies of those children would be discarded. The decision to eliminate such a large proportion of relevant data is not well founded. Indeed, in the most recent edition of his book, Conture (2001) includes monosyllabic word repetition as stuttering.

Meyers (1986) divided the nine disfluency types in her scheme into four *stutter types* and five *normal types*. Again, the problem with these labels is the implied clear-cut dichotomy. In the *Systematic Disfluency Analysis*, Campbell and Hill (1987) distinguished between the class of *more typical* (normal speech) disfluency (six types) and the class of *less typical* (normal speech) disfluency (five types). This terminology appears to be a reasonable alternative, although we have reservations about using normal speakers as the frame of reference. This may imply that stuttering is simply more of what normal speakers do, as opposed to stuttering as a disorder. To us, what drives the interest in disfluency is what the person who stutters does when he or she talks. Questions are also raised concerning Campbell and Hill's use of qualitative judgment. It appears that, regardless of the basic classification, when disfluency is judged as "tense," it is regarded as less typical, thus reducing the value of the system's objective descriptive basis. Additionally, they suggest that repetition with three extra iterations is more typical. Several studies, however, have shown that a disfluency of this length is far from being typical.

In our own classification (Ambrose & Yairi, 1999; Yairi & Ambrose, 1992a), we used stuttering as the reference while attempting to cope with the reality that there are disfluencies that are neither exclusively stuttering nor exclusively normal. We accomplished this by recognizing the greater statistical probability of occurrence of several disfluency types in the speech of one group. Therefore, we advocate two global disfluency classes applicable to all children: *Stuttering-Like Disfluencies* (SLD) and *Other Disfluencies* (OD). The scheme includes the six different types of disfluency described earlier in this chapter. Three of the six types occur more frequently in the speech of people who stutter: part-word repetitions, single-syllable word repetitions, and disrhythmic phonation. Because these are typical, but *not* exclusive, to people who stutter, they were labeled "Stuttering-Like Disfluencies." The other three types—interjections, multiple-syllable word and phrase repetitions, and revision or abandoned utterance—are typical of normally fluent people, and also are found at comparable levels in those who stutter. They were labeled Other Disfluencies.

As can be seen, the various proposed global schemes are quite similar, reflecting a general agreement in the field about the nature of the different types of disfluency. Still, they seem to convey the realization that a distinction between what is stuttering and what is normal is not always possible. We are aware of these limitations and their implications for the data that they generate. Practically, one may assume that some errors occur in both directions: counting as stuttering some disfluencies that actually were normal, and counting as normal some disfluencies that were stuttering. We agree with Conture (2001) that, for the time being, it might be necessary to recognize and accept a relatively small percentage of error. As the state of knowledge about stuttering increases, and with the development of more sensitive, automated technology (Howell et al., 1997), it should become possible to derive more accurate measures.

More on Stuttering-Like Disfluency

To be sure, Stuttering-Like Disfluency is not "pure" stuttering, if something like that can ever be defined. This is why we include the word *like.* Although Wingate (2001) unfortunately interpreted our use of "like" as "resembling," concluding that it is impossible to study something that resembles the phenomenon under study, we maintain that the term is appropriate. By "like," we mean "characteristic of," reflecting an assumption that what the listener hears as "stuttering" is, after all, but the surface aspect of the disorder. Second, we use "like" because judgments of overt speech behavior as "stuttering" are made perceptually by listeners, and these judgments are fluid and change under the influence of many factors (Curlee, 1981; Curran & Hood, 1977; Williams & Kent, 1958). Also, contrary to Wingate (1964, 2001), we recognize that the underlying experience of a stuttering block may sometimes be manifest in all kinds of behaviors, interjections included (Cordes & Ingham, 1995; Hegde & Hartman, 1979a, 1979b; Martin & Haroldson, 1981). The observations made by these authors reinforce our position that, for research purposes, the link between disfluent events and "stuttering" must be in terms of what is statistically most probable to reflect both frequency of speech output and what listeners perceive as stuttering (Bloodstein, 1970; Yairi, 1996), and not based on a rigid theoretical notion of what "stuttering" must be. Therefore, we count disfluencies, and our SLD is an *index* that quantifies the most common disfluencies produced by children who stutter and are also the most likely to be perceived as stuttering.

Another issue is the composition of SLD. Wingate (2001) insists that only syllable repetitions and sound prolongations constitute stuttering. The evidence, however, is overwhelming against his position in that (a) not all stuttering involves syllable repetitions or sound prolongations; (b) not all syllable repetitions and prolongations emitted by people who stutter are perceived consistently, if at all, as stuttering; and (c) syllable repetitions and sound prolongations are also produced by normally speaking children (Ambrose & Yairi, 1999; Hegde & Hartman, 1979a, 1979b; Hubbard, 1998; Johnson et al., 1959; Williams & Kent, 1958; Yairi, 1981; Yairi & Lewis, 1984). Our SLD class includes monosyllabic word repetitions, to which Wingate (2001) objects. Holding to his argument may lead to rather strange conclusions that a disfluent event such as "a-a-a-a boat" (word repetition) *would not* constitute stuttering, whereas "a-a-a-about" (syllable repetition) *would*. Such a position grossly disregards fundamentals of speech production. Speech is not produced in either strings of isolated syllables or word units, but is coarticulated across syllables and words. We must acknowledge the actual ways in which syllables and monosyllabic words are articulated and reiterated. Whether a speaker says "a-a-a-a-bout" (sound repetition) or "a-a-a-a boat" (monosyllabic word repetition), the fluency breakdown of the coarticulated speech string is similar. Or consider "i-i-i-icicle" (sound or syllable repetition) versus "I-I-I-I-I said call" (monosyllabic word repetition). The unit of speech rhythm reiterated and the nature of the fluency breakdown is similar in both cases (Yairi et al., 2001).

Additionally, Wingate (2001) developed his case against counting monosyllabic words as stuttering, arguing that English monosyllabic words are predominantly closed syllable, which makes them markedly different from syllable repetition. This argument, however, also does not hold. The fact is that normal phonological development of young children includes a phase characterized by numerous final consonant deletions. Moreover, words commonly initiating sentences in the speech of young children are monosyllabic with open syllables (*he, she, we, I, you, the,* etc.), and these are the ones that are often repeated by children who stutter.

Our data reveal that monosyllabic word repetitions, like syllable repetitions, do differentiate stutterers from nonstutterers, especially in early childhood. Monosyllabic word repetitions are frequent contributors to the disfluency and stuttering of preschool children. We have reported that, in preschool children who persisted in stuttering, monosyllabic word repetition varied between 33% and 39% of their SLD. It was the second largest element in their total disfluency—two to five times larger than the percentage of disrhythmic phonation (Throneburg & Yairi, 2001). Furthermore, our studies show that the proportion of single-syllable word repetitions in the speech of preschoolers who stutter was four to five times larger than the respective proportion in the speech of normally speaking children (Ambrose & Yairi, 1999; Yairi & Lewis, 1984). Most important, we reported statistically significant differences in the frequency of monosyllabic word repetition between children who stutter and normally fluent children at three different age groups from 2- to 4-year-olds (Ambrose & Yairi, 1999). Curran and Hood (1977) reported that syllable repetitions and word repetitions received very similar ratings whether judged as normal or as stuttering. Quite likely, such disfluencies are not the same in the speech of stuttering and normally fluent children, not only in terms of frequency of occurrence, but also number of repetition units per instance, durational features, speed of repetitions, and other characteristics. Repetitions of normally speaking children typically consist of one extra production of the repeated segment, whereas children who stutter tend to repeat more times per disfluent event (Ambrose & Yairi, 1995; Yairi & Hall, 1993). Thus, "and-and-and-and" (monosyllabic word repetition) is more likely to be perceived as stuttering than "a-and" (syllable repetition). Finally, Zebrowski and Conture (1989) demonstrated that mothers perceived most monosyllabic word repetitions as stuttering. In short, Wingate (2001) ignored several elements that have been scientifically established as critical to the stuttering "formula." Not surprisingly, many researchers have taken a stand similar to ours. The guidelines for identification of stuttering published by the American Speech-Language-Hearing Association's Special Interest Division for Fluency and Fluency Disorders include the following: "Stuttering refers to speech events that contain *monosyllabic whole-word repetitions,* part-word repetitions, audible sound prolongations ..." (1999, p. 31, emphasis added). Likewise, in his recent book, Conture (2001) defined stuttering as typically involving, among other disfluencies, monosyllabic whole-word repetitions.

Factors Influencing Disfluency Analysis

Considering the prominence of disfluency counts in quantifying stuttering, investigators and clinicians should be cognizant of several factors that can significantly influence their research data and clinical reports. Lack of appreciation and control of these can result in inconsistent, questionable results.

Disfluency Types

The number of disfluency types employed can influence the total count. Sometimes, a larger number of types results in a larger amount of disfluency identified in a speech sample because more speech characteristics are included. For example, if tense pause is included in the analysis, more disfluencies will be identified. In other instances, however, a larger number of types does not alter the total count but changes the pattern of the data, such as when part-word repetitions are split into sound repetitions and syllable repetitions. The total number of disfluencies remains the same, but the breakdown provides more detailed information. Similarly, there is a change in the pattern but not in the total count when prolongations are lumped together with broken words to form a single category of disrhythmic phonation. Therefore, comparisons among results of different studies or clinical reports should carefully consider the composition of the disfluency systems employed. Although the number of recognized disfluency types has increased from a mere 3 in early investigations to as many as 11 in later systems, as of today, no disfluency system has become the standard.

Multiple Disfluencies

How a system treats multiple disfluencies occurring on the same word may have considerable impact on the results of the analysis. For example, the word "a-a-a→nother" contains one event of part-word repetition and one event of sound prolongation (indicated by the arrow). The question is often asked: Should only one of the two different events be counted? The strategy in many studies (e.g., Ambrose & Yairi, 1999; Johnson et al., 1959) has been to view multiple disfluencies as separate events, although a few investigators either counted or have advocated counting only one type per word (e.g., Meyers, 1986; Ryan, 2001b). The confusion on this issue has not been completely resolved, as seen in the discussion by Onslow et al. (1992) and Cordes and Ingham (1994). In our opinion, counting only one disfluency type or event per word or syllable where two or three actually occurred is a misrepresentation of the speech phenomena under study. Important information is lost when "Ha-ha-hammm→burger" or "bu-bu-bu→-but" is counted only as a single stuttering event or a part-word repetition when, in fact, in each of these examples, sound prolongation was also produced and perceived. Some disfluency events are quite complex. For example, the word "a-a-a-aaa→and-and" contains one event of part-word repetition, one of prolongation, and one of word repetition.

Age

Like other aspects of speech and language development, disfluency data for young children should be derived for narrow age groups. Clinicians working with language and phonological development would not use normative data that are not specific for discrete age ranges. Because of fast and great changes in speech and language skills during childhood, merging data for children who are 5 years apart in age makes no sense. Why, then, should those of us who specialize in stuttering be less precise? Past observations regarding age-related variations in stuttering from stage to stage, as described by Bloodstein (1960b), and more recent findings of rapid changes in stuttering during the first few months and years of stuttering (Yairi & Ambrose, 1999a; Yairi, Ambrose, & Niermann, 1993) make it clear that disfluency data obtained for children who spread in age by more than a year or two should be questioned. This concern is particularly true for very young children whose language advances rapidly, because of the apparent relationship between language complexity and the rise in disfluency in children who stutter (Logan & Conture, 1995). The age factor is one reason why the well-known disfluency study by Johnson et al. (1959), which used speech samples of children from age 2 to nearly age 9, is significantly weak. In our opinion, for children under age 6, the maximum age span for group disfluency data is 2 years; however, 6-month or 1-year brackets provide a much more accurate picture. This argument is even stronger when the relation between disfluency and language or phonological skills is explored, as these two domains appear to be quite sensitive to small age differences.

Length of Speech Sample

Because disfluencies are separated by segments of fluent speech, the size of a speech sample influences estimates of the child's disfluency. Speech sample size used in research, however, has varied greatly across studies, as well as among subjects in the same study. Johnson et al. (1959) included samples that ranged in length from 31 to 2,044 words, whereas H. D. Schwartz and Conture (1988) used 85 to 650 words. Many studies in the past two decades were based on samples of 300 to 350 words (e.g., Conture & Kelly, 1991; Meyers, 1986). Some samples have been even smaller, with Yaruss (1997) employing 200-syllable samples, and Onslow, Costa, and Rue (1990) using samples as short as 1 minute. Several concerns can be raised about such short samples.

1. They may contain mainly the peaks or the valleys of a child's fluctu-ating disfluent output, providing a skewed picture of his or her speech.
2. They may contain very few occurrences, if any, of certain disfluency types. For example, the 200-syllable samples studied by Yaruss (1997) contained, on the average, a total of six instances per 100 syllables of the "less typical" disfluency types, or 12 in the entire sample. That is, each of the five different disfluency types included in this category was sampled only 2.2 times on average. Similarly, the chance to sample long disfluencies, such as 5-unit syllable repetition (bu-bu-bu-bu-bu-but), more than once is small. Overall, with few entries of each disfluency type or length, the representativeness of the be-haviors measured is questioned.
3. Other measures of disfluency, such as the mean duration or cluster-ing, are also affected by the small number of entries.
4. When speech samples of greatly different sizes are used in the same study, the group data represent children with the greatest verbal out-put rather than those with lower output. Thus, a few children's ex-pressive language skills and motivation to speak may bias the group's disfluency data.

The question, then, is what is a minimal practical size of speech sample for the purpose of disfluency analysis? Although 1,000- to 1,500-syllable samples have been used in our research, we suggest 600 syllables (about 15–30 minutes of talking time for many preschoolers) as a *minimum.* In many cases, a sample of this size adequately taps the less frequent types of disfluency in children's speech. Disrhythmic phonation generally occurs at a much lower frequency than repetitions and is rare in normally fluent speakers, and multiple-unit repetitions may occur only occasionally for some children who stutter. It is advisable to have at least three tokens (representations) of any given type of disfluency: One could be random, two are insufficient to identify a pattern or obtain a mean, but three indicate that the behavior is more than a fluke, presenting some semblance of pattern or typicality. A disfluency that occurs once per 100 syllables (frequency 1.00) would not be difficult to sample even in a relatively short sample, and a 300-syllable sample could yield three tokens. A disfluency that tends to occur only once per 1,000 syllables (frequency .10) will be difficult to sample under any circumstances, and at that level would not appear to make a significant contribution to stuttering unless that one instance, by itself, is very severe. Our data, however, show that important but often less frequent disfluencies, such as disrhythmic phonation and multiple-unit repetitions, are present in children who have just begun to stutter at frequencies between these levels, that is, between .10 and 1.00 per 100 syllables, as well as above them. These stuttering-like disfluencies also occur occasionally in the speech of normally fluent children, but from a frequency of 0 up to a maximum of .49. This would indicate that it is important to "catch" these disfluencies at frequencies of .50 (.5 in 100 syllables or 5 in 1,000 syllables) and up. To obtain three tokens of a disfluency at that rate, a 600-syllable sample is required to provide comfortable assurance that unusual disfluencies are likely to be sampled. Interestingly, data that we have obtained but not yet published (Sawyer & Yairi, 2003) provide strong support to our logical and experience-based opinion just expressed. Comparing the frequency of SLD per 100 syllables in four consecutive 300-syllable segments taken from long speech samples of our subjects, we found that the number of disfluencies tended to systematically increase as the sample got longer. Using information from the first 300 syllables alone would have resulted in underestimates of the frequency and severity of stuttering, especially in mild cases. Speech samples of 600 syllables provided more valid and reliable data.

The issue is not merely sample length, however, but keeping the child talking until whatever stuttering there is may be exhibited. If a child is clearly stuttering throughout the sample, and the parent states that the sample is representative of the child's stuttering, then sample size is less crucial. But many children may talk for quite a while with little or no stuttering, only to move into considerable stuttering later in the sample when a particularly interesting topic is brought up. For young children, then, a short sample may easily miss some stuttering behaviors.

Number of Samples and Home Recordings

Disfluent speech of people who stutter, including young children, and those who are normally fluent, tends to fluctuate in the frequency of its occurrence (Silverman, 1972; Yaruss, 1997). Therefore, the full extent of stuttering could be misjudged if only a single sample is taken on a "good" day when the individual happens to be more fluent. We are not at all concerned, however, if a single sample is recorded on a "bad" day, reflecting the child's potential stuttering severity, because the interest is in what the child does when he or she is stuttering. Of course, periods of fluency, whether during one session or on different days, are also important to note. The variability of stuttering appears to be influenced by numerous immediate factors such as situation, listener, task, fatigue, and others. When certain consistency is detected, clinicians can use the information in counseling parents. What determines larger cycles, however, such as good or bad days, is not yet understood.

Although fluctuations in disfluency have been commonly observed, data about the number of speech samples needed to provide an accurate representation are not available, and that number may not be possible to determine. Several investigators (e.g., J. C. Ingham & Riley, 1998; Onslow, Andrews, & Lincoln, 1994) have advocated obtaining samples recorded in different situations, such as at home, at school, and in the clinic. Yaruss (1997) reported significant differences in five speaking situations recorded during the initial evaluations of preschool children. Inspection of his data, based on very brief 200-word samples, shows that the differences in SLD in the five situations were rather small in magnitude. The differences ranged from about 0.5 to almost 2.0 disfluencies per 100 words, and would quite unlikely alter the overall severity rating. Meyers (1986), on the other hand, reported remarkably consistent disfluency levels of stuttering for children in several interactions with parents. In our opinion, although multiple speech samples probably add information, their practical importance has been greatly exaggerated and the impracticality of obtaining them unduly minimized. The reliability and validity of samples recorded in outside-the-clinic situations is also questioned. Our extensive experience indicates that when parents record at home, they may be quite selective of when and what they record and their own behavior might differ from usual. Few, if any, parents provide clinicians with speech samples recorded during unpleasant family situations. In addition, parents sometimes do not make the recording immediately following the clinic visit, but wait several weeks or months, at which point the home sample does not correspond in time to the clinic sample. Even when recordings are timely, home samples are frequently shorter and of poorer quality than clinic samples.

At present, the question of how many home samples are needed to provide a "true" picture of the child's stuttering has no clear answer. We have obtained a large number of home speech samples, and although some provide data that are somewhat different from those recorded in the clinic, the clinic sample usually exhibits more disfluency. As mentioned, the sample that reflects the more severe stuttering is the more important one. Most significantly, in our experience, home samples rarely, if ever, change the overall diagnosis or severity level of stuttering. We have found that the combination of two large samples, each of 500 syllables or more, taken in the clinic a few days apart, during interaction with two or three people, in most cases provides a good representation of the child's stuttering. On occasion, however, if, in spite of parents' claims, the child stutters very little, if at all, while in the clinic on his or her first visit or two, we suggest bringing the child on a day that stuttering is more pronounced or we seek a home sample recorded by either parents or by a clinician visiting the home.

Metric

Typically, the frequency of disfluency is expressed per fixed amount of speech. Among the more common metrics are (a) percentage of disfluent words, (b) percentage of disfluent syllables, (c) number of disfluencies per 100 words, and (d) number of disfluencies per 100 syllables. The use of percentage or number per 100 syllables or 100 words is convenient because it allows us to use or compare data that were derived from different lengths of speech samples. Clinicians, however, must be aware of the difference among metrics because they yield different data.

When the metrics of percentage of disfluent words or percentage of disfluent syllables are applied, a substantial portion of the disfluency identified is lost because these metrics disregard multiple disfluencies on a single word or syllable. The metric of number of disfluencies per 100 words, on the other hand, reflects all the disfluencies but disregards differences in word length because short words receive the same weight as longer ones. What this means is that the proportion of disfluency to the actual amount of the speech output is simply ignored. Fifteen disfluencies per 100 single-syllable words is, in reality, twice as much as 15 disfluencies per 100 two-syllable words (200 syllables). The second figure indicates that the speech is considerably more fluent than the first, although the number of disfluencies (15) and the number of words (100) are identical to the first figure. Therefore, we favor the syllable-based metric—disfluencies per 100 syllables—because it more accurately reflects the amount of speech being affected by disfluency. This is especially true for young children, because the length of words used increases substantially from age 2 to age 6. In our experience, approximately 85% of the words produced by 2- to 3-year-olds are mono-syllabic, whereas the figure is closer to 70% for 5- to 6-year-olds.

Unfortunately, the significance of this fact in early childhood stuttering has not been appreciated in many studies that used word counts for different ages within the preschool range. For example, Davis's (1939) study of the changes in disfluencies between ages 2 and 5 years used the disfluencies per 100-word metric, overlooking the fact that 100 words spoken by 5-year-olds undoubtedly consist of more syllables than 100 words spoken by 2-year-olds. That is, the downward slope in disfluency associated with increase in age that she reported would have been steeper had she used the more sensitive syllable metric. Also, other studies of early childhood disfluencies that merged data from children of a wide age range or compared children of different age groups and used the word metric (e.g., Pellowski & Conture, 2002) are likely to contain errors. Clinical reports or therapeutic studies of young stutterers that describe disfluency changes over time must consider this fact. We disagree with Conture and Caruso's (1987) opinion that this is an insignificant issue, especially in evaluating young children.

To illustrate the potential effect of the metric, in a given sample of 300 words containing 400 syllables, if a child has 25 disfluencies on 15 different words, Meyers (1986) and Zebrowski (1991) would report the child as being 5% disfluent, Johnson et al. (1959) would report 8.33 disfluencies per 100 words, and Yairi and Lewis (1984) would report 6.25 disfluencies per

100 syllables. Consider another example of a study comparing disfluency development of 2-year-olds with that of 4-year-olds. Typically, words produced by 4-year-olds are, on the average, longer than words of 2-year-olds. This is part of normal language development. Thus, 10 disfluencies in 100 monosyllabic words (10% of the total of a 100-syllable sample) spoken by a 2-year-old are considerably more, in relation to the total amount of speech, than 15 disfluencies in 100 bisyllabic words (7.5% of the total of the 200-syllable sample) in the speech of a 4-year-old. Thus, without taking into consideration how much speech is included in 100 words, there is a "visual illusion" that disfluency has increased with age from 10 to 15, whereas in reality there was an appreciable *decrease* from 10% to 7.5%.

The crux of the matter is how stuttering occurs per *opportunity* to stutter. There is a strong tendency for stuttering to occur at the beginnings of words, but it is not unusual to observe stuttering in later syllables. For example, if a child were to say, "Billy ate all the potato chips before me," how many opportunities to stutter exist? Stuttering is highly unlikely on the second syllable of "Billy," which is unstressed, but quite likely on "–ta–" in "potato," unlikely but possible on "–to" of "potato," and quite possible on "be–" and/or "–fore" in "before." In fact, children often reduce syllables and may say "tato chips," and they may think of "before" as "be" + "for." Based on these considerations, the weight of the evidence favors the perspective that counting the syllables in the speech sample more closely represents disfluency on stuttering opportunities than does counting words. The use of smaller units to achieve accuracy is well recognized in measuring articulatory rate, in which the standard metric is syllables, or even phones, per minute, not words per minute.

Disfluency Norms

In spite of the wide clinical and research usage of information concerning disfluency, until recently, a normative disfluency reference for preschool children in the early stage of stuttering did not exist. The main source used for this purpose was the single large study by Johnson et al. (1959), which featured data for 89 stuttering children and an identical number of normally fluent controls. Although in many ways this famous study charted the territory for study of children's disfluent speech behavior, it contained two significant drawbacks that weaken the status of its data as "norms." First, the children ranged from ages 2 to 8. Treating such a wide age range as a single group is not compatible with what is conventionally viewed as normative speech and language data for young children. Whereas our main interest lies with 2- to 5-year-old children, the typical age range for stuttering onset, some participants in the Johnson et al. study may have been in the third grade. Second, the interval between the onset of stuttering and the recording of the speech samples was as long as 3 years ($M = 18$ months). The long delay between onset and the recording of speech samples also precludes the data from being considered *early* stuttering. This is especially true in view of strong evidence that rapid changes occur in the stuttering of many children shortly after the disorder begins (Yairi et al., 1993).

As pointed out earlier, between 1959 and 1999, many research contributions enriched the field's understanding of the general characteristics and specific aspects of disfluencies of young stuttering children and their normally fluent counterparts. An extensive review of this work can be found in Yairi (1997a). The studies conducted during that period had their own limitations, however, in terms of one or more of the following: (a) a small number of children, (b) the inclusion of children within a wide range of ages, (c) insufficient disfluency data due to short speech samples, (d) speech samples recorded at varied intervals postonset, and (e) inconsistent separation of males and females. To illustrate the point, Yairi and Lewis (1984) used only 10 two- to three-year-olds, Meyers (1986) used speech samples of only 10 minutes in length, and H. D. Schwartz and Conture (1988) reported on 43 children spanning a wide range from almost 4 to 9 years of age. Furthermore, not all studies provided actual frequencies of specific disfluency types, and only a few presented disfluency data uniformly recorded reasonably close to the beginning of stuttering. Because of these constraints (widespread diversity in methodology across studies, and varied or unknown reliability), none of the studies that immediately followed those of Johnson et al. (1959) can be construed as a normative reference for early stuttering. Furthermore, almost all of the aforementioned studies focused on the frequency–type metric, or investigated length or duration of disfluency separately from frequency. These two very important dimensions of disfluency have not been studied combined within a single metric until recently.

Good disfluency norms are important for developing, refining, and answering theoretical questions concerning early childhood stuttering, and to provide a basis for the clinical needs of differential diagnosis. One objective of the University of Illinois Stuttering Research Program was to provide such normative data for preschool children near the onset of stuttering. We sought to obtain data from long speech samples taken from a sufficiently large sample of children representing the population variability of very early stuttering. In addition to providing normative data for disfluency types for early stuttering and normal disfluencies, we also addressed questions regarding possible gender and discrete age differences within the preschool range. Because stuttering is markedly gender-biased, the gender factor was also considered as possibly informative. Our data were reported in an article by Ambrose and Yairi (1999). Since then, the data pool has been expanded and additional analyses performed. The updated findings are presented next in this chapter.

Procedures Employed in Obtaining Normative Disfluency Data

Participants

To overcome shortcomings of past research concerning disfluency in the early stage of stuttering, we adhered to more restrictive criteria in selecting a subset of children from the stuttering group whose data were included in this analysis. To narrow the age range, we used in the normative disfluency study only children who were 60 months of age or younger and whose stuttering history was no longer than 6 months. As a result, the experimental group consisted of 103 children. For the purpose of this analysis, all control group children of comparable ages who were judged by their parents and by us as normally fluent were included. This group consisted of 52 subjects. No limit, however, was set on the number of the disfluencies in their speech because one of the purposes of the study was to determine whether and how the two groups, which were differentiated perceptually, also varied in the characteristics of their disfluent speech. Detailed information on the gender and age distribution of the participants is presented in Table 4.1. The groups include almost all of the children reported by Ambrose and Yairi (1999).

As can be seen, the mean age of the groups varied narrowly from 36 to 39 months; the control group was slightly older than the experimental group. Within each group, the mean age of males and females was close. The male-to-female ratio was a little over 2:1 for both groups, consistent with that found for the entire sample of participants in the University of Illinois Stuttering Research Program for young stuttering children as indi-

Table 4.1
Ranges, Means, and Standard Deviations (*SDs*)
for Age (in Months) at Recording, Age at Onset, and Postonset Interval
for Experimental and Control Groups

Group	n	Age at Recording			Age at Onset			Postonset Interval		
		Range	M	(SD)	Range	M	(SD)	Range	M	(SD)
Experimental										
Male	69	23–59	36.42	(7.77)	22–53	33.57	(7.11)	0–6	2.83	(1.70)
Female	34	25–59	36.97	(8.71)	22–56	33.91	(8.75)	1–6	3.06	(1.61)
Total	103	23–59	36.60	(8.06)	22–56	33.68	(7.65)	0–6	2.90	(1.67)
Control										
Male	36	27–56	39.56	(8.54)						
Female	16	29–58	37.25	(8.21)						
Total	52	27–58	38.85	(8.43)						

cated in Chapter 2. In the experimental group, the age of the children at stuttering onset was also similar for males and females. In this group there was 1 child just under age two, 54 two-year-olds, 37 three-year-olds, and 11 four-year-olds. In the control group, there were 20 two-year-olds, 22 three-year-olds, and 10 four-year-olds. All children who stuttered were recorded within 6 months of stuttering onset; of these, 70 children were recorded within 3 months of onset.

Recording and Speech Samples

As described in Chapter 2, conversational speech samples were audio- and videotaped during approximately 40 minutes of somewhat structured interaction between the child and a parent and between the child and one investigator. These took place during two sessions approximately 1 week apart and held in a sound-treated recording suite while the child was playing with clay. The protocol also included several standard, open-ended questions posed to the child (i.e., questions about favorite toys, TV shows, etc.). With a few exceptions, speech samples ranged from about 1,000 to

2,000 syllables. When samples were formally analyzed, those that were longer than 1,500 syllables were shortened by excluding portions from the beginning or the end.

Frequency and Proportion of Disfluency

By far the most common measure of disfluency is its frequency distribution across the various types counted in ways discussed earlier. Table 4.2 presents our most updated information regarding the frequency, type, and proportion of disfluencies for the two groups of children.

A multivariate analysis of variance indicated statistically significant differences between the groups in part-word repetitions, single-syllable word repetitions, and disrhythmic phonation. [The respective F values were 73.07, 72.12, and 41.43 ($df = 1, 153, p < .001$).] Thus, the total SLD is also significantly different. Similarly, the two groups differed significantly with regard to Other Disfluencies [$F(1, 153) = 8.42, p = .004$], although the two means were closer than those for SLD.

The results to be emphasized are the mean of 11.30 total SLD per 100 syllables for children who stutter versus a mean of 1.41 for their controls; the first mean is almost eight times greater than the second one. Individual children who stutter, however, vary greatly in SLD frequency from just under 3 per 100 syllables to almost 40. Such a wide, though even, distribu-

Table 4.2

Mean Frequency and Standard Deviation (SD) of Disfluencies per 100 Syllables for Experimental and Control Groups

Disfluency Type	Experimental Frequency (SD)		Control Frequency (SD)	
Stuttering-Like Disfluencies				
Part-word repetitions	5.64	(4.28)	0.55	(0.43)
Single-syllable word repetitions	3.24	(2.01)	0.79	(0.74)
Disrhythmic phonations	2.42	(2.62)	0.08	(0.12)
Total	11.30	(6.64)	1.41	(0.96)
Other Disfluencies	5.79	(2.75)	4.48	(2.41)

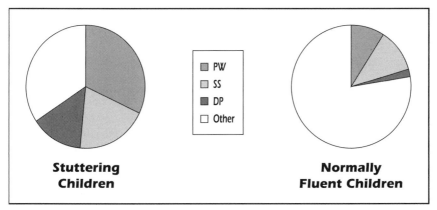

Figure 4.2. Proportion of disfluency types. PW = part-word repetitions; SS = single-syllable word repetitions; DP = disrhythmic phonations. These three categories make up the Stuttering-Like Disfluencies.

tion, with the median close to the mean, makes it difficult to set up expectations for a given child.

An interesting illustration of the differences between the stuttering and normally fluent groups can be seen in Figure 4.2, which displays the proportional relationships of disfluency types. Note that SLD contribute 66% of the total disfluencies for children who stutter, whereas they contribute only 28% for controls, clearly confirming Yairi's (1997a) conclusion. Part-word repetitions are clearly the most frequent disfluency type in children who stutter, but single-syllable word repetitions and disrhythmic phonations are not far behind. In contrast, the data for the control group corroborate Yairi's (1981) findings that, for normally speaking children, repetitions are not a frequent behavior and disrhythmic phonation is rare. Also note that Other Disfluencies do not contribute meaningfully to the differentiation. Overall, considering our method in selecting subjects, recording speech samples, and reliably identifying disfluencies, we are confident that the data are representative of early stuttering. This being the case, it is important to note here that they support our long-held proposition that distinct differences from the disfluency of normally speaking children are present right from the emergence of stuttering.

Similar patterns can be observed in the results of several previous investigations, keeping in mind their various limitations as discussed previously. In the classic Johnson et al. (1959) study, a mean total for all disfluencies was 17.91 per 100 words for the stuttering boys and 16.25 for the girls. Both of these figures were nearly 2½ times larger than the disfluencies for the nonstuttering controls (7.28 for boys, and 7.90 for girls). Emphasizing extensive overlap between the two groups, the investigators stated that one third of the control subjects had more total disfluencies than one third of the stutterers. Vastly reduced overlap, however, emerged from our reanalysis of their data when the focus was placed on disfluencies most relevant to stuttering. When we calculated the SLD (adding together sound and syllable repetitions, word repetitions, broken words, and prolonged sounds), the stuttering children in the Johnson et al. study averaged 11.02 SLD per 100 words (63% of the total disfluencies), whereas the control children exhibited only 1.96 per 100 words (26% of the total disfluencies). Again, as shown in the Illinois study, not only is the frequency greater, but the *proportion* of SLD in the total disfluencies also is greater for the stuttering children than for the normally fluent children. Furthermore, according to our analysis of the Johnson et al. data, the more disfluent the child, the greater the proportion of SLD. As shown in Table 4.3, a number of more recent studies, which focused on children closer to the onset of stuttering, all support the same trend.

Although the numbers vary across the studies, what is striking is that the proportion of SLD is above 65% for stuttering children and below 50% for normally fluent children. This observation of a basic characteristic or "rule" of early childhood stuttering was first made by Yairi (1997a). The consistent, large difference between groups in means and proportions makes it clear that SLD, as a measure of early stuttering, has great differentiating power. Recently, Pellowski and Conture (2002) supported our conclusion in this regard, although their percentage of SLD was even higher than ours.

Extent of Repetitions

Although frequency of occurrence has been the most researched dimension of disfluency, the extent of repetitions, or the number of times that a segment is repeated in *addition* to the intended segment, is also a key distinction for groups as well as individuals. It is a rather straightforward matter: A child repeating a single syllable 10 times is bound to attract more attention and be suspected of having more abnormal speech than the one who repeats only once on each of two or three words. However, when the focus in research or in clinical situations is limited to frequency, the sen-

Table 4.3

Postonset Interval, Mean, and Proportion of Stuttering-Like Disfluencies (SLD)
for Experimental and Control Groups in Previous Studies

Study and Group	Postonset Interval (in Months)	N	Mean SLD	Proportion of SLD to Total Disfluency
Yairi & Lewis (1984)	≤2			
Experimental		10	16.43	.77
Control		10	3.02	.49
Hubbard & Yairi (1988)	≤6			
Experimental		15	16.88	.75
Control		15	2.59	.43
Zebrowski (1991)	≤12			
Experimental		10	9.63	.78
Control		10	1.83	.37
Yairi & Ambrose (1992a)	≤12			
Experimental		27	10.87	.73
Yairi, Ambrose, & Niermann (1993)	≤3			
Experimental		16	11.99	.69
Ambrose & Yairi (1999)	≤6			
Experimental		90	10.37	.66
Control		54	1.33	.24

tence "I-I want t-to p-play a ga-game now" and the sentence "I-I-I-I-I want t-to p-p-p-p-play a ga-g-ga-ga-game now" yield the same count—four instances of repetition— and something is wrong. Should these two linguistically identical sentences be equal as far as the amount of disfluency goes? The answer is a resounding "no." Undoubtedly, the number of iterations has a unique impact not reflected in the frequency formulas. Investigators of early stuttering have reported observations regarding the number of times children repeated words or syllables. Darley (1955), Johnson (1942), Van Riper (1971), and Yairi (1983) found that repetitions at the time of onset, as described by parents, often consisted of three iterations. In our experience, however, parents frequently have counted the number of times, with statements similar to "On Saturday he said 'I' 16 times!" or "Last month she was constantly repeating the beginning of her brother's name; once she said it at least 10 times." The exact accuracy of the count is not the issue; it is clear that repetitions exceeded what would be considered "normal" by parents.

In 1955, Branscom, Hughes, and Oxtoby began quantifying repetition units in the speech of normally disfluent preschool-age children. They found that almost 80% of repetitions had only one unit (iteration). Forty years later, Ambrose and Yairi (1995) provided similar results, with 87% of the repetitions of normally fluent children having only one extra unit. In addition to percentages, Wexler (1982) and Yairi (1981) reported mean units of repetition, averaging 1.10 and 1.13, respectively, for several groups of nonstuttering preschoolers. In other words, these children had slightly more than one extra production of the segments that they repeated (e.g., "bu-but"). This is an extremely important feature, if not a rule, of normal disfluency. It is interesting to note, however, that although Johnson et al. (1959) also reported data on the extent of disfluency, they failed to appreciate the important differences between stuttering versus nonstuttering children along this dimension. This failure can be traced to as early as 1942, when Johnson's initial concepts of stuttering as diagnosogenic were published. Attempting to portray the normalcy of disfluencies at the time of onset, he wrote that parents' descriptions indicated that the child was producing "brief" disfluencies. Oddly enough, he characterized "brief" as "2 to 4 iterations." In our opinion, Johnson did not realize that his cursory comment, if valid, was sufficient to undermine his own concept of normal disfluency being shaped into stuttering via parent reactions, because 2 to 4 iterations of a sound, syllable, or word, are greatly above normal and even above the mean for children who stutter. If, indeed, the parents in Johnson's study were correct in reporting two to four iterations at the time of onset, their children were exhibiting full-fledged stuttering right from the starting point of the problem. Indeed, when Johnson et al. (1959) finally analyzed speech samples, they found that the mean number of repetition units (iterations) was 1.46 for the stuttering group and 1.09 for the control group. Although this difference was statistically significant, Johnson et al. continued to press the ideas of "overlap" and lack of meaningful difference because the groups differed by less than 1 unit on the average. Later research, however, showed that the difference between 1 and 2 repetition units is very significant, causing listeners' judgments to change from normal disfluency to stuttering (Sander, 1963).

Three recent investigations also dealt with the dimension of extent of disfluency in preschool-age children. Two Illinois studies (Ambrose &

Yairi, 1995; Yairi & Lewis, 1984) yielded significant differences between experimental (stuttering) and control groups. The mean number of repetition units for the normally fluent children was approximately 1.10 in both studies, whereas the mean for the stuttering children was 1.53 in one study (Yairi & Lewis, 1984) and 1.70 in the other (Ambrose & Yairi, 1995). The third (Zebrowski, 1991) was the only study, so far, to report no significant differences between repetition units of stuttering and normally fluent children. Mean repetition units (recalculated to adjust for Zebrowski's different measurement technique) for stuttering and control children were 1.35 and 1.15, respectively.

Current data from the 103 stuttering children and 52 controls in the University of Illinois Stuttering Research Program, displayed in Table 4.4, reveal similar data to those reported in our previous studies. The group difference was statistically significant [$F(1, 153) = 33.36, p < .001$]. Overall, the data verify that normally fluent children typically repeat once (e.g., "but-but") and seldom repeat more, whereas those who stutter repeat, on average, more than 1.5 times, with some children occasionally repeating in excess of 10 times per instance. In other words, many repetitions by children who stutter contain two iterations or units (e.g., "but-but-but") or more. On this basis it can be concluded that measures of repetition units also discriminate between the two groups, as does the frequency of specific disfluency types. The following example serves to illustrate the point: A relatively disfluent nonstuttering child who repeats "and" an additional time on each of five different occasions in a 100-word speech sample will produce "and" five extra times, whereas a moderately severe stutterer who repeats "and" three additional times on the same five different occasions will produce "and" 15 extra times. Such a disparity in production also has great impact on listeners' perceptions of normalcy, as stated above.

Table 4.4

Range, Mean, and Standard Deviation (*SD*)
for Repetition Units of Stuttering and Normally Fluent Children

Group	Range	*M*	*(SD)*
Stuttering	1.03–5.34	1.56	(0.53)
Normally fluent	1.00–1.76	1.13	(0.16)

There is more to the dimension of extent and its differentiation significance. Although the mean number of repetition units per instance indicates significant group disparities, the groups still show some overlap, and the mean does not indicate much about the occurrence of repetitions with 1, 2, 3, or 4 and more units. Is the mean number of units for children who stutter greater based on many of their repetitions having just 2 units? Are instances of more than 2 units common? Is there a point along this parameter where overlap ceases? To answer these questions, one must examine both the frequency and the proportion of disfluent segments with different numbers of units. Figure 4.3 provides a graphic representation of the frequency per 100 syllables of repetitions according to their extent, that is, their number of repetition units. These data validate the finding first reported by Ambrose and Yairi (1995) that there is little overlap between stuttering and normally fluent children in the number of instances, per 100 syllables, of repetition of syllables or words that contain

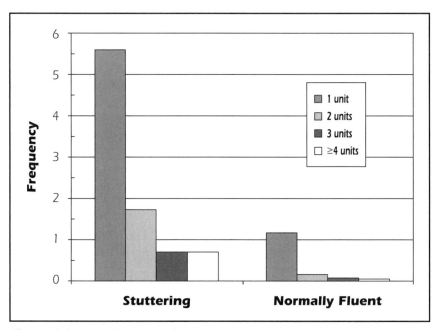

Figure 4.3. Mean frequency of part-word plus single-syllable word repetitions with 1, 2, 3, and 4 or more units, per 100 syllables, for stuttering and normally fluent children.

2 or more extra units. The stuttering group, on average, produces 3.12 multiple unit repetitions per 100 syllables (SD = 3.28), with a range of 0.10 to 21.64. For the control group, the figure is 0.19 (SD = 0.26), with a range of 0 to 1.29.

Besides the obvious conclusion that children who stutter have many more repetitions than the controls, the groups' distributions are different. For the stuttering group, 1-unit repetitions contribute 70% of their total repetitions, 2-unit repetitions contribute 18%, and 3- and 4-repetition units are clearly present at 7% and 5%, respectively. For the control group, 89% of the repetitions are 1 unit and 10% are double unit. Three- and 4-unit repetitions are virtually nonexistent (together, less than 2%) in this group. Therefore, not only is there a large difference in the frequency and proportion of SLD during the early period of stuttering, but there is also marked differentiation in several measures of the extent of repetitions.

Frequency, Type, and Extent Combined

As discussed earlier, a number of measures of disfluency have been employed over the years, including frequency of occurrence of each disfluency type, or all types combined, per unit of speech (word, syllable); frequency of occurrence per unit of time; proportion of each type; ratios between different types; proportion of whole classes of disfluency (e.g., SLD); and extent of disfluency. In spite of this rich variety, no single measure is adequate in reflecting the different dimensions of the disfluency phenomenon: frequency, extent, duration, tension, and so on. Undoubtedly, the coeffect of all the various dimensions leaves its mark on the listener because the whole is more than the sum of its parts. As already pointed out, a count of 3 instances of repetition provides only a portion of the true picture of a person's disfluent speech. It does matter whether, for example, these were 3 instances of "but-but," totaling 6 "buts," or 3 instances of "but-but-but-but," totaling 12 "buts," in 100 syllables. Likewise, to state that 5 instances of sound prolongation were present without specifying whether they were 1 second each (for a total of 5 seconds of elongated speech) or 2½ seconds each (for a total of 12½ seconds of elongated speech) amounts to withholding important information.

We believe that researchers' failure to appreciate and adequately convey the coeffects of even just two dimensions, frequency and extent, has unfortunate consequences. Differences in the disfluent output, as illustrated previously, are known to influence listeners' perceptual judgments of normalcy versus stuttering, and should be reflected in any objective analysis. A widely used clinical tool, the *Stuttering Severity Instrument* (G. D. Riley, 1994), does just this, and has been used in many studies to define subjects as people who stutter or to document changes in stuttering over time. However, the factors that go into the rating are not well researched and frequently are ignored in other studies. It is indeed surprising that such coeffects are not more directly addressed in the theoretical, research, and clinical literature.

A good case in point is the historically key issue of the degree of group overlap between beginning stuttering children and normally fluent children, an issue for which significance has been greatly exaggerated. Although the purported clinical problem of cases at the borderline between normal and stuttering has been considered critical, the fact is that even data from Johnson et al. (1959) indicate the overlap is relatively slight. They showed that only 10% of the nonstuttering children had 3.0 or more SLD per 100 words, whereas 80% of the stutterers had at least 2.6 SLD per 100 words. Yairi and Lewis (1984) and Ambrose and Yairi (1999) also found limited overlap in SLD. Although we have just shown that the dimension of extent is a powerful discriminator between stuttering and normal disfluency, a measure that combines the coeffect of frequency, extent, and duration would seem even better for enhancing the information obtained in disfluency analyses and in helping resolve the overlap issue.

There are many possible ways to combine various measures to create an index that, in a single score, is more representative of the child's stuttering as a whole than are individual measures. For example, the *Stuttering Severity Instrument* (G. D. Riley, 1994), a primarily clinical tool, combines scores assigned to frequency of stutterings, to duration (in seconds) of stuttering events, and to secondary characteristics. Another example is H. D. Schwartz and Conture's (1988) Sound Prolongation Index (SPI), which is based on the proportion of prolongations to stutterings (comparable to our SLD). This index played a major role in their attempt to identify subgroups.

We developed an even more complex measure, the *weighted SLD* (Ambrose & Yairi, 1999), to reflect three dimensions of disfluency—frequency, type, and extent—in a single score. It is calculated by adding together the frequency of part-word and single-syllable word repetitions per 100 syllables (PW + SS) and multiplying that sum by the mean number of repetition units (RU), then adding twice the frequency of disrhythmic phonation (DP) (blocks and prolongations) per 100 syllables. Because in normally fluent speakers disrhythmic phonations are absent or rare, as well as very brief, their presence is a strong indicator of stuttering. We thus doubled their number for the weighted measure. The overall formula is [(PW + SS) × RU] + (2 × DP). Using this formula, one can more clearly distinguish mild but obvious stuttering from normal disfluency.

To illustrate how the weighted SLD can be used, we examine speech samples from two different children. Child 1 has a speech sample of 100 syllables in which there are four SLD: one part-word repetition of four units, one single-syllable word repetition with two units, and two prolongations. These disfluencies occurred in the following utterances of the sample (the remainder of the utterances were fluent):

*Mmmmmm*ake a snake.	(1 DP)
Sitting on *the the the* couch.	(1 SS with 2 units)
*Lllll*ike *th-th-th-th-that.*	(1 DP and 1 PW with 4 units)

Using the conventional count, the frequency of stuttering (SLD) would be only 4 per 100 syllables. This number alone does not necessarily indicate whether the child is mildly stuttering or at the disfluent end of normally fluent. In contrast, the sample from Child 2 also contains 4 SLD: two part-word repetitions of one unit each, two single-syllable word repetitions of one unit each, and no disrhythmic phonations, as shown in the following utterances:

I I smushed *th-the* TV.	(1 SS with 1 unit and 1 PW with 1 unit)
M-make a remote.	(1 PW with 1 unit)
Not *like like* that.	(1 SS with 1 unit)

The calculations would be as follows:

Child 1
$$[(PW + SS) \times \text{units/rep}] + (2 \times DP) = [(1 + 1) \times 6/2] + (2 \times 2)$$
$$= (2 \times 3) + 4 = 10$$

Child 2
$$[(PW + SS) \times \text{units/rep}] + (2 \times DP) = [(2 + 2) \times 4/4] + (2 \times 0)$$
$$= (4 \times 1) + 0 = 4$$

Table 4.5

Mean (and Standard Deviation) and *t*-Test for Weighted Stuttering-Like
Disfluency (SLD) of Stuttering and Normally Fluent Groups

Group	N	Weighted SLD	t	df	p
Stuttering	103	20.40 (17.62)			
Normally fluent	52	1.72 (1.25)			
			10.71[a]	104.02[a]	>.001[a]

[a]Homogeneity of variance not assumed.

Thus, the weighted SLD clearly differentiates the first child from the second.
For the children in our study, we calculated the weighted SLD, which
clearly differentiates the stuttering and normally fluent groups. The mean
scores and results of a *t*-test are presented in Table 4.5. The test shows a statistically significant difference between the stuttering and normally fluent
groups, meaning that the scores of each group are clustered around a different mean (higher for the experimental group; lower for the control group).

The ability of the SLD and the weighted SLD to differentiate the groups
is presented graphically in Figure 4.4. The figure shows the relationship
between the two measures for each child in the two groups. To highlight the
area of potential overlap more clearly, we do not show extreme scores
(outliers) for the stuttering children; all scores, however, are shown in the
inset graph. It is rather widely agreed among experts on stuttering that
3 SLD is the approximate division between stuttering and normally fluent
children; indeed, in our study, only 6 normally fluent children fall above
this limit and 1 stuttering child falls below it. Using a score of 4 as a bound-
ary for weighted SLD, as discussed in Ambrose and Yairi (1999), only 1
stuttering child still falls below and 3 normally fluent children fall above.
Thus, although the weighted SLD measure can be useful in sorting cases
with similar frequencies but varying extent and proportion of DP, in our
experience, these cases are infrequent close to the onset of stuttering. Although the weighted SLD's special power for differential diagnosis of stuttering from normal disfluency may be needed in only a few cases, its usefulness goes beyond the differentiation task. In the main, it provides a
much more comprehensive reflection and quantification of children's stuttering in *all* cases than any other single measure. In our opinion, possible

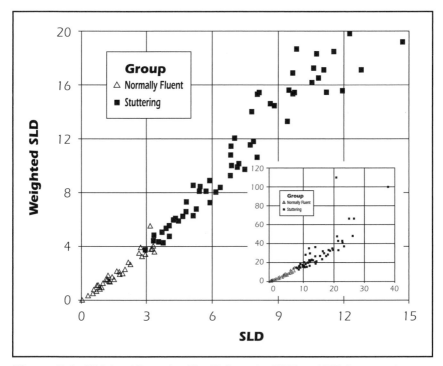

Figure 4.4. Weighted Stuttering-Like Disfluencies (SLD) and SLD for stuttering and normally fluent children in the region of potential overlap. (Inset shows the entire range, including outliers.)

overlap is more of an issue in determining *recovery* of normal speech than in *diagnosing* stuttering.

Spatial Distribution

The Phenomenon and Past Research

As we have demonstrated, efforts to characterize and quantify disfluent speech have been partial to the frequency–type distribution—that is, how many disfluent events of what kind occur in a given speech sample. Van Riper (1982), however, commented that stutterers often produce repetitions in strings. This spatial grouping—the tendency to occur in clusters—is another dimension of disfluent speech output. A cluster can be defined as two or more consecutive disfluencies that occur within the same word, on adjacent words, or on a word and an adjacent between-word interval. One might say that clusters express the density of disfluency. A related question involves perception: Do five disfluent events, randomly distributed within 100 words, leave the same effect on listeners as do five identical events occurring in two clusters, one of three and one of two disfluencies, or in a single cluster of five? This concept of density is potentially significant both for the understanding of the dynamics involved in emitting disfluencies and for the differentiation of stuttering from normal disfluency.

To date, limited efforts have been invested in studying clustering in the speech of people who stutter. Clustering of disfluency has been examined in adults who stutter, yielding conflicting or ambiguous results (Fein, 1970; Still & Griggs, 1979; Still & Sherrard, 1976; I. Taylor & Taylor, 1967). Two studies of disfluency clusters in normally fluent preschool children revealed that disfluencies occurred in clusters more often than would be expected by chance (Colburn, 1985; Silverman, 1973). The percentages of clustered disfluencies were 36% and 38% in the two studies, respectively. Wexler (1982) also reported clustering but did not calculate percentages or chances of occurrence.

The first study of the clustering phenomenon in young children who stutter was conducted in our research program by Hubbard and Yairi (1988). Although the 2- to 4-year-old children who stutter and normally fluent children exhibited clustered disfluency above chance expectations, a rather sharp distinction was indicated between the groups. For the children who stuttered, 57% of disfluencies occurred in clusters, whereas the control children produced 66% of their disfluencies in isolation. Compared with normally fluent children, the stuttering children had more than six times as many clusters. Furthermore, their clusters were frequently longer, with 30% consisting of three or more consecutive disfluencies, compared with only 19% in the controls. A few years later, a second study in preschool stuttering children, reported by LaSalle and Conture (1995), confirmed our findings. These investigators also found that stuttering frequency and severity were positively correlated with the number of clusters.

Theoretical Considerations

In addition to diagnostic purposes, information about clusters could be applied for theoretical purposes. Still and Sherrard (1976) and Still and Griggs (1979) framed theories of stuttering into mathematical models by breaking stuttered speech into sequences of stuttered and nonstuttered words. Whether a stuttered segment was followed by another was used to evaluate the theories of conflict, anxiety, and feedback. For example, according to Sheehan's (1958) conflict theory of stuttering, stuttered segments should be immediately followed by fluent segments because of the sharp drop in anxiety during moments of stuttering. This was mathematically contrasted with Mysak's (1966) feedback model, which implies that stuttered segments tend to appear in clusters during periods when the speaker is monitoring speech feedback. Hubbard and Yairi (1988) took a different approach, suggesting that the occurrence of clusters could be explained by Zimmermann's (1980b) model of disfluency as a motor control problem. That model postulates that when the speech musculature exceeds certain movement thresholds, afferent feedback to the brainstem throws the speech system into oscillation or tonic behavior (disfluency). If the speech system is not stabilized, then the stimulation from the tonic activity causes more maladaptive, hypertonic escape behaviors. Disfluency clusters, especially those involving SLD, could be the result of such behaviors.

LaSalle and Conture (1995) attempted to explain frequency and type of clusters based on the covert repair hypothesis (CRH) of stuttering (Postma & Kolk, 1993). The CRH assumes that stuttered speech is the byproduct of covert self-repair of speech errors, representing the children's attempts to adapt to their slower phonological encoding. Although LaSalle and Conture were able to use the data to support the tenets of the CRH, the results were insufficient to explain the occurrence of clusters. Obviously, considerably more research on the spatial distribution of disfluency is needed to advance the field's understanding of the dynamics of disfluent speech.

Duration of Disfluencies

Disfluency alters the temporal characteristics of speech, in which duration is a prime factor. Whereas it might be hypothesized that the length of disfluent events reflects the relative strength of the underlying disorder, it is clear that longer disfluent events leave stronger impressions on listeners than shorter ones. Earlier, we discussed the dimension of length of disfluency as reflected in extent, that is, the number of iterations of discrete disfluencies. Duration specifically addresses the time domain of length: How long do these disfluencies last? The shift from extent to duration allows inclusion in the data pool of nonrepetitive types of disfluency, such as sound prolongations and silent blocks. Data can also be obtained for duration of entire moments of stuttering, which may contain both repetitive and disrhythmic elements, instead of being limited to the count of isolated specified disfluencies. Two directions in the research of disfluency duration can be distinguished: (a) the total duration of each disfluency type or the overall mean duration of all types and (b) the duration of specified intervals or segments within disfluencies.

Total Duration

Bloodstein (1944) was among the first to study total duration of stuttering events in adults, reporting a range from 0.50 to 3.70 seconds, with a median of 0.90 seconds. By looking at the extreme ends of the range, however, additional information is gained. Johnson and Colley (1945) reported that the mean of the 10 shortest blocks was 0.41 seconds, whereas the mean of the 10 longest was 4.10 seconds. In general, overall duration of disfluencies, especially those that we have labeled as Stuttering-Like Disfluencies, have been considered in the differential diagnosis of stuttering from normal speech (e.g., Curlee, 1980; Van Riper, 1982), as well as in determining the severity of stuttering (G. D. Riley, 1972, 1980). Clinical information, mostly from subjective reports, suggests that disfluencies longer than 1 second are perceived as stuttering (Johnson, Darley, & Spriesterbach, 1963; G. D. Riley, 1980; Van Riper, 1982). These observations are supported by perceptual studies. Lingwall and Bergstrand (1979) reported that prolongation exceeding 913 msec were most likely to be perceived as stuttering. Zebrowski and Conture (1989) showed that, on average, mothers of stuttering and normally fluent children increased their judgments of sound prolongations as "stuttering" from 25% when the prolongations were 258 msec in length to 68% when the prolongations were 1,254 msec long.

Until the 1990s, however, little research activity was devoted to actually measuring the duration of preschool children's disfluencies, a parameter amenable to objective quantification. The few past studies used diverse subject ages and measuring techniques. Furthermore, there was overlap among several of these studies because data were used from identical subjects. Therefore, it has been difficult to make comparisons. Conture and Kelly (1991), for example, measured duration of within-word disfluencies of 2- to 6-year-old children who stutter using the number of videotape frames to derive the data. The accuracy of the technique is limited in that each frame represented a 33-msec time segment, masking smaller differences. Four other studies (Kelly & Conture, 1992; Throneburg & Yairi, 1994; Yairi & Hall, 1993; Zebrowski, 1991), which compared preschool children who stutter with control groups, employed more sensitive computer-based acoustic analyses to extract duration, and used children within a narrower age range and with a greater proximity to the time of stuttering onset. In the first and last studies, the experimental children were within 1 year postonset, and in the other two they were within 3 months postonset.

The results indicate that most repetitions of syllables and single-syllable words, as well as sound prolongations, vary in length from 0.5 second to 1 second for both stuttering and nonstuttering children depending on the particular study. Direct comparisons, however, among studies reporting mean duration data for stuttering and nonstuttering children are not always possible. Whereas Zebrowski's (1991) and Kelly and Conture's (1992) studies yielded no statistically significant differences, our early findings (Throneburg & Yairi, 1994), limited to repetitions of syllables and monosyllabic words, showed overall durations of stutterers' disfluencies to be significantly *shorter* than those of controls. This is important. Apparently, as discussed later, children who stutter repeat faster, making the entire duration of repetition events shorter. What is surprising is that the research of other investigators cited above suggests that sound prolongations of stuttering children are no longer than those of normally fluent children. Louko, Edwards, and Conture (1990) took a different angle in their research by comparing the disfluency duration of two subgroups of stuttering children: those who had disordered phonology and those who had normal phonology. No significant differences were found.

In our most recent investigation of the durational characteristics of disfluency, data were gathered from speech samples of 30 stuttering children: 22 boys and 8 girls, from 27 to 59 months of age ($M = 34$ months; $SD = 3.74$). All were within 3 months of stuttering onset at the time of recording, and none had received any form of direct clinical intervention prior to recording. The children were divided into three groups of 10 according to stuttering severity (based on SLD frequency). The mild and moderate groups each included 8 boys and 2 girls; the severe group included 6 boys and 4 girls. The ranges and means of SLD for these three groups are presented in Table 4.6.

Recording procedures were identical to those described earlier for the entire project, and instances of SLD were identified from the transcripts. As described previously, we defined single-unit repetitions as one extra production of a segment (e.g., "bu-but"; "and-and"), double-unit repetitions as two extra productions of the segment (e.g., "bu-bu-but";

Table 4.6

Range, Mean, and Standard Deviation (*SD*) of Stuttering-Like Disfluencies
for Three Severity Groups of Children Who Stutter

Group	Range	*M*	(*SD*)
Mild	3.28– 4.79	4.09	(0.51)
Moderate	7.15–10.52	8.99	(1.07)
Severe	13.07–37.70	20.19	(7.85)

"and-and-and"), and so on. Because some children had many single-unit repetitions, up to 10 instances of part-word and whole-word repetitions of single units were analyzed per child. All suitable events with multiple-unit repetitions, as well as disrhythmic phonations, were measured.

Disfluencies free of interfering noise were low-pass filtered at 7.5 kHz and digitized at 20,000 samples per second. Durational measurements were made from a Fast Fourier Transformation (FFT)–based spectrogram display using the CSpeech program (Milenkovic, 1987). Part-word repetitions with one repeated unit (e.g., "o-on") were measured from the initial sound to the beginning of, but not including, the final consonant ("n"). For prolongations, cursors were placed at the initiation and termination of the spectral energy of the prolonged sound. For each child, we first calculated the mean duration (in milliseconds) for all disfluent events classified under each disfluency type and each category of each type. Then, we derived group means by averaging the means of all children. A child who did not provide at least two measurable disfluencies of a particular type was excluded from the group's mean for that type. The results are summarized in Table 4.7.

A number of observations can be made. First, it is logical and obvious that as the number of units increases, the duration increases. The increase is smaller for part-word than for single-syllable whole-word repetitions because, as would be expected, single-syllable words are typically longer than parts of a word. What is more interesting is that for part-word repetition, the duration of one- and two-unit repetitions is similar across severity levels, although for three-unit repetitions, the severe group presents a shorter mean duration. For all word repetitions, however, children with severe stuttering present shorter durations than children with mild and moderate stuttering; that is, they repeat faster. Disrhythmic phonation,

Table 4.7

Means and Standard Deviations for Duration (in milliseconds) of Different Disfluency Types for Stuttering and Control Groups

	Group									
	Mild		Moderate		Severe		Total Stuttering Group		Control	
Disfluency Type	M	(SD)	M	(SD)	M	(SD)	M	(SD)	M	(SD)
Part Word										
1 unit	612	(148)	609	(132)	617	(127)	613	(131)	890	(278)
2 units	940	(71)	949	(161)	951	(250)	948	(190)	*	
3 units	*		1,792	(576)	1,248	(424)	1,451	(513)	*	
4 units	*		*		1,536	(221)	2,101	(856)	*	
Whole Word										
1 unit	785	(141)	764	(236)	682	(182)	744	(191)	1,024	(218)
2 units	1,430	(382)	1,514	(748)	1,174	(360)	1,366	(506)	2,028	(651)
3 units	*		1,514	(458)	1,330	(294)	1,452	(357)	*	
4 units	*		*		1,424	(123)	1,755	(747)	*	
Disrhythmic Phonation										
	646	(375)	724	(206)	857	(311)	720	(293)	701	(300)
Mixed										
	1,353	(389)	1,872	(685)	2,061	(387)	1,811	(582)	*	
All Disfluencies										
	960	(430)	1,252	(778)	1,113	(512)	1,120	(607)	1,117	(987)

*Because 2 or fewer subjects exhibited this disfluency type for this group, a mean is not reported. These numbers are included, however, in the average of All Disfluencies.

however, becomes longer as severity increases. Thus, the overall impression of severe stuttering as rapid-fire repetitions and pronounced prolongations receives the support of objective measures. At present, however, no information is available concerning the possible separate and combined effects on listeners of duration and the number of units.

Interval Duration

A handful of investigators took a different approach to the temporal characteristics of disfluency with the view that information regarding duration of substructures, such as the silent intervals within a disfluent event, might be more revealing than the event's total duration. Perhaps this notion has been influenced by early clinicians' observations that the repetition rate of children who stutter rises above the normal tempo of speech (e.g., Froeschels, 1921). If true, the perception of faster repeating rate must be caused by shorter intervals between the repetition units, by reduced length of the unit being repeated, or both. Accordingly, the duration of the words in "but-but" and/or the silent interval between them is shorter. We believe that research along this dimension has yielded promising findings. For example, Howell and Vause (1986) showed that the duration of vowels produced by children during stuttered speech was significantly shorter than the duration of vowels produced during their fluent speech. Similar findings were reported a year later by members of this group from the United Kingdom (Howell, Williams, & Vause, 1987).

A few years later, members of our team (Yairi & Hall, 1993) used computer technology for measuring visual displays of sound spectrograms to determine the duration of 55 monosyllabic word repetitions of young stuttering children within 3 months of onset and those produced by normally fluent controls. Most interestingly, we discovered that the lack of significant group differences in total duration of disfluencies masked the stuttering children's tendency to exhibit considerably shorter silent intervals between the repeated words than those of the controls. It meant that children who stutter do repeat *faster* than normally fluent children. In a large follow-up study, Throneburg and Yairi (1994) included 20 preschool children within 3 months after onset and analyzed 571 disfluent events of single-unit part-word repetitions and single-syllable word repetitions with one and two repeated units. The 20 controls contributed 149 such events for analysis. Using a similar technique, we measured the duration of the spoken repetition units, the intervals between units, and the total disfluency. A portion of the data is presented in Table 4.8.

Clearly, the duration of the intervals between repeated units is much shorter for children who stutter than for controls. Our statistical analyses revealed that interval duration alone was sufficient to differentiate stuttering from nonstuttering children with 72% to 87% accuracy, depending on disfluency type. The interval between the repeated units was the shortest

Table 4.8

Mean Duration (in milliseconds) and Standard Deviations of Silent Intervals
Between Repetition Units for Stuttering and Normally Fluent Children

	Group			
	Stuttering		Normally Fluent	
Disfluency Type	*M*	*SD*	*M*	*SD*
Part-word single unit ("bu-but")	135	76	418	222
Monosyllabic-word single unit ("but-but")	160	89	494	199
Monosyllabic-word double unit ("but-but-but")				
First interval	227	178	569	441
Second interval	194	168	491	299

element in the repetitions of young beginning stutterers; it was the longest
element in the repetitions of nonstuttering children. Contrary to earlier
speculations that repetitions are initially of normal tempo, becoming faster
as the disorder of stuttering progresses (Froeschels, 1921; Van Riper, 1971),
these data give additional credence to our contention that, from the very
early stages of the disorder, children who stutter tend to repeat faster than
normally fluent children, and offer a clue as to why their disfluencies are
recognized as stuttering. In a later study (Amir & Yairi, 2002), we digitally
manipulated the length of different segments within disfluencies. Among
other results, we found that, indeed, as intervals between repetition units
were shortened, the disfluent event tended to be judged as stuttering.
When intervals were lengthened, the event tended to be judged as normal.

Associated Physical Behaviors

Although stuttering is first and foremost a disorder of speech, just prior
to or during speech disfluency, many adults and older children who stutter
display visible tension in parts of the speech system or the face, or movements of the head, neck, eyes, or other parts of the body. Although these
movements, referred to as *secondary characteristics,* are not viewed by
many as an integral part of the original core stuttering (repetitions and

prolongations), they can be observed frequently and have even been included in some definitions of stuttering (e.g., Wingate, 1964). With the exception of a few studies of parental perceptions of early stuttering reporting occasional comments about physical tension and body movements associated with stuttering (Johnson et al., 1959; Yairi, 1983), until recently this phenomenon has received little attention in research of early stuttering, perhaps because traditionally it has been regarded as late developing, a characteristic of more "advanced" stuttering.

Conture and his coworkers were among the first to conduct direct studies of secondary characteristics in very young children. Using frame-by-frame videotape measurements of 10 instances of stuttering for each subject, the different movements were classified with a modified version of the *Facial Action Coding System* (Ekman & Friesen, 1978). In the first study, H. D. Schwartz and Conture (1988) found that all 43 participants, ages 3 to 9, exhibited eye, torso, and limb movements while stuttering. H. D. Schwartz et al. (1990) confirmed these findings in 10 younger children, ages 2 to 5, who were within 1 year of onset. Finally, Conture and Kelly (1991) found that 30 stuttering children from 3 to 7 years of age had significantly more nonspeech movements than did normally fluent controls. The mean number of movements per instance of stuttering was 1.48, whereas the control children had 0.63 movements per fluent word. Additionally, the two groups differed in types of movement. The age range of the children, however, suggests that for many of them the data were obtained long after stuttering onset.

We have investigated secondary characteristics in our program using two different procedures: objective counting and perceptual ratings. In an early study (Yairi et al., 1993), we focused on very young children as close as possible to the beginning of their stuttering and were able to analyze videotapes of 16 children, all within 3 months of onset ($M = 6$ weeks). The results showed that the mean number of movements per instance of disfluency for individual subjects ranged from 0.8 to 5.9, with a group mean of 3.18, twice as many as reported by Conture and Kelly (1991).

Over the years, as more children entered the study, we noted that physical movements were present more often than not, and even pronounced movements were observed early in the course of some children's stuttering. In 1997, Throneburg reported an extensive longitudinal investigation that tracked changes in head and neck movement of stuttering children in our program. For the purpose of this chapter, we extracted data from the first speech samples of a subset of 20 children: 13 boys and 7 girls, 25 to 49 months of age (M = 34.8), recorded within 6 months of onset (M = 2.8). For each child, 10 instances of stuttering-like disfluencies were analyzed, frame by frame, from videotapes taken at 30 frames per second. After determining the initiation and termination of the disfluency by means of a time code display, we tallied the frequency of occurrence of each of 19 different types of head and facial movements selected from the *Facial Action Coding System* (Ekman & Friesen, 1978). These included movements of the eyebrows, eyelids, nose, lips, jaw, head, and eyeballs. Movements that were necessary for normal articulation (i.e., lip pucker associated with the normal production of /w/; lips tight for production of /p/ or /m/) were not included. However, if an abnormal amount of tension was obvious visually, the movement was included.

In this study, we introduced new control procedures. To minimize confounding of the data with apparently normal movements during interaction (e.g., moving the head or eyes to look at a parent or a toy), each disfluent instance was matched with a fluent segment in the child's speech that was equal in the number of video frames and had a similar sentence position and grammatical function. The matching for time rather than for the identical word is the most conservative approach to counting secondary characteristics. Previous studies did not take into consideration that some, or many, movements may be present in the stuttering child's fluent speech. Thus, the difference in the number of movements between the two matched segments was calculated. Pearson product-moment correlation coefficients revealed high intrajudge and interjudge reliability for counting movements at .95 and .91, respectively. The group data presented in Table 4.9 show that the mean number of movements in disfluent segments was 4.8, compared with 3.9 for the fluent segments. Head, eyeball, and eyelid were the most common types of movements.

Although the group means indicate a rather small difference between movements during disfluent and fluent segments, the individual data showed that 7 children exhibited more than one extra movement early on. One child had 4.0 extra movements per disfluency, 3 children had 2.0 to 3.0, and 3 had 1.0 to 1.8 extra movements. Ten children had fewer than a single extra movement, and 3 had more movements in fluent than in disfluent speech.

Perceptual data for secondary characteristics are available for all 103 stuttering children discussed in this chapter. The children were rated by

Table 4.9

Mean Number of Head and Facial Movements in Disfluent
and Matched Fluent Speech Segments for 20 Children Who Stutter

Movement	Disfluent Words	Fluent Words	Difference
Head	16	15	1
Eyeball	11	10	1
Eyelid	16	13	3
Eyebrow	1	1	0
Nose	0	0	0
Lip	2	0	2
Jaw	2	0	2
Total Movements	48	39	9
Mean Movements	4.8	3.9	0.9

the investigators as part of the clinicians' evaluation of stuttering severity,
using the following scale.

0.00	None
0.25	Mild, very few, infrequent, minimal; not noticeable unless looking for it
0.33	Mild, few and occasional; barely noticeable
0.50	Moderate, few and sometimes; noticeable
0.67	Moderate, some and/or often; obvious
0.75	Severe, many and/or frequent; distracting
1.00	Severe, many and frequent; severe and painful looking

Table 4.10 gives a breakdown of the percentages of children rated at
each level. Almost 75% of the children evidenced some degree of physical
characteristics during stuttering, and these were observed without the aid
of slowed-down video. They included lip pursing, eye blinking, foot stomping, head turn, and raised pitch, among others that appeared in various
combinations. Our impression is that children exhibit these movements as
part of their stuttering, without conscious thought of coping or adapting
mechanisms. Some behaviors appear to be part of the involuntary motor
control producing the disfluencies, whereas others may be natural reac-

Table 4.10
Number and Percentage of Children
at Each Severity Level of Secondary Characteristics

Severity of Behaviors	Frequency	Percentage
0.00 (none)	27	26.2
0.25	19	18.4
0.33	19	18.4
0.50	25	24.3
0.67	12	11.7
0.75	1	1.0
1.00	0	0.0

tions to "being stuck." For example, when pronounced eye blinking accompanies stuttering, the movement does not appear to provide assistance to moving forward in speech. However, pitch raising, downward head movement, and jaw and lip tension could be conceived as natural accompaniments to attempts to push through a stuttering disfluency and, as such, could be considered unconscious coping mechanisms. Whatever explanation proves to be valid, it is obvious that the issue of secondary characteristics in children beginning to stutter is much more complicated than was originally thought.

Conclusions and Clinical Implications

It is patently clear that speech disfluency lies at the core of the disorder of stuttering. Without disfluency, even if successfully avoided or modified or otherwise uttered, there is no stuttering. This is not to diminish the importance of the emotional experiences and reactions of people who stutter or to deny that similar phenomena, such as repetition, occasionally occur in nonverbal communication. Rather, our intention is to underscore that disfluency is the essence of the disorder in its widely understood conventional sense and is central to its definition.

As in research concerning many other phenomena, the scientific investigation of speech disfluency began with relatively simple techniques, such as online handwritten speech transcripts and the marking of only three disfluency types that could provide only crude, incomplete, inaccurate, and unreliable information. With the growing power and precision of research technology, especially audio–video recordings and computer-enhanced analyses, and with the growing sophistication of the relevant experimental variables, recent investigators have been gathering objective speech data of considerably higher quality obtained from groups who were more convergent in age, as well as much closer to the time of stuttering onset, than in past investigations. More research is needed, however, to discover and evaluate the optimal metric that combines both high sensitivity and clinical applicability.

Various analyses of our and other investigators' data have led to our cardinal conclusion: *From the time when stuttering is said to begin in preschool children, their disfluent speech is markedly different from that of normally fluent children.* Thus, there is sufficient information for clinicians to make reliable differentiation in the vast majority of cases, as discussed in more detail in Chapter 10 pertaining to the evaluation of stuttering. A derivative of all this is that in normally speaking preschool children, particularly those between ages 2 and 3 years (also the most typical ages for stuttering onset), disfluency is an ordinary characteristic that, although varying individually, stays at low levels. Thus, a second conclusion relevant to clinicians follows: *Although normal disfluency is common, it does not mean that it is frequent.* The total number of part-word and single-syllable word repetitions is, on average, fewer than two per 100 syllables, whereas disrhythmic phonation (prolongations and blocks) are either absent or rare. The presence of larger amounts of these types of disfluency is unusual and should not, in most cases, be viewed as normal, as suggested by past investigators. In many cases, such departures signify the onset of stuttering.

A third important conclusion is that the departure from normal is more than just a rise in frequency. *Disfluent speech at the early stage of stuttering is characterized by a complex pattern of disfluency types and their frequency, proportion, extent, and duration.* Interactions among these factors magnify the distinction from normal disfluency. For example, although frequency of repetition may often be sufficient to differentiate the two, the multiplication of a greater number of repetitions by a greater number of units per repetition, as incorporated in our weighted SLD, yields a powerful coeffect of larger quantities of repeated speech segments in the verbal output of children who stutter that normally fluent children do not even approximate. The conventional disfluency quantifications limited to frequency have failed to capture this coeffect. Another coeffect that has been shaping up as almost a rule of early stuttering is the combination pattern of disfluency types: approximately two thirds of the disfluencies of children who stutter are composed of stuttering-like disfluencies, whereas nearly two thirds of the disfluencies of normally fluent children are composed of other disfluencies. Fourth, *various aspects of disfluency, such as duration, clustering, and associated secondary characteristics, are valuable for differential diagnostic purposes.* Thus, objective evidence from disfluency analyses leads us to the fifth conclusion, which negates Wendell Johnson's theory: The data leave little doubt that, in most cases, *parents who believe that their child has begun stuttering do not exercise erroneous judgment but are reacting to real changes in the child's speech* (Yairi & Lewis, 1984).

Scientific research of early speech characteristics of stuttering reflects an evolution from the stereotypic concept of gradually emerging, simple, effortless repetitions to recognition of heterogeneity of stuttering characteristics at onset that may include severe and complex symptomatologies. On this basis we reach our sixth conclusion that *clinicians should rid themselves of outdated ideas, and their implications, that stuttering develops gradually out of normal disfluencies.* In evaluating young children whose stuttering has only recently emerged according to parents, if disfluencies are within normal levels, there is no need for concern. If there are abnormal levels of disfluencies, particularly in SLD, then stuttering is present. At this point, concerns that stuttering might develop out of these "normal disfluencies," and the beliefs that such a process may be prevented, are misplaced because it is already there. Of course, in some children early stuttering may be mild and may be developing gradually, and these cases are more difficult to differentiate from normal disfluency. However, if it is unclear whether the disfluency is stuttering or not, there is no objective basis for great concern at that moment. The fact that children may be exhibiting the higher end of normal disfluency levels does not mean that stuttering is about to develop, although in the cases of gradual onset, clinicians may be witnessing it. If it is not yet diagnosable, whether it is absent or subclinical and developing, close monitoring will soon reveal its true nature. As we discuss in the next chapter, as stuttering continues, the difficulty lies not in correct diagnosis of stuttering, but in correct diagnosis of its recovery. Although fluency-enhancing strategies may be beneficial, they should not be thought of as means of preventing the emergence of stuttering. Regardless, early identification of the disorder enhances optimal clinical decisions.

Chapter 5

Development of Stuttering

Traditionally, stuttering has been portrayed as a unitary disorder that typically increases in severity through certain stages that most children who stutter follow. Several developmental schemes depicting this view have been offered over the years. On the other hand, there has been growing realization that a large percentage of stuttering cases exhibit the opposite developmental course and exhibit natural (spontaneous) recovery during childhood. Several sources of scientific data have supported this assertion, and more recent models depict heterogeneous developmental pathways. Nevertheless, some researchers have questioned the level and very concept of recovery. Past longitudinal studies that indicated recovery levels between 65% and 80% were marred by a variety of experimental weaknesses. The University of Illinois Stuttering Research Program's longitudinal studies, which were large in scale and carried out with considerably improved procedures than past studies, have yielded many findings reported in this chapter. Our research has confirmed high levels of recovery, provided data on the characteristics of recovery, and identified several factors that influenced this phenomenon. Several types of data supported the same conclusion. Among factors that should be considered in understanding recovery are age at onset, gender, disfluency profile, and familial history of stuttering.

Study Questions

1. What are the essential features of traditional developmental schemes of stuttering? Compare them with those that emphasize developmental heterogeneity.

2. What types of evidence have supported the presence of a large factor of natural recovery? Discuss.

3. What is the theoretical, research, and clinical significance of natural recovery?

4. What are the developmental changes that occur in frequency, type, and length of disfluencies in the speech of children who persist in, and recover from, stuttering?

Background

Stuttering as a Unitary and Progressive Disorder

Although traditional accounts depicted early stuttering as simple, easy repetitions without tension, secondary physical components, awareness, or emotional reactions, previous chapters in this book document a great variety of characteristics, as well as a full range of stuttering severity at or close to onset. The question now is what happens next with the newly emerged stuttering? Is it static, or does it undergo minor or even considerable changes? Do symptoms become less varied and more homogeneous, or do they begin to clearly separate into specific subtypes? Does the nature of the disorder change? Is there any pattern at all? Is stuttering a lifelong disorder, or is it only episodic or a temporary condition?

Whereas in recent years these questions have stirred considerable controversy, for a long period the answers seemed to be fairly clear and widely accepted. Simply stated, stuttering was portrayed as a generally unitary, progressive disorder that develops from normal disfluencies—a disorder that begins as mild and proceeds in a relatively uniform, linear, prescribed stepwise succession, gradually increasing in severity and abnormality with the passage of time. Robinson (1964) wrote a good example of such descriptions:

> Stuttering seldom remains static. It grows. And as it grows, it tends to change form and severity. Early patterns are replaced, obscured, or supplemented by more pronounced and abnormal behavior. Repetitions or prolongations become troublesome "blocks." Tremors may appear in certain oral structures ... (p. 47)

If stuttering proceeds out of normal disfluency, then there exists by definition a critical period during which the change occurs. A young child who exhibits what might be considered borderline stuttering, then, is considered at risk for developing stuttering. Intervention, so it has been proclaimed (e.g., Guitar, 1998, p. 368), is crucial to divert the child's speech path from stuttering back into normally fluent. A child with moderate or severe stuttering, according to this traditional model, has already crossed the Rubicon. Unfortunately, although for many years it has been known that many individuals, especially young children, cease stuttering without intervention, such knowledge seems to have been often repressed to the edge of awareness under the influence of lively descriptions, such as cited above, fueled by powerful theoretical motivations, that highlighted the permanence and additive nature of stuttering.

Sequential Stages of Stuttering

The idea of sequential stages, or phases, of stuttering has been particularly popular. This mindset appears to have underlined much of the current thinking about the nature and treatment of stuttering. Over the first half of the 20th century, the concept drew heavily from subjective observations and clinical impressions by several talented and influential clinicians.

Early Sequential Models

Froeschels (1921) was among the first to attend seriously to the task of charting the developmental course of stuttering, describing it as a process in which simple repetitions of syllables and words change in a progressive fashion, with the speed (rate) of the repetitions being an important factor. At the initial stage, repetition is perceived to be at a normal tempo without tension. Next, an element of tension is added. Later, a faster than normal tempo arises along with the tension. Then, tension is increased while the tempo of the repetitions decreases to below normal. Finally, prolongations of sounds and articulatory fixations arise. The tempo is still slower than normal and the marked tension continues to hold. Froeschels believed that all stuttering individuals follow this sequential pattern, with exceptions attributed to the effects of therapy.

Later developmental schemes described more defined global stages of stuttering, each of which could span several years. Typically, disfluency characteristics were the central element undergoing change, but emotional aspects were also given some attention. Short-term variations and subgroup differentiation were overlooked. Mentioned in Chapter 3 was Bluemel's (1932) two-phase scheme: primary stuttering, with its easy repetition of syllables or words, and secondary stuttering, which involved the addition of marked tension to the disfluency, awareness of the difficulty, and the appearance of fear of speaking. The speaker is conscious of the disfluency and exerts physical effort to either avert the speech block, force it to end, or conceal it altogether. Onset of primary stuttering and the development of secondary stuttering may be separated by a period of several years, but all stutterers follow a similar developmental pattern.

Although we agree that in many cases there are substantial differences between early and advanced stuttering, Bluemel's position that there is a sharp dichotomy between the two stages is unfortunately extreme and has been negated by available data. We most certainly disagree with the implication that all early stuttering is "simple" repetitions. An attempt to correct this unrealistic and artificial depiction of the disorder can be seen in Van Riper's (1954) modification, which included an intermediate stage. According to Van Riper, the primary stage consists of simple repetition at a normal tempo, as well as prolongations. Awareness, however, is lacking. Next, there is a transition stage characterized by faster, longer, and less regular repetition, as well as sound prolongations, with occasional reactions of brief awareness, surprise, and struggle. Finally, secondary stuttering follows, characterized especially by full awareness, fear, and avoidance.

Later Sequential Models

The most well-known stuttering developmental sequence, and the first to be based on research data, not merely clinical intuition, was suggested by Bloodstein (1960a, 1960b, 1961). Using a cross-sectional investigation, he analyzed initial speech evaluation reports that were kept in the Brooklyn College Speech and Hearing Center's clinical records of 418 stuttering children who were evaluated at different ages. Thirty files were selected to represent each age group at 6-month intervals between ages 2 and 16. Then, the degree to which nine preselected features of stuttering were evident in the children's diagnostic reports was determined.

Bloodstein appeared to assume that the characteristics exhibited by the age-sequenced groups reflected the course of the disorder that children typically go through. In other words, the assumption in a cross-sectional study is that a group of 16-year-olds represents the group of 2-year-olds as they would stutter years later when they grow up. When the research was conducted, however, the investigator did not take into account the reality that many children stop stuttering at different points in time after the onset of the disorder, and that only a few of them advance through all these stages, if indeed they go through them. This phenomenon was already known then, but its implications were not fully recognized. It is quite certain that the older children in Bloodstein's study represented a very small minority of those who had ever stuttered. It is also important to recall that the evaluation reports had been generated by many different clinicians over a period of 6 years. We suspect that their clinical diagnostic standards and procedures were far from being uniform and controlled.

Nevertheless, based on this information, Bloodstein (1960b) proposed a four-phase sequence of stuttering development. The essential features are summarized here.

Phase I: The preschool period (2–6 years of age)

a. The dominant symptom is repetitions of words and syllables; some prolongations and secondary characteristics are possible.
b. Stuttering events occur primarily on function words ("but-but"; "and-and"; "he-he") at the initial position in phrases.
c. Stuttering is cyclic and variable: It increases and decreases in frequency and severity.
d. Stuttering is intensified under communication pressure (e.g., when a child is excited or telling a story).
e. Mostly, there is little evidence of the speaker's concern about his or her speech.

Phase II: Elementary school children

a. The dominant symptom varies and may consist of repetitions, hard contacts, and others.
b. The locus of stuttering changes to chiefly content words (nouns, verbs, adjectives, adverbs); it occurs throughout the sentence.
c. Stuttering is essentially chronic, but it still increases under conditions of excitement or when speaking rapidly.
d. The child regards him- or herself as a stutterer but typically has little or no concern about his or her speech.

Phase III: Late childhood

a. The overt symptomatology is fully developed, complex stuttering.
b. Stuttering varies in relation to specific situations, as well as certain words and sounds.
c. Anticipation of stuttering and some negative emotional reactions (e.g., word substitution and circumlocution) begin, but there is little or no fear or embarrassment.
d. Although stuttering may be unpleasant, emotional reaction is limited; the person tends to speak despite his or her stuttering.

Phase IV: Adolescence and adulthood

a. Strong emotional reactions take over; there is fearful anticipation of stuttering in general.

   b. The individual fears certain words, sounds, and situations, and makes frequent word substitutions and circumlocutions.

   c. The individual exhibits avoidance of speaking situations, and demonstrates shame and embarrassment.

   d. The speaker expresses strong sensitivity to listeners' reactions; stuttering becomes a personal and social problem.

As we see it, essentially Bloodstein's system delineates changes in five parameters: (a) type of disfluency, (b) loci of disfluency, (c) physical tension, (d) cognitive awareness, and (e) emotional reactions. To his credit, Bloodstein viewed his phase system as a general outline that recognizes individual differences, particularly in regard to the age at which the person exhibits the various characteristics of stuttering prescribed for each stage. Nevertheless, the overall uniformity and linear directionality of the disorder dominates the model in that only one sequence was recognized.

Whereas all of the sequences mentioned so far were rooted in symptom changes, Brutten and Shoemaker (1967) used a different principle for the staging of stuttering. They advocated a developmental scheme driven by their two-factor learning theory of stuttering, a scheme that reflected the causative elements and dynamic features of the theory. The first stage of the disorder is viewed as normal speech with occasional sporadic "fluency failures," a term that referred particularly to repetitions and prolongations. During the second stage, there is an increase in fluency failures due to internal and external stressors (termed "noxious stimuli") that affect sensitive, fine motor acts. Such failures of speech can become associated with, and thus conditioned to, various stimuli. The third stage is characterized by the development of conditioned negative responses to speaking situations and specific words.

In describing his developmental stage system, Guitar (1998) stated that interplay between constitutional physiological conditions, such as brain organization, and environmental factors, is the cause of stuttering. Similar to the Brutten and Shoemaker (1967) model, Guitar's system explains that stuttering develops through classical and instrumental conditioning. Guitar's scheme of developmental/treatment levels envelops five stages: (a) normal disfluency; (b) borderline stuttering—frequent but "loose and relaxed" disfluency occurs with no secondary characteristics present; (c) beginning stuttering—repetitions are tense and rapid, laryngeal tension and prolongations are apparent, and the first blocks and secondary characteristics appear; (d) intermediate stuttering (occurs between 6 and

13 years of age)—blocks are the most frequent characteristic and appear along with occasional prolongations and repetition; fear, avoidance, and secondary characteristics are common; and (e) advanced stuttering (occurs at age 14 and above)—blocks become longer, tremors of speech organs may be evident, and avoidance of specific words and speaking situations is extensive. According to Guitar, although not all children advance through all five stages, the stages represent the most typical development. These stages were constructed not only to suggest a possible sequence of stuttering development, but also to help clinicians choose the appropriate treatment for clients of various ages.

All of these developmental models of stuttering have portrayed it as a progressively worsening disorder. Although some individual differences were recognized (e.g., by Bloodstein, 1960a), the overall uniformity of the disorder appears to have an overriding effect, reflected in the basic assumption that stuttering begins similarly and most, or all, people who stutter progress through the respective sequence. Little provision was made for alternative sequences, such as for those children who show a static pattern, or those evidencing cyclic fluctuations. Reversed sequences, in which complex, severe initial stuttering is accompanied by sharp awareness by the child and then gradually changes into mild stuttering, were not even entertained. The outlook presented in these models is remarkable in view of the long-available evidence indicating that the classical progression concept is applicable to only a small proportion of stuttering cases. The underlying philosophy, however, can be explained. Wingate (1976) opined that the philosophy was strongly influenced and motivated by learning theories or any theory that views stuttering as a psychological problem. If stuttering is learned, then it must be reinforced in order to "worsen." The clinical implications of the models were also apparent, providing the basic rationale for clinicians to pursue early preventive intervention: If stuttering evolves from normal disfluency and undergoes a developmental process from normal to abnormal, then perhaps such a process can be stopped.

Developmental Heterogeneity Tracks

In a departure from traditional views, Van Riper and Conture each proposed a developmental track that recognized heterogeneity in the course of stuttering. In 1971, Van Riper abandoned his original staging system, summarized earlier, in favor of multiple pathways. His new system, however, was derived by studying long-term clinical records of 44 children, data that were not obtained in a controlled scientific procedure. Nevertheless,

Van Riper was able to use the information to chart four alternate tracks that stuttering may follow from its inception.

▶ *Track I.* Onset is gradual at a young age of 30 to 50 months, following normal fluency. The main symptom is easy repetitions, which later become irregular and faster, and then change into increasing numbers of prolongations associated with physical tension. Awareness, fear, and avoidance appear late. Stuttering can be cyclic and remit for short periods.

▶ *Track II.* Onset is gradual but at a somewhat older age in children with delayed speech development and poor articulation. Stuttering begins when phrases and sentences emerge. Early symptoms are hurried, irregular repetitions, which later are supplemented with more hesitations, revisions, and more false starts, while prolongations are few. Speech is generally disorganized, and stuttering is steady with no intermittent remissions. Awareness and emotional reactions are slight and appear slowly. Little avoidance behavior is exhibited.

▶ *Track III.* Onset is sudden following trauma, and occurs at a later age than Track I. The main symptom is unvoiced prolongations. Soon, laryngeal blocks and much tension appear, followed by respiratory irregularities. Later, fixation spreads to other articulators. Awareness and frustration are quick to appear, followed by intense fear and avoidance. This track represents the most morbid and severe form of stuttering. There is little or no natural remission.

▶ *Track IV.* Onset is sudden and unusually late, between ages 5 and 9. The main characteristics are deliberate repetitions of whole words and phrases, although some children show only gaps and pauses. Over time, frequency may increase, but the patterns remain stable. There are no interruptions or forcing, and there is little evidence of fear or avoidance behaviors.

Van Riper (1971) reported that Track I represented 48% of the 44 children; Track II, 25%; Track III, 11%; and Track IV, 9%. Only a small proportion, 7%, did not fit into any of the tracks. Van Riper indicated, however, that not all of the individuals in any one track followed its sequence exactly. Our analysis of his track scheme reveals that, in effect, it is based on four variables or risk factors: (a) age at onset (early–late), (b) type of onset (gradual–sudden), (c) pattern of stuttering (repetitions–blocks–tension), and (d) concomitant speech–language problems. For example, children exhibiting early and gradual onsets with repetitions as the dominant symptom (Track I) had better chances for recovery than those exhibiting sudden onsets, blocks, prolongations, and physical tension (Track III). Children with delayed speech (Track II) were also slower to improve or recover than those with otherwise normal speech. Some support for this differentiation scheme was reported in two studies with older subjects (Daley, 1981; Preus, 1981).

The last scheme presented here is a three-track system offered by Conture (1990), utilizing four potential stages. Children may begin at different stages and may progress through some or all of them at different rates. Thus, the tracks are described as "possible developmental sequences" and are in part defined by "speculations regarding chronicity/recovery with and without therapy" (p. 25). In other words, these were not based on systematic research and rely on low figures for natural recovery (40%–50%), which we think is incorrect. The first subgroup (40%–50%) Conture suggested comprised children who had brief, subtle inefficiencies in speech production leading to repetition. They were thought never to develop tense, fixed speech production or emotional reactions to speech, and were likely to recover without therapy. The second group, also comprising 40% to 50% of children, first had subtle speech production inefficiencies that developed into repetition. Blocks and prolongations, as well as verbal and nonverbal reactions to disfluencies, appeared later. These children were likely to recover only if they received speech therapy. The third group, 5% to 10% of children, exhibited a sudden onset of stuttering. The initial stage of easy repetition was not evidenced, and the children almost immediately exhibited advanced stages, including blocks and prolongations, with associated nonspeech behaviors. Conture suggested that this group receive psychosocial evaluation and counseling before speech therapy.

Conture's (1990) distinction of tracks reflects the belief that proper intervention is the main reason why almost all children who stutter might be able to recover. We certainly hold that the course of stuttering is diversified but that natural recovery is a major developmental path. We agree that treatment can be effective, to various degrees, in some and perhaps many children. Although Conture's scheme represents a move in a desirable direction, his descriptions of the dynamics within each track and estimates of natural recovery were not quantified via systematic research data. Conture and his associates' more recent writings (Conture, 2001; Yaruss, LaSalle, & Conture, 1998) have placed more emphasis on predicting who will be most or least likely to require therapy to improve or recover, based on specific features of stuttering. Estimates were derived from diagnostic records and therapy recommendations, but not on therapeutic outcomes. As we discuss later in this chapter, our data are at variance with much of the symptomatology that Conture ascribed either to children who recover or to those who persist. For example, we show that children who recover initially exhibit stuttering that is not less severe than those who persist.

Natural Remission: The Phenomenon and the Evidence

The University of Illinois Stuttering Research Program data reported in previous chapters have definitively and objectively illustrated that early stuttering generally does not follow a rule, but may begin as sudden or gradual, mild or severe, with or without disrhythmic phonation and accessory physical characteristics, and with or without emotional reactions to it. As a matter of fact, even Wendell Johnson's data showed considerable variability in early stuttering, although he apparently overlooked much of it, and Van Riper's four tracks of stuttering clearly acknowledge, even emphasize, the heterogeneity observed in stuttering. Great variability is also the hallmark of the further development of stuttering, beyond the point of onset. As the traditional model of its course flourished for decades, a body of evidence was growing that strongly contradicted the concept that the disorder *always* steadily increases in severity. Indeed, one of the most fascinating features of the course of childhood stuttering, widely recognized by clinicians but barely mentioned in several well-known developmental sequences (e.g., Bluemel's and Bloodstein's), is that the most typical developmental trend of early stuttering is a decrease in severity. However, the methodologies employed have influenced the different pictures. For example, Bloodstein employed cross-sectional techniques, and Van Riper's tracks were based on 44 subjects who "represent clinical failures" (1982, p. 93), whereas our studies were longitudinal and focused on a sample population representative of *all* those who ever display stuttering. It is no wonder there are differences in the portrayals.

Remarkably, the process of amelioration leads to complete recovery, without clinical intervention, in a majority of children who ever stutter. Just as overwhelming evidence indicates that the majority of cases begin stuttering during early childhood, substantial evidence also shows that this is the period when natural remission has its peak. As we explain later, for a considerably smaller subgroup of children, stuttering persists into adolescence and adulthood and may become more severe. In some children, perhaps a third subgroup, stuttering continues at a very low level that does not present a clinical problem either for the person or for listeners.

It is this phenomenon of diverse developmental pathways, which has become a focal point of research, theory, and treatment of the disorder, that led us to track and compare stuttering characteristics over a long time span to obtain more precise estimates of the magnitude of recovery and persistence, and to discover if any clues exist from early on that could help predict eventual outcomes. Much of this chapter is devoted to reporting our longitudinal investigation. First, however, let us briefly review the scientific literature pertaining to natural or spontaneous recovery, sometimes referred to as "unassisted recovery" or "recovery without treatment." These terms have been applied interchangeably, but there are obviously some differences in meanings. Although "spontaneous recovery" has been the most commonly used term, we prefer "natural recovery."

Indirect Studies

Natural recovery has been documented with two principal types of evidence. First is the population-wide estimate of the incidence–prevalence discrepancy. Estimates of the incidence of stuttering (how many people have ever stuttered) are usually less credible than are those of prevalence (how many people stutter at a given time). This is because prospective studies that follow a large, representative sample of children during the period when most stuttering onsets and remissions occur are essential to obtain valid data on the lifetime incidence and other pertinent epidemiological information of a disorder in a population. Most of the data on epidemiology of stuttering, however, including incidence, come from cross-sectional questionnaires or interview studies that rely on various informants to report whether they or members of their family currently stutter or have ever stuttered. The accuracy of such data is compromised by their secondhand nature, informants' use of different diagnostic criteria, lack of knowledge about familial history of stuttering, lapses in memory, and, in a few cases, fabrication.

Until recently, incidence data have been relatively scant, the best source being a longitudinal study of stuttering conducted in Britain by Andrews and Harris (1964) that reported 4.9% incidence. Although some of their results have been challenged, they were recently supported by a study carried out in Denmark by Mansson (2000), who had access to the birth records of all children born over a 2-year period on the Danish island of Bornholm, which has a low-mobility population of 45,000. Mansson and a team of four other clinicians conducted individual, face-to-face speech, language, and hearing screening of the entire population of 1,040 children born over 2 years (98% of the recorded births), within a month or two following their third birthday. Mansson reported that 4.9% of the children exhibited stuttering, a figure identical to that found by Andrews and Harris (1964) in a British sample of a similar size. Mansson also reported that the figure rose to 5.09% after two follow-ups were conducted several years later. In general, when the broad literature is reviewed, although estimates of the lifetime incidence and prevalence of stuttering in the United States and western Europe vary greatly (Bloodstein, 1995), considerations of the central tendencies of the various reports, as well as their scientific merit, would seem to indicate that about 5% of the general population of these parts of the world has ever stuttered.

To obtain valid data about prevalence—that is, the percentage of people who stutter at any given time—researchers should use cross-sectional studies of large, representative samples of a population, who are assessed by trained examiners using standardized diagnostic procedures and criteria. In reality, however, a diverse collection of samples, procedures, and criteria has been used to gather such data. A review of the literature (Bloodstein, 1995) shows that a substantially lower percentage of the general population stutters at a given time. Most estimates of prevalence are either a little over or under 1.0%, including those for Grades K through 12 in a nationwide study of over 30,000 school-age children conducted in 1976 by Hull, Mielke, Willeford, and Timmons. Thus, there is general acceptance of the incidence and prevalence estimates just presented in spite of a variety of weaknesses in data collection. Now, if the "true" percentage of people ever affected by stuttering (incidence) is close to 5%, and the percentage currently affected (prevalence) is about 1%, then it is mathematically transparent that stuttering ceases, for whatever reason, for about 80% of all who begin. Or, conversely, it appears that the discrepancy between incidence and prevalence clearly indicates that the disorder persists in only the minority of all cases involved. In cases where no clinical intervention has occurred, we refer to such recovery as "natural." What is responsible for this high rate of stuttering remission is not clear, however, and is a key issue in dispute.

The second type of evidence for natural, unassisted recovery has been based on clinical experience and studies that were aimed at direct estimation of the phenomenon through immediate observations or secondhand procedures specifically designed to tap the rate of recovery. Three types of sources can be distinguished: (a) subjective clinical impressions based on extensive experience with large caseloads, (b) studies that used a single sample at one point of time, and (c) studies that employed longitudinal methodology in following a sample of participants for several years. As early as 1934, Johnson made a general estimate, apparently based on clinical observations, that 30% to 40% of children who stutter outgrow their stuttering by age 8 or 9. Shortly thereafter, he was echoed by Bryngelson (1938), also one of the pioneers in the modern era of speech pathology, who stated that approximately 40% of children affected by stuttering would not need the services of the speech clinician because their stuttering would subside prior to age 8. In 1938, Bryngelson provided documentation from 1,492 case files from the University of Minnesota Speech Clinic that supported his conclusion of about a 40% natural recovery rate.

More than 60 years since these early publications on natural recovery, the clinical and research literature has provided a good number of recovery estimates in different age groups of people who stutter. Unfortunately, the more direct estimation studies also generated their data largely by means of retrospective techniques applied to high school students and adults who were former stutterers (e.g., Dickson, 1971; Sheehan & Martyn, 1966) or to parents who reported about their children's progress. Typically, these studies lacked speech-based data to verify the initial diagnosis and remission, as well as tight criteria for "stuttering" and "recovery." A good example is the 1971 Dickson study where, using a sample of almost 4,000 children in Grades K through 9, parents were asked to respond to questionnaires regarding their child's speech history. Of the 42 children identified by their parents to have stuttered at the time, or to have had a history of previous stuttering, 58% were reported to have recovered naturally. In the 1966 Sheehan and Martyn investigation, self-reports by adults, ages 17 to 56 years, were used to determine past stuttering of those identified as "recovered" at the time of the survey. The investigators found a recovery rate of 80%. Many more investigations concerning schoolchildren and adults can be found in the literature, and a good number of them were reviewed and summarized by Wingate (1976). He calculated that the overall recovery rate is approximately 43% by age 14 (p. 113). Wingate, however, offered several reasons for believing that the recovery rate may be well above that composite value, a point on which we elaborate later.

Most pertinent to our work is the research that dealt with preschool-age children. For example, Johnson (1955) followed 46 preschool-age stuttering children for up to 5 years (median = 30 months). The children's mean age was 50 months, with 75% of them having stuttered for less than 1 year at the time the study was initiated. The parents were interviewed at the beginning of the study and 1 to 18 additional times later on to inquire about the children's stuttering. None of the children received speech therapy for their stuttering during the course of the study. The parents were asked to describe the characteristics of their children's speech that they labeled as stuttering. At the end of the study, Johnson again determined the children's stuttering status based on parental reports. Stuttering severity decreased in 85% of the children, with 72% evidencing complete recovery. Johnson attributed the improvement to a shift in parental attitudes resulting from an initial single counseling session.

The absence of systematic research methods for assessing recovery is also seen in a later study by Johnson et al. (1959), reporting on 150 stuttering children 2 to 7 years old. Based on reviews of clinical files of 118 of these children, parental judgments, and, in a few cases, brief observations of the children at a 2½-year follow-up, this team of investigators found evidence of improvement in 88% of the children, with 36% exhibiting complete recovery. We suspect that the older age of the children in this study, which must also reflect children with longer histories of stuttering, was an important factor for the lower overall percentage of recovery; that is, younger children who had already recovered were not well represented. Regardless of the specific percentage of complete recovery, it is of special interest that only in 4% of the cases did the stuttering severity increase—a far cry from the traditional view that stuttering continuously grows in complexity and severity.

Another well-known study from that era was carried out by Glasner and Rosenthal (1957) by means of interviewing the parents of 996 children ages 5 and 6. They found that slightly more than 15% of the children had evidenced a period during which they stuttered. This figure was consistent among the 25 schools that participated and for the different interviewers. Parental reports indicated that 54% of the stutterers experienced complete recovery, about 16% stuttered only occasionally, and 30% continued as habitual stutterers at the time of the study. Of special interest is that only 2.6% of the parents of children who ever stuttered sought any type of professional help for the stuttering.

Longitudinal Investigations with Speech-Based Data

Considerable improvement to the body of knowledge concerning the development of stuttering has been made by several longitudinal studies that enabled closer monitoring of children's stuttering from near onset, and thus have provided more reliable and valid information because the same children were observed for a period of time in some systematic manner. Even these studies, however, had drawbacks: They either were limited in scope, were short-term, or did not employ objective speech data. Other problems include relatively late starting points in relation to the onset of stuttering and intervals between observations that were too long to provide data concerning the timing of changes in the various aspects of stuttering, such as type, frequency and loci of disfluency, accessory behaviors, awareness of stuttering, and affective reactions.

The most famous investigation was carried out by Andrews and Harris (1964), who followed 1,000 children in the English city of Newcastle upon Tyne. The children were visited by health workers and speech therapists at periodic intervals from birth to age 16. Of the 43 children identified as exhibiting stuttering, a total of 79% recovered without treatment: 39.5% recovered within 6 months of stuttering onset, 25.5% within 2 years of onset, and 14% by age 12. Only 9 children, 21%, were still stuttering at age 16.

Panelli, McFarlane, and Shipley (1978) reported similar results for 15 children, all diagnosed as exhibiting stuttering by their parents and by a speech pathologist when they were under age 5. Several years later, at ages 7 to 14, when the children were reevaluated and tape-recorded for the second time, 80% were judged independently by three clinicians as being nonstutterers. None received therapy.

A small longitudinal study that included a group of 22 children between ages 2 and 3 was reported by Ryan (2001a). The children were tested and recorded eight times, at 3-month intervals, over 2 years. More than 68% recovered without treatment within this period.

Three European investigations were reported more recently. Rommel, Hage, Kalehne, and Johannsen (2000) provided an interim progress report for a relatively large study in progress. Sixty-five German-speaking stuttering children were first examined at approximately age 5 and subsequently tracked at 6-month intervals for several years. As of the sixth data collection point, roughly 3 years into the study, Rommel et al. reported that nearly 71% (46 children) of the group recovered and 29% (19 of the original 65) persisted. According to Johannsen (2001), the percent of recovery increased to 77.4 by the ninth data collection point, 4.5 years into the study. A weakness of this study is the late starting point of the observations. Because the first examination takes place between ages 4 and 5 years, a significant number of children who began and stopped stuttering at younger ages are not included, making the report of recovery an underestimated figure. A second prospective longitudinal study, conducted in the Netherlands by Kloth, Kraaimaat, Janssen, and Brutten (1999), followed 93 children born into families with a stuttering parent. Two years into the 6-year project, 23 children were identified as stuttering. At the completion of the study, 70% had recovered naturally. A third European longitudinal study, mentioned earlier, was reported by Mansson (2000). He assessed the incidence of stuttering in all 1,040 children who were born on the Danish island of Bornholm during 2 consecutive years; individual screenings were conducted at age 3. Having identified stuttering in 5.09% of the children, the investigator also reported that a 2-year follow-up yielded 71.6% recovery. By 5 to 6 years after the initial identification, recovery reached 85%. Possible intervention, however, was not clear. Another European study, by Frittzell (1976), that found nearly 47% recovery is hopelessly at fault in that children were first observed between ages 7 and 9.

In this group of investigations, we also list our own pilot longitudinal study (Yairi & Ambrose, 1992a), which reported, for the first time, systematic, long-term, speech-based data on the development of childhood stuttering. This small-scale project was aimed primarily at developing the mechanism and procedures for longitudinal investigations of stuttering, and was not intentionally planned to study recovery. Nevertheless, the data indicated a large reduction in disfluencies over time. At the beginning of the study, the 27 young participants ranged in age from almost 2 to 4½ years, with a mean of 3 years. Their mean months since onset of stuttering was 6½ months. They were tape-recorded during spontaneous conversation at the first visit and repeatedly at 6-month intervals over a 2-year period. For 21 of the children, there was an additional recording several years later, ranging from 3 to 12 years after onset of stuttering. Eighteen children were exposed to minimal therapy for stuttering (up to 10 sessions), whereas 9 received no therapy. The longitudinal results showed marked deceleration in the total count of Stuttering-Like Disfluencies (SLD), especially during the first 18 months postonset, for both treated and un-treated children. By the end of 2 years, exactly 33% of *each* of the treated and untreated groups continued to stutter, and 67% of *each* of the groups had completely recovered. At the final later visit during elementary school years, a few additional children had recovered.

A second preliminary report by several members of our research group (Yairi, Ambrose, & Niermann, 1993) presented longitudinal data on varia-tions in five measures over a 6-month period during the earliest stage of stuttering for 16 very young children. Members of this group ranged in age from 2 to 3 years (25–39 months), with a mean of 2 years, 9 months, and were first evaluated within 12 weeks of stuttering onset. None received ther-apy. Speech samples were taped upon entry into the study and again 3 and 6 months later. Many of these children evidenced moderate to severe stutter-ing and high disfluency levels at the earliest stage of the disorder and confirmed a trend for quick, sharp reduction in disfluency. Mean SLD de-clined from nearly 12 to 4.5 per 100 syllables during the 6-month period. Furthermore, this sharp trend was associated with a decline in mean facial and head movements from 3.18 to 1.91 per disfluency. Corresponding mean stuttering severity ratings, using a 7-point scale, also fell from 4.43 to 1.99. Within this 6-month period, which ended no longer than 9 months after onset, 63% of the children were judged as exhibiting much improve-ment: 19% of the children were judged as recovered, and another 44% were judged as "possibly" recovered. Improvement and recovery included cases of initial severe stuttering. Subsequent follow-ups at 6-month intervals over 2 years indicated that none of the children experienced a relapse and that most subjects who had stuttered at their 6-month visit had continued to stutter less. There was a general tendency for boys' stuttering to persist longer than that of girls. We concluded that the peak of stuttering for many children is reached during the first 2 to 3 months following onset, just prior to a sharp decline.

In summary, the few longitudinal studies that were conducted over several years yielded consistently high figures for unassisted recovery, ranging from 68% to 85%. High recovery levels have been indicated in studies that tracked stuttering during shorter periods. Although caution must be exercised in view of the limited number of children involved, or the absence in several studies of speech samples to verify stuttering and recovery, the accumulated evidence from the more reliable studies appears to favor substantial unaided recovery. What is important to point out is that these studies indicate remission levels commensurate with that inferred from the incidence–prevalence discrepancy data discussed earlier. Thus, we have a reasonable level of validation for the rate of natural recovery and persistence. Furthermore, there appears to be good evidence that recovery without treatment includes severe cases of stuttering and that a substantial proportion of the cases that remit do so during the first year after onset. In spite of reservations about less than desired methodologies, the sheer number of reports about recovery resulting from different methodologies, and coming from different countries and from investigators of different theoretical orientations, would lead many to conclude that the weight of evidence provides ample justification for more comprehensive research of this phenomenon.

Spontaneous Recovery Questioned

Despite the mounting evidence for a substantial recovery factor in stuttering, several experts have expressed skepticism and even outright objections to these reports. Their criticism has been directed to several issues. First, and quite justifiably, questions have been raised concerning methodological aspects of past research, particularly the indirect procedures (questionnaires, relatives' reports, etc.) used to acquire information, as well as the lack of hard evidence for either the presence or remission of stuttering. Another procedural matter criticized was the emphasis on a child population, which may have minimized the phenomenon of recovery in adulthood (R. J. Ingham, 1983). The second cause for attack was the high level of estimated recovery reported in several studies, especially the nearly 80% found by Andrews and Harris (1964). M. A. Young (1975) concluded from his analysis of the literature that the rate of recovery is only between 40% and 50%. Wingate (1976) concluded that the average recovery is approximately 43% by age 14, but stated that there are grounds to believe that the recovery rate is well above this value.

   Perhaps the most serious challenge has been to the very concept of "spontaneous" recovery. Several writers advocated that the observed recovery could be the result of informal treatment activities that, in the main, are carried out by parents of the stuttering children. (R. J. Ingham, 1976, 1983; Martin & Lindamood, 1986; Wingate, 1976). As already mentioned,

Johnson (1955) felt that recovery resulted from a single parent-counseling session, and R. J. Ingham and Bothe (2001) expressed similar views. Additionally, information obtained from parents in several studies indicated that a good number of them tend to advise their children about ways of controlling the stuttering, such as slowing down the speaking rate, taking a breath, and so on. In adults, Martyn and Sheehan (1968) found that 62% of those who proclaimed themselves to be recovered stutterers attributed their progress to taking action to help themselves.

Responding to the Criticism

As we see it, much of the skepticism is not justified. Although the methodologies employed in early studies, often relying on secondhand data, were indeed weak, the brief review of the literature has shown that they were gradually replaced with longitudinal investigations that provided considerably more valid and reliable data. In response to the criticisms regarding estimated high recovery rates, we point out that the best studies, those that employed direct longitudinal observations, are the ones that reported the highest levels of recovery: from 65% to above 80%. Those are the actual data reported, not estimates based on various assumptions. We go even further by stating that there are grounds to suspect that the true rate of recovery has been underestimated, not overestimated, even in studies reporting high levels.

The problem with critics suggesting that recovery rates must be lower than reported is that they have failed to consider the epidemiological complexity of stuttering in their analyses. Two factors to keep in mind are age and gender, as well as the interaction between them that influences recovery figures in a substantial way. There have been strong indications that much of the recovery occurs by age 5, and that quite a few children demonstrate even earlier recovery within a few months after onset (Yairi & Ambrose, 1999a; Yairi et al., 1993). Thus, with each successive year along the age range, the composition of any sample of individuals who stutter gets increasingly loaded (and biased) with greater percentages of cases that will eventually become chronic stutterers. In other words, developmental studies of stuttering composed of samples of older participants can be expected to erroneously yield smaller percentages of recovery. Additionally, simultaneously with aging, there is an increase in the proportions of males in samples of people who stutter because females tend to recover at earlier ages and in larger proportions than males. Keeping in mind these facts, older samples present not only the age factor but also the gender factor, both of which tend to result in biased smaller recovery figures.

The upshot of all this is that research that intends to explore the true magnitude of recovery must begin at very early ages and very soon after onset, before early recovery in general, and recovery of females in particular, alters the subject sample and thus distorts recovery figures among the remaining subjects. Studies that overlooked these epidemiologic characteristics and used older children (Dickson, 1971; Johanssen, 1998; Ramig, 1993) or adults (Sheehan & Martyn, 1966; Wingate, 1964) employed such a late starting point in terms of the developmental course of stuttering that one can assume with a high degree of certainty that much of the phenomenon under investigation—recovery—was simply bypassed by the investigators. The older populations prevented them from observing and reporting a large proportion of children who exhibited early recovery.

A good example is a study reported by Ramig (1993) in which 14 of the 17 stuttering subjects were considerably older than the children included in the Illinois studies. Those 14 children ranged in age from 4 years 9 months (4-9) to 8-6. Although no data were provided concerning the length of their stuttering histories at the time of the initial evaluation, based on what is known about the typical age at onset, one can assume that the children had stuttered for more than a year or two, if not several years. In other words, Ramig's sample appears seriously biased because it consists of children who at first assessment in the study had already passed the period at which much of natural recovery occurs. No wonder he concluded that recovery had been overestimated in previous studies. His conclusion, however, overlooks the most pertinent scientific considerations for this kind of research. As we already stated, in our opinion, current figures of recovery probably err by underestimating. Furthermore, Ramig's findings support our conclusions that chances for persistent stuttering increase approximately 15 months after onset.

The important point here is that accurate data on recovery can be obtained only when sampling begins close to stuttering onset so as to include the maximum possible population of those who ever stutter. The following analogy to infant mortality research serves to further drive the point home. Reasonable investigators of the incidence of infant mortality would not conduct their surveys using a sample of children who are older than 1 year, after the majority of infant deaths had already occurred. The earlier deaths would not be in the sample, and the results would be inaccurate to a great degree. Although environmental forces are likely to influence recovery from stuttering, we maintain that the argument about the powerful influence of parents' informal intervention, although an interesting hypothesis, is far from presently receiving credible experimental support. In fact, if a single parent-counseling session were so effective (Johnson, 1955), it would obviate the need for treatment.

Why Is Information on Persistence and Recovery Important?

Theoretical and Research Significance

Theoretically, information about percentages and timing of recovery gives rise to important questions pertaining to the nature of stuttering and the nature of the differences between persistent and recovered stuttering. Although arguments in favor of environmental factors, such as parental intervention, have been entertained (e.g., R. J. Ingham, 1983; Wingate, 1976; Zebrowski, 1997), a study by Ambrose, Cox, and Yairi (1997) provided evidence suggesting that the two subsets of children who stutter, those who persist and those who recover, have different genetic liabilities for stuttering. Such unrecognized heterogeneity may explain many previous ambiguous or contradictory results regarding characteristics of speech, physiology, home environment, and other parameters. By this we mean that different types or subgroups of stuttering may have been mixed together in many studies and thus blurred the findings. If researchers can separate (a) those who will eventually persist in and (b) those who will recover from stuttering, researchers could increase precision in experiments concerning various aspects of the disorder in childhood, and provide data-based grounds for modifying traditional views of stuttering as a unitary disorder (St. Onge, 1963) toward recognition of subgroups.

Clinical Significance

Although information on the development of stuttering is important to the overall understanding of the disorder and to theoretical formulations about its nature, such information is particularly useful for clinical purposes. In fact, as the evidence for a large number of young stutterers who recover without therapeutic intervention mounts, there have been a few attempts to identify prognostic indicators of future recovery or persistence (chronicity). These began with various isolated ideas that were based on clinical hunches but later replaced with more systematic instruments. One of the pioneers in this area was Glyndon Riley who, in 1981, published the

Stuttering Prediction Instrument for Young Children. Another instrument was published by Cooper and Cooper (1985). These efforts are discussed in more detail in Chapter 10.

Reliable estimates of the probability and timing of natural recovery, or of the risk of developing persistent stuttering, have direct implications for clinicians' ability to discriminate among subgroups and make individual prognoses for each child regarding the risk for chronic stuttering. Based on the scientific merit of projected risks, these prognoses will significantly impact the overall intervention strategies, such as choosing between a waiting period or immediate therapy. When therapy is recommended at a particular point in time, it will be possible to select intervention programs relevant to the progress of the disorder in each subtype of stuttering. The character of parent counseling will be changed. Instead of providing standard advice, counseling will become more specific to parents of children with high risk and those with low risk for chronic stuttering. Another major implication relates to clinical efficacy research. Information about developmental diversity has already forced questions and a debate about the need, usefulness, and cost-effectiveness of early clinical intervention in early childhood stuttering (Andrews, 1984; Curlee & Yairi, 1997, 1998; R. J. Ingham & Cordes, 1998; Packman & Onslow, 1998). As a result, treatment efficacy studies for early childhood stuttering would be expected to become considerably more rigorous by better isolating the true treatment effects from natural recovery.

The Illinois Longitudinal Study

Having discussed the various views on the development of stuttering and tremendous importance of such information, we are now ready to present the longitudinal portion of the Illinois studies that deals directly with this aspect of the disorder. An interesting point is that our research on the development of stuttering did not begin with any specific motivation to study natural recovery. Being influenced by traditional views, we were planning to quantify detailed changes in disfluency over time, expecting to find the predicted upward curve. The realization of what appears to be a high rate of natural recovery occurred later, when only a few instances of disfluencies typical to stuttering were left in the speech of many children after a relatively short follow-up period. The results of this initial experimentation with the small number of 27 children were published by Yairi and Ambrose (1992a). This observation led us to look more closely at recovery and to begin experimenting with procedures and criteria for studies with more focus on this phenomenon.

Four experimental questions, all related to important theoretical, research, and clinical issues are raised regarding natural recovery: (a) What is its actual rate? (b) When does it occur? (c) Who will recover? (d) What factors govern recovery and persistence? The first question deals with a fundamental issue of the persistence–recovery phenomenon. In our main investigation, we were able to secure a much more accurate estimate of recovery than in past research because we followed three basic rules for such research, as discussed previously: (a) we examined stuttering from very close to onset, (b) the children were very young, and (c) cases were closely followed for several years. As explained, even a short delay in recruiting stuttering children for any developmental study of stuttering may cause significant errors in estimates of recovery and its characteristics because those who have already recovered would never be referred, reported, and counted. Obviously, accurate overall recovery–persistence data are also necessary to answer our second and third questions. Without maximum inclusion of all children who stutter, it would be impossible to determine when many recoveries occur. Similarly, it would be impossible to determine accurately who recovers (e.g., boys versus girls). Finally, maximum inclusion in research on persistence and recovery rates is needed for full examination of each of the factors that may control these developmental paths, such as stuttering severity, physical and emotional characteristics, and genetic components. Furthermore, the relationship between overall magnitude, timing of recovery, who recovers and who persists, and factors that seem to influence this diverse development, could provide (a) the means for making early identification of young beginning stutterers as being at high risk, low risk, or no risk for developing a chronic problem, and (b) clues regarding differential strategies for clinical intervention decisions. Although these issues rank high among research priorities for early childhood stuttering, data on factors that govern recovery are particularly scant.

Criteria for Persistence and Recovery

Let us look at a common health problem: a cough. A cough that keeps an individual up at night for 7 to 10 days is tiring and unpleasant, but such a cough lasting considerably more than 2 weeks is considered persistent and a sign of the need for medical attention and possible serious concern. How do we know when stuttering is persistent? What is it that might be different about children who persist and children who recover? We will now examine more closely how the overt symptoms of stuttering wax and wane over time for these two subgroups. One of the first steps in undertaking our research was the setting of a clear understanding of definitions of *persistence* and *recovery*. This is not as simple a task as it might seem because when stuttering is considered to be persistent (chronic) or naturally recovered is, to a large extent, a matter of a somewhat arbitrary definition. Is 2 years of stuttering history long enough for us to consider the problem as persistent? Is 5 years long enough? Until adulthood? Until death? These are not merely rhetorical questions in light of the fact that some individuals may recover at just about any time along the age range, after very different lengths of stuttering histories, and many seem to recover only to relapse later. So at what point does one enter the category of "persistent"? It was necessary to come up with a reasonably practical solution. Using 4 years postonset of stuttering as the minimum observation period, we considered whoever continued to stutter throughout the study as persistent. This meant that any child classified as exhibiting persistent stuttering must have stuttered for at least 4 years. When stuttering lasts for only 1 or 2 years in 2- to 4-year-olds, the impact on their lives, and any possible long-term effects, are most likely minimal. When a stuttering problem lasts for 4 years or more, the chance is greater that it could have negative impact on communication experiences and overall social and emotional development. The older the child, the greater is the self-awareness of stuttering and the potential for emotional reactions.

Persistent Stuttering

We defined *persistent stuttering* as that which continued to be present for the duration of the study, with a minimum time period of 4 years from the onset of the disorder. Presence of stuttering was indicated by *any* of the following criteria: (a) parental description of stuttering episodes, (b) parental severity rating of stuttering of higher than 1 on the rating scale described in Chapter 2, (c) investigators' observation of speech characteristics judged as stuttering, and (d) investigator severity rating of stuttering of higher than 1 on the Clinician Stuttering Severity Scale (see Figure 2.1). Because any single criterion precluded classification as recovered, the definition as used here minimized false negatives, that is, classification of a child as free of stuttering who actually still stutters. Any single indication of continuing stuttering had an overriding effect on imposing the persistence classification, even when little supporting evidence was available or when other indications suggested essential recovery. For example, a child might exhibit normally fluent speech during any examination based on SLD count and investigator rating, and parents might state that their child had basically "normal speech." Yet, if the parents also state that at times, "about once a month or so," the child stutters when very excited, and their description or imitation represents stuttering behavior (multiple-unit sound or syllable repetitions, or blocks or prolongations), then the child was classified as persistent. In other words, even if a child appeared to be clinically normal for all practical purposes, but occasional "real" stuttering was reported, the child was classified as persistent.

Recovered Stuttering

The goal of minimizing false negatives was applied to recovered stuttering in the reverse direction; that is, to be considered recovered, a child had to meet *all* of the following criteria: (a) clinician general judgment that the child did not exhibit stuttering, (b) parental general judgment that the child did not exhibit stuttering, (c) parent rating of stuttering severity of less than 1, (d) clinician rating of stuttering severity of less than 1, (e) SLD observed and reported as fewer than 3 per 100 syllables, and (f) no stuttering present for the remainder of the study, for a minimum of 12 months, as judged both by parent and clinician. In the vast majority of cases, this time limit was exceeded considerably. In a few cases, at any given visit, no overt stuttering was reported or observed, but parents or investigators rated a child's fluency as borderline (1.00) because the child's speech appeared somewhat "choppy" or "hesitant." Such cases continue to be observed until positive classification can be made.

Contrary to the opinions expressed by a few writers (e.g., Onslow & Packman, 1999) that the Illinois studies used "very liberal" criteria that inflated the number of recovered children, our method does the reverse. We employed strict *multiple* criteria that included cross-validation by several observers who had to pass a judgment on stuttering as well as its severity, in addition to more objective counts of certain disfluency types, to unambiguously identify recovery while using any indication of even mild occasional stuttering for classification of persistence. As mentioned previously, children had to have ceased stuttering for at least 12 months to enter the category of "recovered." Once in this category, they had to maintain the classification through the minimum time period of 4 years *and* to the end of the study. Without the additional 4-year criterion, some children could have entered the recovery group in less than 4 years. For example, if a child had stuttered for, say, 16 months and stopped, 12 months later would be a time period of 28 months, considerably less than 4 years. Such recovered children could potentially be included in the data set before persistent children were eligible. Thus, the ranks of the recovered group could be disproportionately larger. To eliminate this bias, all children were followed for a minimum of 4 years before being placed into either group.

Children in the Longitudinal Study and Follow-Up Schedule

All of the children in our program whose data are reported in this section were first examined within 12 months of stuttering onset and participated for at least 4 years; a large majority participated for a longer period. It is imperative to state from the outset that *none* of the children who were later identified as recovered received therapy for their stuttering. On the other hand, 17 of the 19 children who eventually persisted received therapy for their stuttering. For comparisons, normally fluent children were also followed for a minimum of 4 years. Their data, however, are pertinent for some analyses but not for others. More information about the children in the stuttering and control groups is presented in Table 5.1.

Table 5.1

Mean Age (and Standard Deviation) at Onset, Age at Initial Evaluation, and Postonset Interval (in Months) for Experimental Group, and Mean Age at Initial Evaluation for Control Group

Group	n	Age at Onset Range	M	(SD)	Age at First Visit Range	M	(SD)	Postonset Interval Range	M	(SD)
Experimental										
Male	64	22–51	33.36	(6.56)	23–59	38.55	(7.96)	0–12	5.19	(3.66)
Female	25	22–55	33.24	(8.53)	25–65	37.36	(9.69)	1–11	4.16	(2.87)
Total	89	22–55	33.33	(7.12)	23–65	38.21	(8.44)	0–12	4.90	(3.47)
Control										
Male	29				27–56	41.59	(8.49)			
Female	13				29–63	39.62	(11.40)			
Total	42				27–63	40.98	(9.39)			

Summary of Procedures

Speech samples, severity ratings, and other measures were collected as described in Chapter 2. All 89 children were seen at the following intervals after the first visit: 6 months later, 1 year later, 18 months later, 2 years later, 3 years later, and 4 years later. A final exit visit was conducted several years following the 4-year visit for some children. As mentioned, for all children the first visit occurred within 12 months of their stuttering onset. However, a fair number of children were seen particularly close to onset, within 3 months; they received an extra follow-up visit that took place 3 months after the first visit.

Findings: Duration of Stuttering and Timing of Recovery

Percentage of Recovery

The duration of stuttering for the 89 children, all followed for 4 to 12 years after stuttering onset, is the basis for determining incidence of recovery and persistence. Identification of persistence or recovery necessitated careful review of disfluency data and parent and clinician severity ratings. Using the criteria given previously, the duration of stuttering was charted for each child. Figure 5.1 reveals a distinct pattern. Most children who completely stopped stuttering (gray bars) did so within the first 3 years (36 months) following onset. After this sharp drop in the recovery rate, some children continued to recover from 3 to 5 years following the onset of their stuttering. Of the children who persisted in stuttering for at least 5 years, as shown by the black bars, none, to date, have recovered completely. Between 49 and 60 months of stuttering, however, some children continued to stutter and some recovered. This overlap is indicated by the adjacent gray and black bars in the graph. Children represented by the gray bars did not stutter further. Those represented by the black bars had been stuttering for that long, but later data points have not yet been collected for them. Once they are observed for another year or two, it will be clear whether they continue stuttering for 5 or more years, or recover very late.

At the 4-year point, when all children had been observed for a minimum of 4 years following their stuttering onset, the rate of recovery was 74%. Table 5.2 shows the recovery rates, given the observation period; the recovery rate drastically increases during the first 3 years, then increases more slowly up to 5 years following onset, after which time no further recovery has been observed. Given a child who has just begun stuttering, we

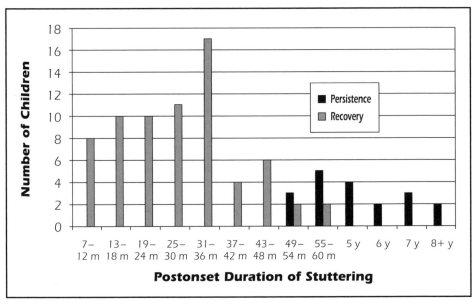

Figure 5.1. Duration of stuttering in months (m) or years (y) for all children followed for 4 to 8+ years postonset of stuttering.

Table 5.2
Rate and Chance of Recovery at Different Times Postonset of Stuttering

Time Postonset	Rate of Recovery by This Time	Remaining Chance of Recovery	Rate of Continuing Stuttering
2 years	31%	47%	21%
3 years	63%	16%	21%
4 years	74%	5%	21%
5 years	79%	0%	21%

can thus say that he or she has about a 65% to 80% chance of natural recovery by 3 to 5 years after onset, or a 20% chance of persistence. Conversely, as shown in the middle column of the table, after 36 months of stuttering, there is only about a 16% chance of recovery, and after 48 months, only a 5% chance, because most recovery occurs earlier. Unfortunately, we cannot tell parents for certain if their child will be one of the 80% who recover or the 20% who continue to stutter.

Our persistence rate of over 20% continues to uphold our previous findings, which include many of these same children (Yairi & Ambrose, 1999a). The fact that the percentage remains about the same even with a larger, more controlled sample indicates that the rate is quite robust. We must caution, however, that the 70% to 80% recovery rate applies to children seen *early* in the course of their stuttering. Evaluation of children who have already been stuttering for 1 to 3 years must take into account the considerable bulk of children who have already recovered.

Another important aspect of documenting recovery in our study is the length of time that we followed children after their recovery to verify that stuttering did not recur. For the persistent children, the duration of their stuttering equals the total time they were followed in the study. The persistent group had been stuttering for a range of 51 to 107 months, with a mean of 70.63 months ($SD = 18.11$), considerably longer than the 48-month minimum. Our classification criteria also specify that recovered children were followed for a minimum of 12 months following their complete recovery, in addition to having been followed for a minimum of 48 months past their onset of stuttering. This postrecovery observation period of 12 months was exceeded for a majority of these children. The mean postrecovery observation period was 40.77 months ($SD = 23.08$), ranging from 15 to 129 months. In fact, over 80% were followed for an additional 2 to 3 years, and close to half were seen for an additional 3 to 4 years. This long-term follow-up provides powerful support for the completeness of early, natural recovery.

The Age Factor

The age at which the persistent and recovered children entered the study was another point of interest. The 19 children who eventually persisted in their stuttering were, on average, a little older when they started stuttering than the children who recovered, and their postonset interval was also longer, as shown in Table 5.3. It is not clear why parents of children who became persistent first sought contact with us later than parents of the children who recovered. A few had already pursued evaluation and treatment, but without success, and were not referred to us until later in the course of their stuttering. Parents of several children in both persistent and recovered groups were advised by pediatricians or speech–language clinicians

Table 5.3

Age at Onset (in Months) and Months Postonset (with Standard Deviations), and *T*-test Results, for Persistent and Recovered Groups

Group	Onset Age*	Months Postonset of Stuttering**
Persistent	36.05 (7.93)	7.11 (3.26)
Recovered	32.59 (6.75)	4.30 (3.30)

$^*p = .059.$ $^{**}p < .001.$

Table 5.4

Distribution of Boys and Girls into Persistent and Recovered Groups

		Persistent		Recovered	
Group/Gender	N	n	%	n	%
Males	64	15	23.4	49	76.6
Females	25	4	16.0	21	84.0
Total	89	19	21.3	70	78.7
Male-to-Female Ratio		3.75:1		2.33:1	

that their child's stuttering was a "normal stage" and that they should not be concerned. The months postonset of stuttering interval was statistically significantly different (see Table 5.3) for the two groups. The age of onset difference bordered on statistical significance (see Table 5.3), which means that children who persisted in their stuttering tended to have slightly later onsets. We wonder whether this finding suggests that the two groups represent different subtypes.

The Gender Factor

The long-known gender effect in stuttering is also reflected in our longitudinal study. The distribution of the 89 children according to gender in the two developmental categories, persistent and recovered, is presented in Table 5.4. The rate of recovery would be expected to be higher for females because the male-to-female ratio is close to 2:1 at onset but is up to 5:1 or 6:1 for adults (Bloodstein, 1995), indicating that more females than males must recover. Our developmental data show that the male-to-female ratio is 3.75:1 for the persistent group and 2.33:1 for the recovered group. Indeed, the recovery rate for females is somewhat higher, at 84%, than for males, at about 77%. The difference, however, is not statistically significantly different [$\chi^2(1)$ = .59, p = .44]. The low number of persistent females, however, results in low power for the analysis, making significance test findings questionable.

The gender factor can be further explored by determining the duration of stuttering for males versus females or, in other words, the timing of recovery. The data, illustrated in Figure 5.2, indicate a clear gender difference. All of the females who recovered, except 2, did so by 36 months after their stuttering onset. Although most of the males also recovered within 36 months of onset, recovery continued up to 60 months. In other words, for males, duration of stuttering ranged from 7 to 58 months, with a mean of 29.45 months (SD = 12.40), and for females, duration ranged from 8 to 45 months, with a mean of 24.19 months (SD = 10.55). This difference, however, is not statistically significant [$t(68)$ = 1.70, p = .09]. Technically, therefore, preschool boys and girls who eventually recover from stuttering have similar durations of stuttering—about 2 years on average—but there may be a trend for girls to recover a bit sooner than boys. Then

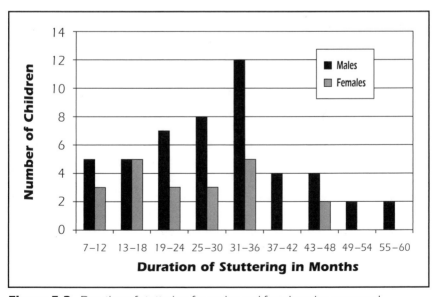

Figure 5.2. Duration of stuttering for males and females who recovered.

again, a child may also be one of the 20% of children whose stuttering becomes a chronic problem. Gender is only one of the many ingredients that controls the course of stuttering.

Findings: Longitudinal Disfluency Data

The primary factor that determines persistence or recovery is the presence or absence of abnormal disfluencies and associated characteristics. In this section, we examine the course of stuttering behaviors for children who persisted and recovered over the 4 or more years that they participated in our study. To examine developmental patterns of stuttering behaviors and trends of persistence and recovery from onset on, we discuss here only those children who were seen initially within 12 months of their stuttering onset, and for a minimum of 4 years at the time of the writing of this text. Children were seen initially within 1 year of onset, and then followed at 6-month intervals for two years, and thereafter seen yearly. Because not all children were seen within 6 months of onset, data points for the 0- to 6-month postonset interval were not available for some children.

Disfluency Profiles

Disfluency analyses of conversational speech samples recorded at each visit during the longitudinal study were performed in a manner identical to that described in the previous chapter. We can compare the frequency of SLD (Stuttering-Like Disfluencies, which includes part-word and single-syllable word repetitions, and disrhythmic phonation) to that of OD (Other Disfluencies, which includes interjections, such as "um" and "uh"; revisions or abandons; and phrase or multiple-syllable word repetitions). Table 5.5 shows the means and standard deviations for SLD and OD for persistent, recovered, and control groups. Standard deviations were rather large through all visits for the groups, and in the persistent group, the standard deviation even exceeded the mean at the 37- to 48- and 49- to 60-month intervals. This indicates that there is high variability within each group at each time period.

Results of a multivariate analysis of variance (MANOVA) revealed interesting patterns. Only at the 0- to 6-month visit were the persistent and recovered groups *not* significantly different in their SLD frequency. For all successive visits, a significant difference existed. By 7 to 12 months postonset, then, the two groups diverged. During the first year of stuttering, the SLD levels of the control group were also significantly different from those of both the persistent and the recovered group. After 2 or more years of

Table 5.5

Mean Stuttering-Like Disfluencies (SLD), Other Disfluencies (OD), and Standard Deviations (in Parentheses) for Persistent, Recovered, and Control Groups of Children

	Postonset Interval						
	1st Year After Onset		2nd Year After Onset		3rd Year After Onset	4th Year After Onset	5th Year After Onset
Subject Group	0–6 mos.	7–12 mos.	13–18 mos.	19–24 mos.	25–36 mos.	37–48 mos.	49–60 mos.
Persistent							
SLD	11.31 (6.12)	9.76 (6.32)	7.82 (5.31)	7.34 (6.75)	7.93 (6.40)	5.85 (8.37)	3.61 (4.42)
OD	4.64 (2.05)	5.41 (2.09)	5.42 (2.48)	5.75 (3.57)	7.49 (4.20)	5.54 (1.67)	6.38 (3.01)
Recovered							
SLD	11.03 (6.74)	5.38 (4.37)	3.01 (2.65)	1.99 (1.51)	1.62 (1.56)	1.18 (0.81)	0.91 (0.64)
OD	5.85 (3.00)	5.21 (2.34)	5.13 (2.92)	4.80 (2.25)	4.93 (2.89)	5.07 (2.06)	5.75 (2.51)
Control							
SLD	1.42 (1.01)		1.11 (0.79)		1.08 (0.97)	0.93 (0.89)	
OD	4.42 (2.27)		4.39 (1.60)		4.67 (2.17)	5.42 (2.02)	

stuttering, the recovered and control groups had comparable SLD levels, both within normal limits.

In stark contrast are the levels of Other Disfluencies. Between all three groups—persistent, recovered, and control—OD levels were not statistically significantly different from one another within any time interval. In addition, for each group, there was no significant change over time. In other words, not only does the OD level remain very static over time, but the groups are indistinguishable. This finding agrees with our previous reports (Ambrose & Yairi, 1999; Yairi & Ambrose, 1999a) and corroborates the conclusion that the OD category is a measure that is *not*, in general, indicative of stuttering severity in young children. There is, however, one exception: During the third year of stuttering, the frequency of OD for the persistent group distinctly rises, and in fact, there is a statistically significant difference between the persistent group and each of the other two groups. At this particular point, several of the persistent children exhibited very high levels of the use of interjections (the highest level was 19.88 for one child), perhaps, in part, as a reaction to their stuttering.

The general measures of SLD and OD provide clear evidence for differences and similarities, and indeed, for OD, there are few differences no matter how the data are examined. However, to measure how the stuttering changes over time, and how and when the persistent and recovered groups diverge, the finer dynamics of SLD changes must be explored. How does each of the three SLD components—part-word repetition, single-syllable word repetition, and disrhythmic phonation—change over time? Do repetition units (the number of extra times a syllable or word is repeated) change over time? As we discussed in the previous chapter, this important facet of disfluency is markedly different for children beginning to stutter and their normally fluent peers. Is it equally distinctive for the speech of persistent and recovered children? Throneburg and Yairi (2001) first reported findings for 20 children that bear on these questions. They found that frequency of disfluencies did not change over time for children whose stuttering persisted, but for those who recovered, frequency and proportion of disrhythmic phonation decreased dramatically. Now, with data for many more children analyzed, the updated information for the three SLD types and repetition units are shown in Table 5.6. Statistically significant differences ($p < .05$) are indicated with asterisks.

Some general trends are evident. First, we compare the persistent and recovered groups for each visit. At the first visit, there are no statistically significant differences between groups for any of the disfluency types. It is

Table 5.6
Means for Stuttering-Like Disfluency and Repetition Units for Persistent
and Recovered Groups Across Time

		Months Postonset						
Disfluency Type	Group	0–6	7–12	13–18	19–24	25–36	37–48	49–60
Part-word repetitions	Persistent	5.18	4.08*	3.36*	3.04*	3.04*	2.30*	1.78*
	Recovered	5.94	2.17*	1.14*	0.86*	0.65*	0.51*	0.46*
Single-syllable word	Persistent	3.53	3.33	2.40*	2.29*	2.67*	1.59*	0.00
repetitions	Recovered	3.20	2.39	1.47*	0.98*	0.84*	0.55*	0.34*
Disrhythmic phonation	Persistent	2.60	2.36*	2.06*	2.01*	2.23*	1.96*	0.89*
	Recovered	1.89	0.82*	0.40*	0.19*'	0.14*	0.13*	0.12*
Repetition units	Persistent	1.39	1.44*	1.42*	1.33*	1.33*	1.22*	1.17*
	Recovered	1.61	1.27*	1.16*	1.14*	1.12*	1.07*	1.06*

*$p \leq .05$.

of interest, however, to note that both part-word repetitions and repetition units are higher in frequency in the recovered group, while disrhythmic phonation is less frequent for the recovered group. At the 7- to 12-month postonset visit, differences are already clear. All of the disfluency types except single-syllable word repetition are significantly different. At each of the following visits, *all* of the disfluency types are significantly different between the two groups.

Second, examining the trends over time provides clear evidence for rapid differentiation between the persistent and recovered groups. Looking at the persistent group, all of the measures either decline gradually or remain rather static and then decline gradually. The disfluency frequencies for the recovered group, however, show a sharp decline as early as the 7- to 12-month postonset visit. For part-word repetitions, the entire range for the two groups for all visits is from 0 to 27. The highest value occurred at the 0- to 6-month visit for a child who later recovered. The levels for the persistent group decline gradually, whereas the recovered group has its greatest drop between the 0- to 6-month and the 7- to 12-month visits. Single-syllable word repetitions look a bit different. The range in frequency was from 0 to 12, and again, the highest value occurred for a recovered child on the initial visit. The decline for the persistent group is quite gradual. For the recovered group, the decline is also rather gradual, with no sharp decreases. For disrhythmic phonation, the pattern looks quite similar to that of the part-word repetitions. The range is from 0 to 17, but the child with the highest frequency is a persistent child at the 37- to 48-month visit. In fact, high levels occur sporadically (and occasionally) at almost every visit. Repetition units also show gradual reduction for the persistent group and rapid decline for the recovered group. The decrease is even steeper than it might seem: Because it is a ratio of total units of repetition over total instances of repetition, it cannot be less than 1.00. The range is from 1 to 5, and the highest frequency occurred at the 0- to 6-month visit for a child who later recovered (not the same child with the highest part- or single-syllable word repetition frequency).

To clarify the degree of the rapid changes during the first year or so of stuttering, the mean percentage of change (up or down) for each disfluency type is presented in Table 5.7. The first column of percentages refers to the change from the 0–6 to the 7–12 months postonset visit; the second column is the change from the 7–12 to the 13–18 months postonset visit. Repeated-measures analyses of variance were conducted for the frequency changes; significance is marked by asterisks. From the very early initial visit (0–6 months postonset) to the second visit (7–12 months postonset), the rapid decline in disfluency for the recovered group is indeed statistically significant for each type. For the persistent group, only disrhythmic

Table 5.7

Mean Percentage of Change (Up or Down) in Stuttering-Like Disfluency (SLD) Types During the First Year of Stuttering for Persistent and Recovered Groups

SLD Type	Group	Change from 0–6 to 7–12 Months Postonset	Change from 7–12 to 13–18 Months Postonset
Part-word repetitions	Persistent	−21%	−18%
	Recovered	−63%**	−47%**
Single-syllable word repetitions	Persistent	−6%	−28%
	Recovered	−25%**	−38%**
Disrhythmic phonation	Persistent	−9%**	−13%
	Recovered	−57%**	−51%*
Repetition units	Persistent	+4%	−1%
	Recovered	−21%**	−9%*

$*p < .01. **p < .001.$

phonation declines significantly. There is no significant change in frequencies of part-word and single-syllable word repetitions or repetition units. From the 7–12 to the 13–18 months postonset visit, the picture is virtually the same. All types are significantly different for the recovered group, and none are different for the persistent group.

It is not known what the level of disfluency frequency may have been if the persistent children had not received treatment for stuttering (all but 2 did receive treatment at some point). What is clear, however, is that even without taking treatment into account, the frequency of disfluency for the persistent group is consistently higher than for the recovered group. The two groups become markedly distinct from one another as early as the 7- to 12-month postonset visit; however, the timing of recovery varies for each child.

Seeing that the trends for the disfluency types are similar within each group, the weighted SLD can be examined to obtain a simpler picture. The weighted SLD (see Chapter 4) is a measure that combines the effects of frequency of part-word or single-syllable word repetitions, the mean number of times a segment is repeated per instance, and the frequency of disrhythmic phonation weighted by a factor of two. Figure 5.3 illustrates the data

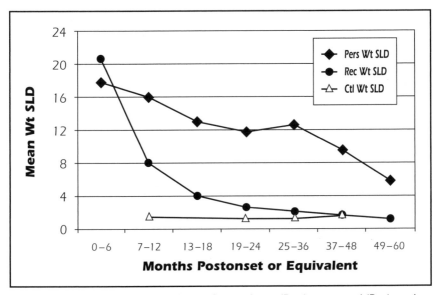

Figure 5.3. Mean weighted (Wt) SLD for persistent (Pers), recovered (Rec), and control (Ctl) groups over time.

for weighted SLD. The trends are apparent. The recovered group begins with a higher weighted SLD than the persistent group, but very quickly drops, reaching the approximate stuttering–nonstuttering border at a weighted SLD of 4. The persistent group remains a bit more stable, with an overall decrease in the weighted SLD score, but not reaching normal levels. As a reference point, the weighted SLD for the control group is also plotted, although these children were seen only four times, each a year apart. The figure well summarizes the data shown in Tables 5.6 and 5.7.

Given that the disfluency levels declined so quickly for the recovered group, one might ask if such a drop is a reliable predictor of recovery. A considerable drop in any of the SLD types may be a good indicator of recovery, but children who persist may also experience fluctuations in the severity of their stuttering. In terms of disfluency counts, then, the best predictor is a decrease in all SLD types, which approach normal limits within 6 to 18 months following onset. In other words, if substantial recovery is not seen within this time period, chances for natural recovery decrease. Early stuttering is highly variable, and predictions of recovered versus persistent pathways, based on disfluency profiles alone, are still difficult to make accurately early in the course of the disorder. The more significant finding, however, is that such recovery shows strong signs within the first 12 months of stuttering. Based on current data, we need to examine more than disfluency levels to obtain optimal early prediction.

Duration

The dimension of length of young children's disfluencies near stuttering onset was discussed in Chapter 4 in relation to two different metrics: the number of iterations, or repetition units, and the duration of disfluencies. Naturally, the findings about the children's declining amount of disfluency, as well as the decrease in the number of repetition units over time, heightened our interest in possible longitudinal changes in the temporal parameter of duration. It is interesting to note that both the *Chronicity Prediction Checklist* (Cooper & Cooper, 1985) and the *Stuttering Prediction Instrument* (G. D. Riley, 1981) specify length of disfluency as a risk factor for chronic stuttering. Thus, additional longitudinal research of the duration of SLD was carried out by Throneburg and Yairi (2001). For this investigation, we followed 20 of the children in the original study, 10 who eventually recovered and 10 who eventually persisted in stuttering, and analyzed speech samples from three testing periods. For both groups, the first samples were taken from the initial visit. At the time, the mean postonset interval was 7 months for those who would persist and 5 months for those who would recover. For the persistent group, a second speech sample was taken at 20 months postonset on average, and a third sample at an average of 32 months postonset. For the recovered group, the second speech sample was taken while the children were still stuttering, with the mean postonset time of this prerecovery visit being 13 months; the third sample was recorded when recovery criteria were first met, at about 19 months postonset, on the average.

Disfluencies were measured according to type and length: (a) part-word repetitions with one unit, (b) part-word repetitions with two units, (c) part-word repetitions with three units, (d) single-syllable word repetitions with one unit, (e) single-syllable word repetitions with two units, (f) single-syllable word repetitions with three units, and (g) disrhythmic phonation (i.e., blocks or prolongations). As described in Chapter 4, durational measures of the selected disfluency segments were performed with a computer software system, CSpeech Version 4 (Milenkovic, 1995), which processed the acoustic signal. For part-word and single-syllable word repetitions, the duration was measured for the entire disfluency, as well as for each repeated unit and each interval between units that constituted the disfluent event.

Although we reported separate measurements for repetitions composed of one, two, or three units, for the sake of simplicity, we recalculated group means for all sizes of each type combined. As can be seen in Table 5.8, at the initial visit, the mean duration values for repetitions tended to be a bit longer for the children who later recovered. The MANOVA statistical tests, however, revealed no significant differences in the mean duration. More important, changes in total duration over time were *not* significant. Similarly, more intricate analyses of duration of segments within instances of disfluency revealed that, over time, the recovered group had a tendency toward increasing the duration of silent intervals between repetition units. For example, the interval within a repeated word ("but-but") increased from 226 msec at the beginning of the study to 370 msec after recovery had occurred; the interval within a repeated syllable ("a-and") increased from 133 msec to 264 msec. This change suggests a normalization process in that longer intervals indicate that the iterations are slower in tempo (Throneburg & Yairi, 1994). Still, the trend was not statistically significant. In regard to disrhythmic phonation, there was a tendency for the persistent group to increase overall duration from 620 msec at the beginning of the study to 886 msec at its end. This change, however, could not be evaluated statistically and should probably be disregarded because of the small

Table 5.8

Mean Total Duration of Disfluencies (in milliseconds), Standard Deviations (in parentheses), and Number of Disfluencies Measured for Children Who Persist in or Recover from Stuttering Over Three Visits

Group/Visit	Part-Word Repetitions		Single-Syllable Word Repetitions		Disrhythmic Phonation	
	Duration	No. Measured	Duration	No. Measured	Duration	No. Measured
Persistent						
<12 mo.	754.17 (346.69)	149	816.86 (358.98)	132	620.30 (376.75)	46
19–24 mo.	732.47 (390.99)	193	941.50 (448.75)	131	779.69 (618.17)	32
31–36 mo.	668.82 (306.18)	114	839.33 (500.80)	136	886.46 (527.74)	35
Recovered						
<12 mo.	873.27 (458.52)	172	1,004.08 (471.06)	157	615.67 (272.72)	12
Prerecovery	650.45 (356.80)	103	973.76 (551.01)	131	619.90 (249.28)	10
Recovered	754.74 (395.14)	47	943.20 (462.22)	66	567.00 (71.53)	3

number of children who contributed sufficient material to the group mean
at all three visits.

All in all, the data on total duration of disfluency at the initial visit
(shorter than 1 second) appear to be comparable to several previous reports and also show that soon after onset there are minimal differences between children who eventually became persistent and those who recovered
from stuttering. The nonsignificant differences between the groups do not
support assumptions made in the literature (e.g., Cooper & Cooper, 1985;
G. D. Riley, 1981) that longer blocks and prolongations serve as warnings
of persistence. Also, the nonsignificant change in the duration and rate of
repetitions over a 2-year period for the persistent group do not agree with
expectations. For the persistent group, the duration of disfluencies remained relatively constant over a 3-year period instead of increasing as
expected according to the conventional assumptions. The data do not uphold the traditional notion that, as a rule, when stuttering continues, repetitions become more rapid, irregular, and longer. Because the total duration
of disfluencies was similar to that found by Zebrowski (1994) for school-
age children who stutter, we see more support for our suspicion that little
change is taking place in this parameter for several years after onset. Nevertheless, one cannot ignore the fact that some children who persist eventually develop more severe problems.

Associated Physical Behaviors

Persons who stutter often display visible tension of the face or movements
of the head or eyes that seem to be associated with their disfluency. Traditionally not viewed as an integral part of the original, or core, stuttering,
these movements have been commonly referred to as secondary characteristics. These movements, however, are so typical and frequent that they
have been included in many definitions of stuttering (e.g., Wingate, 1964).
Although the physical concomitants most often involve parts of the speech
mechanism or related structures (Bloodstein, 1995), they sometimes spread
to other body parts (e.g., hands, arms). For many years, the literature on
stuttering reflected the assumption that secondary characteristics are typically late-developing phenomena acquired in conjunction with increased
awareness of and as a reaction to stuttering. As discussed in Chapter 4,
however, in the past two decades, a few studies have documented the presence of head and facial movements near stuttering onset in a good number
of young children. Furthermore, as discussed later, there have been quite a

few suggestions that the presence of secondary characteristics is a predictor of chronic stuttering.

In relation to the developmental features of this aspect of stuttering, one of our own pilot studies (Yairi et al., 1993) of 16 children seen very close to onset of stuttering, and again 3 and 6 months later, indicated that the number of head and facial movements decreased over time as the frequency of disfluency decreased. In a later investigation, Throneburg, Ambrose, and Yairi (2003) also studied young stuttering children near onset (part of our larger group of children), 10 whose stuttering eventually persisted and 22 who eventually recovered from stuttering as verified through several years of follow-up evaluations. Two measures were employed at 6-month intervals: (a) clinician ratings of the severity of physical concomitants and (b) number of head and facial movements during disfluent and control fluent segments derived from frame-by-frame analyses of videotaped speech.

Physical concomitants were observed near the onset of stuttering for both groups. At the first visit (from 0 to 6 months postonset), the recovered group evidenced a large amount of secondary characteristics, according to both measures. Their mean clinician rating of 0.42 (on a scale from 0 to 1) was higher than that of the persistent group at any time. However, as of the second visit (from 7 to 12 months postonset), those who eventually persisted evidenced more secondary characteristics, rated as .37, than those who eventually recovered, whose rating fell sharply to .08. This statistically significant difference was found for all following visits.

The number of physical concomitants did not increase over the 3-year period examined for the persistent group. At the second visit, the persistent group exhibited a mean of 4.46 movements per disfluency, and at the 3-year postonset visit, they evidenced 3.01 movements per disfluency. The results of this study reemphasize the need for clinicians to monitor children over time. Although a large number of physical concomitants close to the onset of stuttering does not appear to be a warning sign of persistent stuttering, a decreasing trend over time may be a positive sign of recovery, and absence of minimal change of physical concomitants within a year could be a warning sign.

Looking at the data for the group of children analyzed in this chapter, one can see that our current data on the rated frequency or severity of physical behaviors associated with stuttering are in good agreement with our previous findings just described. As part of our clinician severity rating (see Chapter 2), secondary characteristics were rated on a scale of 0 to 1, going from *absent to barely noticeable* to *painful and obvious*. Table 5.9 shows the

Table 5.9

Mean Severity Ratings for Associated Physical Characteristics
for Persistent and Recovered Groups over Time (range from 0 to 1)

	Months Postonset						
Group	**0–6**	**7–12**	**13–18**	**19–24**	**25–36**	**37–48**	**49–60**
Persistent	0.32	0.30	0.35	0.28	0.32	0.21	0.21
Recovered	0.32	0.10	0.06	0.01	0.01	0.01	0.00

mean ratings for persistent and recovered children at increasing intervals after onset of stuttering. Even without any statistical treatment, it is obvious that the initial ratings are identical, whereas by the 7- to 12-month visit, they are distinctly different. Indeed, a multivariate analysis of variance revealed no significant difference for the 0- to 6-month interval ($p = .99$) and a highly significant difference at the 7- to 12-month visit ($p = .003$) and at all later times ($p < .001$). This is another piece of evidence for the very rapid differentiation between persistent and recovered groups.

Severity Ratings

Clinician and parent severity-of-stuttering ratings were obtained at each visit for each child. The 8-point rating scales ranged from 0 to 7 and are explained in detail in Chapter 2. Briefly, they are as follows:

Interval	Stuttering Severity
0–1	Normally fluent speech
1–3	Mild stuttering
3–5	Moderate stuttering
5–7	Severe stuttering

Parents are asked to simply circle or draw a line where their child falls on the scale, and may choose halfway points between the numbers. Parents are instructed to rate the severity of their child's stuttering at the current time—not specifically during the evaluation, but the severity over the last week or so. If large changes occurred between the rating at the previous visit and the current visit, parents are asked to indicate varying ratings for severity between those times. The clinician rating scale involves four

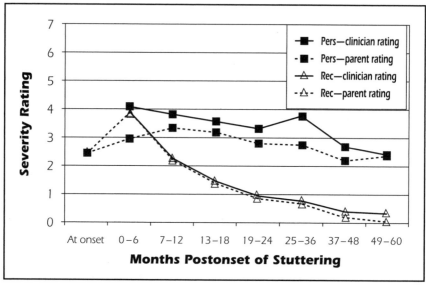

Figure 5.4. Mean parent and clinician severity ratings for persistent (Pers) and recovered (Rec) children over time.

subscales: frequency, duration, tension, and secondary characteristics (see Chapter 2). These are combined to yield a score ranging from 0 to 7, as listed previously.

Means for both clinician and parent ratings are shown in Figure 5.4 for persistent and recovered children. For the parent ratings, an additional rating is shown for the onset of the child's stuttering, as reported by the parents. Clinician ratings for persistent children for all visits ranged from 0 to 6.67. Remember that a persistent child could be rated as 0 by clinicians if there was no stuttering during the evaluation. As long as parents provided evidence that stuttering was still present, children were classified as continuing in their stuttering. Clinician ratings for recovered children for all visits ranged from 0 to 6.32. The ranges for parents were similar: Parents rated persistent children from 0 to 6.5, and recovered children from 0 to 6.

The clinician ratings for the persistent and recovered groups are virtually identical at the 0- to 6-month visit. Ratings sharply divide at the following visit, with the persistent ratings dropping to some extent, and the recovered ratings dropping substantially. Ratings of the recovered group reach normal limits (less than 1) by the 19- to 24-month visit, and remain well within normal limits for the following visits. Because clinician severity is composed in part of frequency and extent of disfluencies, the ratings closely match weighted SLD levels for each group. It is interesting that ratings for persistent children fall only to a small degree, even though all but 2 of these children received treatment for stuttering. The 2 who did not receive treatment had mild–moderate to mild stuttering throughout the study. In this light, the early sharp reduction in stuttering for the recovered group is all the more outstanding.

A most interesting finding is that the mean parent ratings for stuttering severity closely mirror the clinician ratings. Parent ratings are extremely close to clinician ratings for the recovered group, and only slightly lower for the persistent group. Parents are not aware of clinician ratings when they rate their child, and clinicians rate independently of parents. The correlations between clinician and parent scores (as well as frequency of SLD) for all visits were statistically significant at $p < .01$. This provides strong evidence that subjective parental judgments closely parallel the more objective judgments by trained clinicians. It must be remembered, however, that a mean represents the average score, not individual scores. Indeed, some parent ratings differed considerably from clinician ratings, but these were few and far between. To indicate how individuals may vary from each other and across time, disfluency and severity data for 1 persistent and 1 recovered child, chosen randomly, are presented in Table 5.10. Imagine, based on this chart, the amount of data for the other 87 children discussed in this chapter.

CONCLUSIONS

The Course of Childhood Stuttering

Although natural recovery has long been recognized in the clinical and research literature of stuttering, it has had little impact on the traditional conceptualization of the disorder, which has basically ignored and contradicted its existence. Our findings challenge a long-held view of stuttering as a disorder that begins as a "small animal" and gradually transforms into a "big monster." The findings of the University of Illinois Stuttering Research Program indicate that in the majority of cases of early childhood stuttering, the disorder progresses the other way—primarily toward amelioration and resumption of normal speech fluency. The graphs in Figure 5.3 confirm our earlier reports for a smaller number of subjects (Yairi &

Table 5.10
Individual Disfluency and Severity Data for 1 Persistent (Pers)
and 1 Recovered (Rec) Child

| Characteristic | Group | Months Postonset | | | | |
		0–6	7–12	13–18	19–24	25–36
Part-word repetition	Pers	6.15	4.14	1.59	0.80	0.68
	Rec	10.75	3.16	4.22	1.66	0.35
Single-syllable word	Pers	4.37	0.40	2.76	1.94	1.61
repetition	Rec	7.23	3.16	3.46	1.18	0.94
Disrhythmic phonation	Pers	2.37	1.11	2.85	1.47	0.76
	Rec	0.10	0.29	0.00	0.00	0.00
Stuttering-Like	Pers	12.89	5.66	7.20	4.21	3.05
Disfluencies (SLD)	Rec	18.08	6.62	7.68	2.84	1.29
Repetition units	Pers	1.60	1.36	1.12	1.12	1.04
	Rec	1.51	1.62	1.18	1.08	1.00
Weighted SLD	Pers	21.57	8.39	10.57	6.01	3.90
	Rec	27.35	10.82	9.06	3.07	1.29
Other Disfluencies	Pers	2.30	3.94	6.78	3.68	4.41
	Rec	4.49	9.11	4.87	7.34	4.69
Accessory characteristics	Pers	0.50	0.00	0.00	0.25	0.33
	Rec	0.25	0.00	0.00	0.00	0.00
Clinician severity rating	Pers	5.16	2.00	1.92	2.50	3.33
	Rec	4.40	3.00	2.00	0.67	0.67
Parent severity rating	Pers	4.00	1.00	1.00	1.00	2.00
	Rec	4.00	4.50	2.00	0.00	0.00

Ambrose, 1992a, 1999a; Yairi et al., 1993) that, in general, the amount of stuttering and its severity, as reflected in SLD and other measures, reach their peak during the early stage of the disorder. Parent reports also substantiate the conclusion that stuttering frequency and severity increase during the first few weeks or months postonset. After the disorder reaches its peak within this time period, the young children exhibit a strong tendency for substantial alleviation in the overt symptomatology. This tendency is seen in almost all measures employed, be it number of SLD, number of secondary movements, severity rating by clinicians, or severity ratings by parents. A good many children exhibit up-and-down fluctuations in the level of stuttering; these cycles, however, do not restrain the overall downward progress. Only a minority of children depart from the average pattern, maintaining or increasing the level of stuttering as the disorder progresses.

Overall, within the first 4 years after onset, the aforementioned decline in stuttering leads to complete (natural) recovery in approximately 75% of cases, with a few more recovering over the next year, leaving about 20% persisting beyond 5 years of stuttering. These figures are strikingly similar to those obtained nearly 40 years ago in the famous longitudinal study reported by Andrews and Harris (1964), as well as in more recent longitudinal studies (Johannsen, 2001; Mansson, 2000). Furthermore, we are quite convinced that the 25% persistence rate is an overestimate. As explained, children whose parents provided evidence of only rare, mild manifestations of stuttering were kept in the persistent group. For all practical clinical purposes, however, these children would be considered recovered because they would no longer meet the minimal criteria for entry into the study. Five of the children in our study fit this category. Perhaps a third category of "unclassified" or "clinically recovered with traces of stuttering" might be justified. Additional considerations strengthen our conclusion that 25% persistence is an overestimate and 75% recovery is an underestimate for the population at large. There are children whom we refer to as cases of "reported but unverified" stuttering and recovery. Those are the children whose parents call us with vivid descriptions of their child's sudden stuttering onset or a significant surge in his or her stuttering, but 2 weeks later cancel a diagnostic evaluation because the stuttering stopped or was drastically reduced. At other times, we have received calls from various professionals asking if we would be willing to evaluate a stuttering child whom they just saw, but the parents fail to contact us. These cases, not counted in our study, probably represent a general trend in the population.

Another example is that of unreported cases. Because recovery can take place at a very early age and within a few months after onset, it is highly probable that a number of stuttering children go unreported. As adults, these children are often unaware of their stuttering history, even if it was severe. Evidence for such scenarios has been detected in families of participating children when we accidentally and belatedly discovered cases of unreported stuttering among siblings. Unreported cases were not counted in this study and may, we suspect, constitute an even larger group than those reported but not verified.

It is interesting that long-term follow-ups have been advocated as necessary to confirm that recovery occurred (e.g., Onslow & Packman, 1999). Bloodstein (1995) suggested a minimum of 5 years. The logic behind this position is that a longer time will reduce false or temporary amelioration and yield a lower percentage of recovery. It is clear from the data, however, that the opposite is true. Children who recovered early and maintained fluency for at least 12 months did not show relapse. As the observation period extended to 5 years after the onset of stuttering, some recovery continued to occur. It may be that children in our study who continued with traces of stuttering, but appeared clinically normal, may have future episodes of stuttering, further justifying their placement in the persistent group. Thus, our high percentage of recovery remains, even when allowing for some degree of relapse. Additionally, we see no support for the suggestion that the longitudinal evaluations, in and by themselves, could have affected the results, causing reduction in the levels of stuttering. If this were true, we would have discovered a remarkably easy and powerful therapeutic tool. In our humble opinion, our evaluation, initial parent counseling, and follow-up appointments, were not sufficient to eradicate stuttering in over 75% of the children we have seen. Also, the fact that longitudinal observations did not aggravate stuttering might add further weight against Wendell Johnson's theory that attention to stuttering increases it.

In summary, there are good reasons to believe that the true incidence of natural recovery from stuttering exceeds 75% and may reach 85% of all those who ever stutter. Conversely, we believe that fewer than 25% of the children persist. Remember, however, that these numbers refer to children seen close to the onset of stuttering, before children who recover early drop out of the picture. One of the reasons leading to previous erroneous estimates of recovery below the 50% level (e.g., Wingate, 1976) was rooted in neglecting adequate considerations of epidemiology—in other words, the inclusion of data from studies that used samples composed of teens and adults, both groups in which persistent stuttering is prominent, and the lack of cases that had already recovered in early childhood. Unfortunately, the bias toward persistence was not recognized or appreciated by Wingate more than 25 years ago or by many current investigators who commented on the development of stuttering.

Duration of Stuttering and Timing of Recovery

Recovered Children

Although the data show that substantial deceleration occurs in all measures of stuttering during the first year, and that deceleration during this period is a reasonably good predictor of eventual recovery, it does not mean that complete recovery occurs so quickly. For most children, recovery was a quite gradual phenomenon, although some do stop stuttering after a relatively short time and fully recover within a few months postonset. Contrary to doubts as to whether such children have ever really stuttered, all of those in our present study had their stuttering unquestionably identified and verified by several observers and according to all established criteria. Several exhibited severe stuttering, and the overall severity of the recovered group, early on, was equivalent to or higher than the eventually persistent group. This is an important point to repeat: There is no scientific, clinical, or any practical justification for the notion that children who stutter less than 6 months should not be considered as "real stutterers" or that their stuttering was not real. The purpose of epidemiological studies is to account for *all* cases properly identified under any disorder to better understand all of its characteristics. In our study, the duration of stuttering was one of the main independent variables. It would be quite unacceptable if investigators in other health fields decided to discard data for patients who exhibited acute but short-term symptoms of a disorder.

The majority of the children who eventually recover, however, present stuttering for longer periods. For them, recovery is a slow and gradual process that usually begins during the first year, reaching completion at various points in time, mostly within 3 years postonset but occasionally up to 4 or 5 years. Indeed, a fascinating characteristic of the overall course of stuttering is its asymmetry—a brief beginning and ascending phase, followed by a relatively prolonged declining phase. We wonder if it reflects maturational process or adjustment or compensation strategies. In any event, we conclude that natural recovery from stuttering, like its onset, is primarily a phenomenon of early childhood. Clearly, the long accelerating pattern of stuttering, typically depicted in past writings about the course of the disorder, is not fitting for the majority of cases of early childhood stuttering.

Persistent Children

According to our data, only a minority of the children continued stuttering at the end of 4 or 5 years. Even in this subgroup, only a few fit descriptions that inspired past clinicians and investigators to conclude that stuttering continues to grow for years. Such a false generalization for the entire population of those who stutter is predictable when investigators are unaware of, or turn their eyes away from, or fail to track those who recover. What is important for clinicians to recognize, however, is that children who eventually persist exhibit a relatively stable SLD level during the first year. The typical drop seen in the recovered group is missing. A stable SLD curve, as well as stability in other measures during the first year, should be viewed as a warning sign for persistence. This sign, of course, should be considered a matter of probability rather than certainty because a few children who eventually recovered also maintained a stable SLD level during the first year. Clinicians must also be careful to note when a child's stuttering began. A new referral does not necessarily indicate recent onset. Many children who stutter are not seen by a speech–language clinician until they have stuttered for a year or more. In these cases, it is too late for early indications, and the very fact that the stuttering has continued at a level severe enough for them to be evaluated may place them at higher risk of persistence.

There is no question that a few persistent children eventually do develop severe complex stuttering. At times, remarkable changes can take place very quickly, even in those who recover later. The clinician should understand this possibility, be prepared for adverse changes, and adequately inform and counsel parents. There is additional information, however, that the competent clinician should keep in mind. Based on our findings, few extreme alterations appear to take place during the first 2 years or so after onset in the disfluency patterns of the majority of children who persist; in fact, one of our most interesting findings is that, on average, the persistent children progressed in the opposite direction than expected, actually experiencing *improvement* in their stuttering as time passed. The reason for the eventual decline in severity for the persistent group, however, is not clear, but it may at least in part be due to the therapy that many in this group received from outside sources at various times. We cannot help but make the intriguing observation that complete recovery did not occur in the persistent children during the course of the study in spite of intervention, whereas complete recovery occurred in the recovered group in the absence of fluency treatment.

The Validity of the Recovery– Persistence Classification

A frequently asked question is how confident we were about classifying the children as recovered or persistent. Naturally, much of the concern is directed toward the final decision that a child had recovered. If the child stutters, then it is relatively easy. But what if he or she does not stutter during the follow-up? How do we know that the child does not stutter in other situations? Can we trust periodic recorded speech samples obtained in the clinic? There is no simple answer. We believe that securing long speech samples over more than 1 day in each follow-up, and having the child converse with several people, is very likely to reveal at least some indications of existing stuttering. We remind the readers, however, that the classification rested on much more than that. In addition to extensive speech samples recorded with several conversational partners over 2 different days at each visit, there were repeated parent reports, over several years, regarding the presence or absence of stuttering at home. These were accompanied by their severity ratings, along with the experimenters' impressions and independent, online severity rating. All these multiple procedures and criteria greatly reduce the possibility of a child being misclassified as recovered.

One objection to our procedures came from Onslow and Packman (1999), who, fearing that absence of stuttering in clinical samples might result in false negatives, stated that home speech samples must be used to establish recovery. Ideally, developmental research of stuttering should be conducted in conditions that reflect as purely as possible the natural course of the disorder, limiting confounding variables. It is the complex interaction of multiple factors that creates stuttering—it is not a single entity that can be examined in isolation. Stuttering occurs almost exclusively when the affected person is engaged in interpersonal communication involving a wide variety of situations. Our data have shown, however, that home samples have not appreciably differed from clinic samples. We have obtained many home speech samples of children who recovered and who persisted. Inasmuch as the child stuttered, in almost all cases stuttering was more severe in the clinic, and in no case did a home sample change the classification of a child as recovered or persistent. It is important to understand that, if a child stuttered only at home and very rarely, the home speech sample is almost as unlikely to "catch" one of these moments as the clinic sample. We think that Onslow and Packman's (1999) concern is satisfactorily addressed by detailed parent reports at each visit. Whereas it is quite possible for some variations in precise frequency or severity of stuttering to occur from situation to situation (Silverman, 1972; Yaruss, 1997), it appears unlikely that the presence of a stuttering problem, diagnosed at home and confirmed in the clinical environment, will be completely missed by all concerned, parents and experimenters, during formal and informal observations in several environments over a period of several years. This study was not a single-shot experiment, but was based on numerous observations by quite a few people for a long period of time. The very similar, sometimes identical, severity ratings assigned by parents and clinicians for both groups of children would bear out this conclusion.

The Factor of Stuttering Severity

Another issue is the relationship of severity to either persistence or recovery. It is counterintuitive that early severity is unrelated to eventual outcome, but our data undeniably illustrate their independence. It is *not* the case that children with initially mild stuttering are those who recover naturally; wide variation is seen in early severity in both the persistent and recovered groups. Thus, we agree with Wingate (1976, p. 114) that "level of severity does not necessarily limit the expectation of recovery in any particular case." Clinicians must be aware of this phenomenon when making treatment recommendations and counseling parents. Although very early severity is unrelated to outcome, later severity is a primary indication for concern. Why, then, are initial symptoms unable to provide clues as to the future course of the disorder? As the king in *The King and I* (Rodgers & Hammerstein, 1956) stated, "Is a puzzlement."

The Gender Factor

Although the data continue to indicate that the percentage of boys who persist is larger than that of girls, the trend was not statistically significant. The most likely reason is the small number of females. The same gender proportions with a sample twice as large would have yielded significant differences. Indeed, other investigators (Seider, Gladstien, & Kidd, 1983) who examined larger numbers of people who stutter, with a male-to-female ratio almost identical to that reported here, found a statistically significant gender factor. Their sample, however, comprised families of adults with persistent stuttering. In spite of the radically different sampling techniques, females evidence a higher recovery rate than do males.

In addition to the higher chance for females to recover, the influence of gender is also seen in the tendency for females to recover at an earlier age. The gender-modified expression of persistence versus recovery, reflected in the smaller proportion of persistent females, as well as shorter duration of stuttering in females, provides a provocative clue as to the genetic involvement in these two pathways of the disorder (Ambrose et al., 1997). We will discuss this issue in greater detail in Chapter 9 on the genetics of stuttering.

Clinical Applications

As data obtained in research that complies with epidemiological principles solidify, the picture of the disorder's course becomes increasingly clearer. Our special effort to identify all children who ever stutter, close to the onset of stuttering, and to follow them over time, provides an optimal database for our conclusions. Clinicians should know that only a minority of these children persist in stuttering, whereas in the majority of cases stuttering is a temporary, often short-lived disorder that disappears without formal intervention, apparently on its own accord. Improvement and recovery dominate the early stages of early childhood stuttering (Wingate, 1976; Yairi & Ambrose, 1999a). In only a small number of children does stuttering become progressively more complex and severe with time. Of course, this is a group trend, a general frame of reference. Nevertheless, it provides a general optimistic outlook for both clinicians and parents. Also, the majority of natural recoveries occur within 3 years of stuttering onset. Clinicians should also know that, although early stuttering often undergoes quick up-and-down cycles, which are masked by group data, the downward trend becomes overriding sooner or later for the recovered group, and also for a good number of children in the persistent group. It is useful to know, however, that once recovery in young children has been achieved and maintained for 6 to 10 months, chances are very high that it will be permanently sustained. There is no support in our study, nor in Andrews and Harris's (1964) data, for the belief (e.g., Bloodstein, 1995) that reversal of recovery maintained for a substantial period is common at these ages. Furthermore, recovery during early childhood appears to be complete in terms of normal speech fluency. In a perceptual study of the speech of several recovered children, listeners were unable to differentiate at better than chance levels between speech of recovered children and speech of normally speaking control children (Finn, Ingham, Ambrose, & Yairi, 1997). This is quite different from recovery in adults who report residual stuttering (Wingate, 1976) and from the frequent relapses reported for many older children or adults who undergo treatment for their stuttering.

The information is also important for service policies and planning, as well as for counseling parents of young children who exhibit stuttering. The need to focus intensely on early identification of the children who are at higher risk for chronic stuttering is particularly apparent. These are the children who should be identified early and have priority as the recipients of available clinical resources. There are several ways to improve our current ability to assess a child's risk for developing stuttering. The overt symptoms of stuttering described in this chapter, especially the longitudinal trend of SLD during the first 12 to 18 months, may be used by clinicians to determine if a particular child appears to be following a pattern of persistence or recovery. The child's gender and the type of familial history of stuttering are also particularly useful information. These and other practical prognostic principles will be discussed in Chapter 10 concerning the initial evaluation of childhood stuttering. So far, however, none of the items, or combinations of them, has been incorporated into a formal differential diagnostic instrument. Many other factors must be weighed in decisions regarding treatment for each individual child. Future, perhaps computerized, diagnostic instruments may become more sophisticated as we continue to analyze our data.

One of the most important implications of the results pertains to clinical efficacy research in early childhood stuttering. The findings make it amply clear that any claim of successful therapeutic regimen or any clinical efficacy study on preschool children must recognize the strong factor of unaided, natural recovery (Curlee & Yairi, 1997, 1998). In studies of clinical efficacy, it would be ideal to include a nontreatment control group, if ethically possible, but it is also important to strive for unbiased subject samples. Those who insist that every child who begins stuttering should receive immediate intervention, should include in their experimental and control groups children in close proximity to the onset of their stuttering to assess with greater validity the effect of unaided as compared to aided recovery. Clinical studies with older children with a longer stuttering history (e.g., 1 year) can certainly contribute useful information concerning the merit of different treatment techniques, but they cannot isolate the full effect of natural recovery. Finally, we must stress that the recovery factor is critical in evaluating young children who have stuttered only a short time. Once a child has stuttered for several years, complete natural recovery is somewhat unlikely.

Old ideas and established traditions are difficult to alter or abandon, however, even when negating evidence is mounting. Consequently, some reservations, resistance, or even outright objections might be expected. Onslow and Packman (1999) claimed that the recovery reported in our studies could be attributed to a single brief parent counseling session. This is a misguided argument. If, indeed, a single counseling session is so powerful, why is there a need for all the elaborate, sometimes lengthy, treatment programs that they and others have advocated? Should clinicians resort to a single counseling session as *the* treatment of choice for childhood stuttering? Our guess is that answer would be negative. Additionally, there are no credible data to support the contention that a single counseling session is effective in curing or reducing stuttering. In fact, Fortier-Blanc, Labonte, Beauchemin, and Jutras (1997) reported data questioning the effectiveness of indirect intervention with preschool children who stutter.

On the other hand, a measured degree of skepticism is scientifically healthy, and we must be willing to carefully scrutinize new information just as we continuously question the old. Although our main findings may appear challenging, on the whole they are not really all that new. Our historical review of literature has shown that the central ingredients of what we have reported have been known for several decades. Our contribution has been primarily in providing the necessary documentation and scientific support to confirm and further detail that knowledge. Nevertheless, in view of questions and controversies that have sprung in various scientific forums, it is useful to restate the reasons for our confidence in the methods employed in the investigation and its main findings. Finally, the natural question concerning all this research and our findings is why some children recover while others persist in stuttering. Currently, this question is a difficult one to answer.

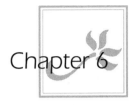

Chapter 6

Development of Phonological Ability

Elaine Pagel Paden

Among speech pathologists it has been common knowledge for many decades that, in children, stuttering is a disorder frequently accompanied by phonological impairment. Although the research literature includes numerous studies that have investigated various aspects of this relationship, scholars typically have not followed the same children for a period of time to see how the relationship progresses. The University of Illinois Stuttering Research Program, therefore, provided a unique opportunity for the longitudinal study of phonological development concurrent with early stuttering. Of special importance, we were able to compare the phonological development of children whose stuttering would later prove to be persistent with that of children in whom stuttering would disappear without therapy. Other aspects of this co-occurrence were also examined. This chapter's focus is on reviewing our findings in the context of preexisting information resulting from other studies in this area.

Study Questions

1. *What chief differences were found between the phonological development of groups of children whose stuttering later proved to be persistent and those in whom it disappeared spontaneously?*

2. *Can the state of phonological development of a child who recently began to stutter predict the future course that his or her stuttering will take? Explain why or why not.*

3. *What relationship does the phonological ability of a child who stutters have with the severity of his or her stuttering and the words upon which he or she stutters? Explain.*

A relationship between stuttering and speech sound production has been suggested in three areas: (a) the frequent association between disordered phonology and early stuttering, (b) the influence of speech sounds on the specific location of stuttering, and (c) the possible impact of central speech planning of sounds on the occurrence of stuttering. In the first area, although stuttering historically has been conceptualized as a single disorder, attention of workers in the field has been drawn to various indications that in young children it tends to be associated with other disorders. Of these, the co-occurrence of stuttering and articulation or phonological difficulties appears to be the most common. In the second area, some of the earliest research in stuttering that attempted to uncover rules of the disorder was aimed at the phonetic characteristics of moments of stuttering, and an interest in this question continues. Concerning the third area, in recent years theories of stuttering have taken a strong interest in phonological encoding processes during central speech planning and the system's attempts to correct its errors as a factor in the occurrence of disfluent speech. In the present chapter, we discuss the research regarding the relationship of phonological ability to stuttering in each of these areas.

General Historical Background

The relationship between stuttering and the ability to correctly produce and use the sounds of speech has been investigated since the 1920s. The continuity of this topic in the literature may not be recognized immediately because there has been a notable change both in the terminology used and in the concept of incorrect speech sound production. Before the 1980s, children who had any difficulty producing or using speech sounds were usually said to have an articulation disorder. Since then, the term most often used is phonological disorder or delay. The change in terminology represents an increasing understanding of the task that children face in acquiring intelligible speech. Early on it was assumed that they simply needed to learn how to *produce* all of the speech sounds appropriately and then practice using them wherever they occurred in the speech stream. In other words, this difficulty was thought to be a disorder of motor execution in that the child had not yet learned to control the muscles of articulation appropriately (i.e., a problem "in the mouth"). The child thus needed to be taught where to place the tongue, for example; or to make a close, rather than a firm contact of the lips; or not to use vibration of the vocal folds for some consonants. Articulation disorders were described in terms of the number of phonemes that were missing or incorrectly produced (e.g., Templin & Darley, 1969).

Beginning in the 1970s, speech–language pathologists recognized that the problem also may be that the child does not yet comprehend all that is required for intelligible speech. Not only must children acquire sufficient motor control for correctly producing increasingly more difficult sounds, but they must also acquire subliminal awareness of classes of sounds and their distinguishing features, of the different syllable shapes used in our language, and of the places in words, or adjacent to what types of sounds, certain others may be used. In other words, they must gradually develop awareness of the *sound system* of the language (Hodson & Paden, 1991). The designation *phonological disorder* (or impairment) is now used intentionally to include any of these central and peripheral abilities. *Articulation disorder,* meanwhile, properly should be reserved to mean only the inability to perform the motoric act of producing typical sounds of American English, whether they have not yet been learned or, possibly, result from a physical handicap, as in the case of a child with cerebral palsy. In this chapter, we use *phonological disorders* as just defined, but we may use *articulation disorders* when referring to research that was done during the era when unintelligible speech was thought to be due only to inability to produce sounds correctly.

Co-Occurrence of Stuttering and Phonological Disorders

Over several decades a good number of studies have reported a high incidence of young children who stuttered and also appeared to be phonologically impaired. This phenomenon is intriguing from both theoretical and clinical considerations. Upon contemplation, such co-occurrence does not seem surprising. As mentioned in Chapter 3, stuttering onset usually occurs during the third year of life, a period when a child's development in almost every capacity is usually advancing very rapidly. Not only are changes in physical growth, motor skills, and cognitive ability observable almost week by week during the ages from 2 to 4 years, but also linguistic abilities in general, including phonological skills, are typically expanding at a rapid pace. The complex interaction and mutual influences of the various domains of speech and language during this period are far from being understood, but it is logical to assume that any interference with normal development or rapid progress in one aspect can have multiple effects. A study by Arndt & Healey (2001) verifies this supposition. Of 457 schoolchildren who stuttered, identified by certified speech–language pathologists in 10 states as widely scattered as Florida and Minnesota, Oregon and Vermont, the researchers found that 33% evidenced both phonological and language disorders, 35% had only language disorders, and 32% had only phonological disorders. Those reported with other deficiencies, however, were not included in the study.

The purpose of most early studies was to determine the percentage of children who stutter and also have speech sound disorders. Some of these reported percentages were as high as the 66% to 71% found by St. Louis and Hinzman (1988). On the other hand, McDowell (1928) identified only 19% of the young stutterers he reviewed as having other speech problems, and G. W. Blood and Seider (1981) reported an even smaller number, 16%. More recently, several investigators have reported the incidence to be between 30% and 40% (e.g., Cantwell & Baker, 1985; Wolk, Edwards, & Conture, 1993; Yaruss, LaSalle, & Conture, 1998). Unfortunately, the sample size, the age and gender distribution of the groups studied, and the procedures and test materials, as well as the specification of "disorder" varied considerably in these studies. All of these factors could have contributed to the large differences in the reported results and are among the important reasons why a firm figure on the incidence of the co-occurrence of stuttering and phonological impairment cannot be established. A few studies were based on rather large numbers of children, for example, 126 by Schindler (1955) and 1,060 by G. W. Blood and Seider (1981). Others employed small samples, only 54 children in the G. D. Riley and Riley (1979) study and 48 in the Thompson (1983) study. The early investigations also differed considerably in the age range of the children surveyed. Although most focused on school-age children, some surveyed children in Grades 1 through 12 (Schindler, 1955) or Grades K through 9 (Williams & Silverman, 1968). Several researchers chose participants based on chronological ages instead of grade, such as from 2 to 14 years (Darley, 1955), 7 to 12 years (McDowell, 1928), and 3 to 6 years (Morley, 1957).

Methods for determining whether the children had articulation deficiencies also differed widely. Some investigators simply based their reports on interviews with parents (Andrews & Harris, 1964; Darley, 1955; Seider, Gladstien, & Kidd, 1982). At least one relied only on speech pathologists' reports (G. W. Blood & Seider, 1981). Others have made a direct, but only very informal, assessment of the children's speech, such as asking them to repeat a number of sentences while the observer recorded articulation errors (McDowell, 1928) or asking them to tell a story (Williams & Silverman, 1968). Schindler (1955) reported using a test but did not name it. Several investigations (Cantwell & Baker, 1985; St. Louis & Hinzman, 1988), however, were based on results from the widely used, standardized *Goldman–Fristoe Test of Articulation* (Goldman & Fristoe, 1972).

In spite of the variety in research designs and methodologies, all but two of the early reports agreed on the general conclusion that larger percentages of children who stutter are found to exhibit articulation impairment than their normally fluent peers. In the more recent surveys, after researchers began using more rigorous research procedures, only one study has been located that failed to find a larger number of children with articulation disorders among those who stuttered than among similar groups of normally fluent children. In that study by Seider et al. (1982), however, the normally fluent controls were siblings of those who stuttered. That similar numbers of children with articulation problems were found in the two groups could have been predicted, in that articulation impairment, as well as stuttering, often runs in families.

Regardless of the exact percentage, there is a general recognition that phonological impairment is the most common speech problem that coexists with stuttering in children. Nevertheless, there have been dissenting voices (e.g., Nippold, 1990, 2002). Also, although the most commonly cited estimate is that about 30% to 35% of children who stutter and are seen in clinics also have phonological disorders, this may not be representative of the larger population of young stutterers. Throneburg, Yairi, and Paden (1994), after studying 24 children selected from 75 young participants in the University of Illinois Stuttering Research Program, noted that the proportion of stuttering children who were in the severe level of phonological error was smaller than 30%, although the specific proportion was not reported. For contrast, one must keep in mind that the expected incidence of phonological disorders in the general population is between 2% and 6% (Beitchman, Nair, Clegg, & Patel, 1986).

Other Areas of Research Focus

Loci of Stuttering and Phonological Difficulty

A question related directly to the stuttering–phonology connection is whether it is revealed by the specific locations where stuttering occurs in speech—that is, the words or speech sounds that are stuttered. Since the 1930s, the point in the speech stream at which stuttering most frequently occurs has occasionally intrigued investigators. Pioneering studies by Johnson and Brown (1935), S. Brown (1938), and Hahn (1942) focused on adults who stutter, and attempted to determine which consonants cause the most difficulty for them. They identified /g, d, θ, l, ʧ/ as those most often stuttered. A few years later, S. Brown (1945) concluded that phonetic attributes are only one factor that determines the loci of stuttering. Although consonants were found to have greater chances than vowels to be stuttered, he noted that word position (early in the sentence) and grammatical factors (content rather than function words) have greater weight in this regard. Forty years after Brown's study, other scholars (Bloodstein, 1974; Bloodstein & Grossman, 1981) raised the question of where stuttering most often occurs in the speech of young children; they implicated syntactic elements as being the most frequent controlling factors of the loci of stuttering in this age group.

More recently, the phonological difficulty of a word has been examined as a possible explanation for triggering a stuttering event. One of the earliest investigations within the University of Illinois Stuttering Research Program dealt with this question. In a study by Throneburg et al. (1994), 24 children, ages 29 to 59 months ($M = 41$ months), were selected from our participants to represent four conditions: severe stuttering/good phonology, severe stuttering/poor phonology, mild stuttering/good phonology, and mild stuttering/poor phonology. Seven categories of phonological difficulty were then identified comprising words with consonant clusters, multiple syllables, or late-developing sounds, and the four possible combinations of these three. Words that are not phonologically difficult (i.e., present none of these difficulties) were also included as the eighth category.

From the approximately 1,000-word sample of each child's conversation recorded at the first visit, all the words he or she used were classified according to type of phonological difficulty. The numbers of words produced by a child within each category were tallied, so that the percentage used within each category by each child could be determined. Then each word on which a child stuttered was noted, and the proportion of words stuttered within each category was determined. From these data, each group's percentages for each category were derived. It was found that the largest proportion of disfluent words (roughly half) used by each group was "not phonologically difficult"; that is, the words were not from any of the seven categories of phonological difficulty. The proportion of stuttered words in each of the seven categories was small and did not match the proportion of the occurrence of that word type in the child's conversation. This was true for each group of participants. We concluded, therefore, that phonological difficulty does not influence the occurrence of stuttering.

Another team of investigators (Howell & Au-Yeung, 1995) essentially repeated the Throneburg et al. (1994) study, but with a somewhat more elaborate design, dividing 31 participants, ages 2 to 12 years, into three age groups (younger, middle, and older). They also observed the lack of association between phonological difficulty and incidence of stuttering in each of their age groups. Even the conjecture that stuttering on a word may result from anticipation of phonological difficulties in the word that will follow it could not be supported by either the Throneburg et al. or the Howell and Au-Yeung research.

A more recent study by Wolk, Blomgren, and Smith (2000) of a small group of 7 males, whose ages were 4 and 5 years, investigated whether the phonological difficulty of a syllable was related to the occurrence of stuttering. The investigators reported that the group's mean frequency of stuttered syllables with phonological errors was not significantly different from the mean frequency of stuttered syllables that were *not* produced with phonological errors. They did find, however, that disfluency on clusters with phonological errors (i.e., with phonemes omitted, substituted, or distorted) occurred significantly more often than on clusters without phonological error. Because of the small sample size, the investigators suggested that their findings be interpreted with caution. Thus, considerable evidence has accumulated that, for children, there is no overall strong relationship between phonological difficulty and the occurrence of stuttering.

Severity of Stuttering and Phonological Ability

Another pertinent research issue regarding the association between stuttering and phonological disorders has been the effect that each of these disorders may have on the other. Inasmuch as the two conditions tend to coexist, the question is whether the children's severity of stuttering is influenced by the level of their phonological ability or, vice versa, the level of phonological development is influenced by the severity of stuttering. In other words, is there a cause–effect relation between the two?

Unfortunately, research in this area also has been sparse. There were only two investigations pertaining to this issue prior to our research. St. Louis and Hinzman (1988) and St. Louis, Murray, and Ashworth (1991) compared the articulation errors of children (ages 6.8 to 17.5 years; $M = 12.6$) exhibiting moderate stuttering severity with those of children at the severe level of stuttering. They found that, although the level of stuttering did not change the types of articulation errors produced, children with severe stuttering did make more errors than those whose stuttering was moderate. Furthermore, the errors were characterized as greater in severity. Yaruss et al. (1998) also dealt with this issue as part of an overall review of the other speech and language characteristics of 100 children (85 boys and 15 girls, with a mean age of 54.7 months) who were examined due to parental concern about their stuttering. The investigators found no significant differences in the fluency of these children related to whether their phonology was normal or disordered.

Our program has also contributed to this research area. At the time of the first visit of the children in our study, they were usually younger than those reported in previous investigations of this issue, and it was worthwhile to study whether any relationship between the two disorders could be observed closer to the onset of stuttering. Gregg and Yairi (2001), therefore, selected for study children who were within the 2-year-old range. They assembled four mutually exclusive groups, each distributed in the male-to-female ratio of 5:2, whose ages were between 25 and 38 months ($M = 32$ months)—one with severe stuttering and one with mild, one with good phonological skills and one with poor. A clear gap was left between the designations of "good" and "poor" and of "mild" and "severe" in forming the groups. Results suggested that even at this age there is little effect of level of stuttering severity on phonological ability or of phonological ability on level of stuttering severity.

Nature of Phonological Differences

Another focus of research has been the study of differences in articulation abilities of children who stutter and their normally fluent peers. Such research has typically been conducted through one-time observation of the articulation errors made by children of comparable ages.

The earliest age at which such differences have been assessed was reported by Bernstein Ratner (1997), who assembled children very close to the onset of stuttering, with a mean age of less than 3 years. They were matched with normally fluent children by age, gender, and socioeconomic status. The articulation abilities of 12 such child pairs were evaluated using *The Goldman–Fristoe Test of Articulation* (Goldman & Fristoe, 1986), on which the stuttering children scored in the 56th percentile and the fluent children in the 63rd percentile, thus showing a slight, but nonsignificant difference in favor of the normally fluent children.

Other studies provided data for greater numbers of older children. Schindler (1955) reported on 126 stuttering children from Grades 1 through 12, compared with a larger, closely matched control group. Schindler's findings showed that children in both groups made the same kinds of articulation errors, but those who stuttered made more of them. St. Louis and Hinzman (1988) and St. Louis et al. (1991) also found that children who stutter make more of the same types of errors than children who do not. Additionally, they identified the most common error as sound substitution, with over half of these occurring in the word initial position.

At the time our project was begun, only two reports had been published that attempted to describe the phonological abilities of young children who stutter. Louko, Edwards, and Conture (1990) compared 30 children who stuttered (28 boys and 2 girls, ages 2 to 7 years) with normally fluent children, by analyzing the phonological processes they used during recorded informal interactions with their mothers. They reported that the stuttering children exhibited a total of 18 different processes, whereas the matched group of normally fluent children used only 11 processes, all of which were among those used by the children who stuttered. The mean number of processes per child in the two groups, however, was similar. One interesting contrast was that consonant cluster reduction was used a total of 18 times by the children who stuttered—more often than any other process by either group—but only once by the control group.

The second study (Wolk et al., 1993) compared the conversational speech of three groups of 7 boys (ages 4 and 5 years). One group stuttered and had disordered phonology, another stuttered but had normal phonology, and the third did not stutter but had disordered phonology. Thus, the researchers were able to observe whether any phonological differences between the groups resulted from co-occurring stuttering. Among other measures of phonological inadequacy, the numbers of occurrences of 27 processes known to be common at this age were tallied for the two groups of children who stutter. Results indicated that the performance of the stuttering/disordered phonology group and that of the normal fluency/disordered phonology group were more similar than different in terms of the phonological processes used and their frequency of occurrence. For both groups, the most frequently occurring age-inappropriate phonological process was cluster reduction. Two atypical phonological processes (velarization and glottal replacement) were found to be more common for the children who stuttered and exhibited disordered phonology than for the disordered phonology group alone. As did Louko et al. (1990), they observed cluster reduction to be the most prevalent age-inappropriate process used by children with disordered phonology, whether or not they also stuttered.

The small number of investigations explains why, when we began investigating the phonological abilities of young children close to the age of stuttering onset, we were pushing into minimally charted territory. Because of the potential to contribute answers to questions regarding the theory of stuttering, we wished to study these children's phonological development in more detail than had previously been attempted.

Theoretical Explanations

Predictably, theories seeking to explain the cause of stuttering have also dealt with the question of why stuttering and phonological disorders may interrelate. Very early, Orton (1937) hypothesized that a single syndrome of basic linguistic deficit manifests itself separately or simultaneously in stuttering and other language difficulties. He classified children who stuttered into four groups: those who had undergone an enforced shift from left to right handedness, those who were slow in selecting a handedness, those with a family history of stuttering, and those for whom other types of language disorders or a tendency toward left handedness was found in the family. West, Kennedy, and Carr (1947) described stuttering as a psychophysical complex outwardly manifested by sudden and frequent tonic and clonic spasms of the face and lips, tongue, larynx, and/or respiratory machinery, which interrupt the flow of speech. Van Riper (1971) believed that stuttering is a common neuromotor deficit that follows one of four tracks of development, only one of which is accompanied by poor articulation and begins at the time the child is producing his or her first sentences. Based on their research, Byrd and Cooper (1989b) proposed that stuttering reflects a central neurological processing deficit, as does apraxia, but exhibits even more disfluencies than that disorder.

A relationship between stuttering and phonology is central to the covert repair hypothesis (Postma & Kolk, 1993), which asserts that speech difficulties of persons who stutter result from problems in premotor phonological encoding wherein the speaker attempts to correct speech errors before they are uttered. Conture, Louko, and Edwards (1993) further speculated that, when children who stutter speak too rapidly for their ability to activate phonological encoding, they may make inappropriate phonological selections, and that correction of these errors results in disfluencies. The research of Yaruss and Conture (1996) suggests that, for children, disfluencies represent by-products from repairs of nonsystematic speech errors (use of unusual or uncommon processes), rather than from those that are systematic (natural processes). Our group (Paden, Yairi, & Ambrose, 1999) entertained the possibility that genetic factors that differentiate subgroups of children who stutter, currently under study in the University of Illinois Stuttering Research Program (Ambrose, Cox, & Yairi, 1997), may also be associated with concomitant speech disorders of these children.

Reservations About Early Data

As mentioned previously, investigators of the stuttering–phonological disorders connection have not reached consensus, and some have expressed strong reservations. A critical review of the early studies in this area was published by Nippold (1990), pointing out methodological flaws, such as a lack of appropriate test–retest data or interscorer reliability measures, and questionable criteria for "articulation errors," including failure to distinguish between articulation differences and disorders. Indeed, we believe that more recent research also needs to be evaluated for possible occurrence of these problems.

Furthermore, new questions and issues have been raised about research in this area. Yairi (1999) noted several epidemiological factors that could have affected past research findings about the stuttering–phonology link. For example, the accuracy of the incidence reported may suffer due to insufficient consideration of gender and age factors. First, before 6 years of age, girls, as a group, are generally assumed to acquire linguistic skills, especially articulation proficiency, more rapidly than boys (Smit & Hand, 1997). In other words, boys are more likely to exhibit phonological deficits at this time. Thus, inasmuch as even at very young ages boys who stutter outnumber girls 2:1, reports of high percentages of phonological deficits in stuttering children might be, in part, a reflection of the skewed gender ratio in the group under study. Moreover, the older the children in the group, the greater is the percentage of boys and, hence, the greater the likelihood of finding higher percentages of phonological problems. Additionally, the nature of the phonological deficits varies with age. Children who are 3 years old typically present quite different phonological abilities from those who are 5. Other conditions that might be taken into account are familial characteristics, such as socioeconomic group, level of education, race, and area of residence.

Early investigators almost always failed to consider three other factors that can strongly influence findings about phonological inadequacy in children who stutter. First, for the most part, they failed to study those who were in the early stages of stuttering. The surveys typically focused on children of school age, so that the youngest were usually in first grade, or sometimes kindergarten, even though the onset of stuttering is most often about 3 years of age. This practice ignored large numbers of young children who stuttered for a few months or years, but then recovered spontaneously. Are the phonological abilities of these children apt to be better developed than those of children whose stuttering will persist? Darley (1955) was one of the few early investigators who included children younger than kindergartners. The children whose mothers he interviewed were ages 2 years 4 months (2-4) to 14-0, but no separate report was made on those younger than 5 years. Cantwell and Baker (1985), in a study of 600 children with speech and language disorders, stated that the majority of their participants were preschoolers, but in summarizing their observations, they did not separate the children by age. They only reported that 40 of the 600 children (up to 16 years of age) stuttered and, of these, 30% also had articulation disorders.

Second, most researchers observed children only once, and thus were unable to report on how phonological development, as well as stuttering, changed in the same children over time. They did not take into account that stuttering, as well as phonological deficiencies, may be quite different at different ages. Morley (1957) was the only early researcher who observed the same children over several years. Thirty-seven youngsters who stuttered were seen three times at about 2-year intervals. Only at the oldest age (6-6) did she report a larger proportion of the group with articulation disorders than in a comparable group of 113 normally fluent children. We can assume that this observation does not mean that the early phonological abilities of the children were actually *better* than at the older age; rather, inappropriate production of phonemes that are known to be later developing would not have been labeled as errors when the children were younger. For example, at age 4 years, the children probably had not mastered liquids, especially /r/, but this would not have been considered a "disorder" in 2- to 4-year-olds, whereas the same performance would be so labeled when a child reached 6 years of age.

Third is the issue of recovery. Only one study of the frequency of coexisting stuttering and phonological deficiency has been found that considered the fact that, for a large number of children who stutter, the condition is not persistent. In 1982, Seider et al. reported that, of 168 children who stuttered and later recovered, 7% had articulation problems, compared with 9% of 667 whose stuttering was persistent; however, the authors did not define what they meant by "articulation problems." In contrast, among the nonstuttering siblings of the persistent group, only 4% had articulation problems, as did 10% of the nonstuttering siblings of the recovered group. This survey was based on interviews with adults who stuttered or parents of children who had stuttered, and therefore it is not surprising that many more children were reported in the persistent than in the recovered group; that is, no interviews were reported with adults who had once stuttered and subsequently recovered. It is of interest, however, that in this study more "articulation problems" were found among the children with persistent stuttering than among those who had recovered (the latter presumably reported by parents of children who had recovered).

The result of the failure to address any of these three areas in past research has been a considerable lack of knowledge about the course of phonological acquisition after stuttering emerges. Information was especially sparse concerning whether there were differences related to the two tracks that stuttering may follow—that is, whether it will become persistent or spontaneously disappear. What influence may each course have on subsequent phonological development? It was thus essential that children's phonological abilities be evaluated as soon as possible after stuttering onset, and then observed over a period of several years. This became the primary goal of the study of the stuttering–phonology connection within the University of Illinois Stuttering Research Program. Previous chapters have recounted our overall plan of recruiting children soon after the onset of their stuttering, determining that they indeed stuttered by using several strictly defined criteria, collecting many kinds of information about them, assessing their language competencies in numerous ways (including phonologically), and reassessing them at regular intervals for several years. Our research plan has resulted in a large body of data, obtained from a previously unmatched large group of children, regarding the phonological development of those who once stuttered but later recovered—an area virtually ignored in previous scientific research—as well as information concerning the early phonological development of children whose stuttering would be chronic. Much of the remainder of this chapter reviews these studies in some detail.

Evaluating Phonological Competency

The phonological development of a young child can be assessed in three different ways. The first is by counting *phoneme errors,* or the number of times a child errs when attempting to produce the phonemes in targeted words. This was the method typically used by early investigators who wished to determine whether more articulation disorders are seen among children who stutter than among those who do not.

The second method, used in a few more recent studies, focuses on the kinds of inadequacies in the child's phonological system, rather than on individual speech sound errors. This is done by observing the *phonological processes* that a child uses—that is, the systematic ways in which he or she deals with specific aspects of the phonological code that have not yet been mastered. Thus, uses of stopping, cluster reduction, velar fronting, final consonant deletion, and other "natural" ways of simplifying the system, as well as unusual ways, are noted. It is then determined how extensively these processes are used and whether they are appropriate for a child of a given age.

The third choice is to determine the percentage of times a child fails to produce an essential *phonological pattern* that is present in the adult version of the words he or she is attempting to say—that is, failures to produce the appropriate sound class (e.g., stridents, velars, liquids), number of syllables, or syllable shape (e.g., consonant clusters, final consonants) (see Hodson & Paden, 1991). The goal is to count all instances in which a target pattern is not used, including those in which a phoneme is totally omitted, a phoneme is substituted that does not contain the target feature, or the appropriate syllable shape is not produced. Thus, this type of study gives an account of the child's overall phonological inadequacy, and makes it easy to compare the child's performance at different ages or with other children.

In the University of Illinois Stuttering Research Program, we were not primarily interested in the number of phonemes not yet mastered or in the phonological processes resorted to by the children when they could not yet produce all of the sounds and syllable structures of English. We were more interested in measuring the extent to which each child had failed to master the ability to use all of the essential characteristics (features) of the American English sound system, and to be able to do this when the child was as young as 2 years, when most of his or her phonological inadequacies would not be considered disorders. We deemed it desirable to be able to express this in a score that could be compared with those of other children who were evaluated at the same time and, even more important, to be able to make accurate comparisons of a child's progress over several years.

Based on the foregoing considerations, we chose *The Assessment of Phonological Processes–Revised* (Hodson, 1986) for evaluating a child's current phonological system. This instrument focuses on the 10 "basic patterns" that are typically acquired between the ages of 2 and 6 years. These are production of (1) nasal, (2) glide, (3) velar, (4) strident, and (5,6) liquid consonants (/l/ and /r/ considered separately), use of consonants in (7) initial and (8) final positions in syllables as required; (9) use of more than one syllable in a word when appropriate; and (10) use of consonant sequences (including clusters). The percentage of a child's failure to produce each pattern in these attempts can be determined, as well as the mean percentage of error on all 10 patterns. On the basis of the latter scores, the mean percentage of error for a group can be derived, and then groups of children can be compared. Furthermore, by using the same test items at each yearly visit, a child attempts each feature the identical number of times and in the same phonetic environments. As a result, there is considerable confidence in comparing a child's performance with that of previous years and with others in a group, as well as in comparing different groups of children. The instrument has been widely used with children of the age of the participants in our program, and guidelines are available for the ages at which each pattern should be essentially mastered (Hodson, 1997; Porter & Hodson, 2001).

The Illinois Studies of Stuttering and Phonology: Longitudinal Phonological and Stuttering Development

One of the important limitations of research on the phonology exhibited by young children who stutter, up to the time our studies began, was that the phonological analyses of such children were conducted at a single point in time; that is, investigators described what was seen of these children at only one age. Although the phonological status on a particular testing date is valuable information, children's phonological abilities change rapidly, and nothing has yet been reported about how their skills may have later improved and at what pace. Therefore, researchers had not addressed such questions as when children who stutter and have phonological deficits can be expected to achieve normal phonological systems.

The main contribution of our studies in this area is that we assessed children at 1-year intervals on several occasions, beginning as soon as they could be seen after stuttering onset. What we found casts a new light on the interaction of the two disorders, and provides a perspective on what can be expected of a very young child who stutters and is also phonologically less advanced than most children at his or her age. A second major contribution results from our knowing whether each child's stuttering would disappear within a few years or sooner, or would eventually become chronic. When we reviewed their initial performance for this study, we had already accumulated the data to know which children would recover from stuttering within 36 months of onset and which would persist 48 months after onset. Thus, we were able to look at these two groups separately to see whether there might be any differences in their early phonological development that could predict what their course of stuttering would be. What we learned through such research is the focus of the rest of this chapter.

Phonology Near Stuttering Onset

Initial Insights

Before our research began, the association between stuttering and phonological disorders typically had been based on surveys and clinical observation of *school-age* children. Whether this co-occurrence would be observed in the earliest months of stuttering usually had not been asked, and we wanted to study this question. We also wanted to know whether the co-occurrence could be seen in children whose stuttering would later disappear spontaneously and, if so, whether children who would recover early from stuttering would have less phonological impairment than those who recovered later. If such information were to become available, especially if it provided a basis for predicting the future of a child's stuttering, this knowledge would be extremely valuable.

Early on, in a small exploratory study within our program, Yairi, Ambrose, Paden, and Throneburg (1996) found that, when children were tested soon after stuttering onset, the mean amount of phonological error was greater for the groups who had continued to stutter longest. When we compared these groups of children with others of the same mean ages who had never stuttered, we found that the phonological ability of each of the normally fluent groups was more advanced than for the age-comparable group that stuttered. Therefore, we had good reason to ask if the same difference would be found if the study were more carefully controlled, especially with more exact pairing of the stuttering children and their nonstuttering peers.

Insights with Closely Matched Nonstuttering Pairs

In our next attempt to answer these questions (Paden & Yairi, 1996), we closely matched both age and gender in pairing the normally fluent children with those who stuttered. Three groups of 12 children who stuttered, none of whom had undergone fluency intervention, were studied: (a) one whose stuttering we already knew would persist for more than 3 years after onset, (b) one who would recover between 1 and 3 years (late recovered), and (c) one whose stuttering would disappear within 1 year after onset (early recovered).

When they were first tested, the mean age of the persistent group was almost 4 years, or about 9 months older than the late recovered group and 11 months older than the early recovered group. In spite of their older age (which should have resulted in better phonological performance), the persistent group showed somewhat more phonological error than either of the two recovered groups, although the differences were not great (see Table 6.1). The performance of each of the stuttering groups, however, was poorer than that of the normally fluent group with whom it was matched in age and gender.

These results confirmed that groups of children who stutter can indeed be expected to progress more slowly in phonological acquisition than groups who do not stutter. Using percentage of phonological error as a

Table 6.1

Means (and Standard Deviations) for Percentage
of Phonological Error and Age for Matched Pair Groups ($n = 12$) at Initial Visit

Group	Percentage of Phonological Error	Age (in Months)
Persistent stuttering	27.5 (11.7)*	47.2 (9.0)
Control for persistent	14.8 (14.6)	46.8 (8.4)
Late recovered stuttering	24.3 (15.6)	38.3 (6.4)
Control for late recovered	17.6 (13.4)	37.8 (6.0)
Early recovered stuttering	21.7 (10.6)	36.7 (6.9)
Control for early recovered	18.5 (13.8)	36.3 (7.1)

Note. From "Phonological Characteristics of Children Whose Stuttering Persisted or Recovered," by E. P. Paden and E. Yairi, 1996, *Journal of Speech, Language, and Hearing Research, 39*, p. 984. Copyright 1996 by American Speech-Language-Hearing Association. Reprinted with permission. *$p < .05$.

measure of extent of phonological acquisition, the group whose stuttering would persist was *significantly* poorer than the paired group of children who had never stuttered. On the other hand, both groups who later recovered were not significantly different from the normally fluent groups with whom they were paired, although their scores were somewhat poorer.

Of additional importance, and of great interest to us, we found no significant difference in the mean level of the scores of the two recovered groups. This indicated that grouping children whose stuttering would disappear on the basis of the length of time it took for recovery to occur provided no information beyond what would be seen if these children were treated as a single group. Therefore, this division was not made again in our research.

What should not be overlooked (and is not shown in Table 6.1) is that the range of phonological acquisition among children within all three groups was similar. In each one, the individual children who stuttered showed mean phonological error ranging from 0% to as high as 45%. Moreover, among the normally fluent groups with whom these children were compared, the range of mean phonological error was virtually as wide. This illustrates, as we said earlier, that individuals in these ages (2 to 5 years) move at very different rates in phonological acquisition, apparently regardless of whether the children stutter or are normally fluent. Unfortunately, this means that the level of phonological ability for a single child is not sufficient for predicting the future course of that child's stuttering.

Even though the differences in amount of error between the persistent and either recovered group were not significant, the group whose stuttering would persist was, on average, 9 or 10 months older than those who would recover. Given this age difference, the older group would be expected to show a distinctly lower percentage of error than the groups who are younger, as is true when our nonstuttering control groups are compared. However, our data did not show how far behind in phonological development the group of children whose stuttering would be persistent actually was compared with those who would no longer be stuttering after 3 years. It was obvious that, in our subsequent research, age must be taken into account when comparing children's phonological progress.

The results of Bernstein Ratner's (1997) study, cited earlier, of 12 pairs of 3-year-olds, tested even closer to stuttering onset than our group (within 3 months), are remarkably similar to our finding that the groups that would later recover from stuttering showed a mean percentage of error somewhat poorer than, but not significantly different from, their age- and gender-matched peers who had never stuttered. Might these data suggest that most of the children in Bernstein Ratner's study would later recover spontaneously from stuttering? Or, because Bernstein Ratner's group experienced stuttering onset so recently, is it possible that the slowdown in phonological acquisition that we seemed to see in children whose stuttering would persist had not yet had time to affect these children? Neither of these studies could answer these questions. The basic similarity in the results, however, adds strength to the conclusion of both: that soon after stuttering onset, children show poorer phonological development than normally fluent children of the same age.

In-Depth Study of Phonological Acquisition

Because we found clear differences between the phonological achievement of children with persistent and transient stuttering in our early studies, it was apparent that more extensive observation of phonological acquisition by children who stutter could be profitable. A much larger group of children first seen close to stuttering onset was now available in the University of Illinois Stuttering Research Program, for whom it was already known whether their stuttering would later disappear or persist. These were 62 children who had been found no longer to stutter within 4 years after onset (the recovered group), and 22 who still stuttered after 4 years (the persistent group). The distribution of 18 boys and 4 girls in the persistent group and 41 boys and 21 girls in the recovered group reemphasized that many more boys than girls stutter, but it also emphasized that more girls who stutter will recover (33.9% of our group) rather than persist (18.2% of our group). Although we do not claim that the proportion of girls we had in each group is exactly what would be seen if more children who stutter were surveyed, the fact that we found almost double the proportion of girls in the recovered group clearly illustrates that girls have a better chance of recovery than boys. The children in both groups were 2 to 5 years old at this point, but the mean age of the persistent group was about 4½ months older than that of the recovered group.

In contrast with our exploratory study, three changes were made in the next study, which we describe here. First, we now knew that the children's mean phonological error scores need to be slightly weighted for age when young children are compared to reflect the fact that better scores are expected from somewhat older children. Thus, a small fraction of a point was added to a child's score for each month his or her age exceeded 36 (Paden et al., 1999). Second, all of the children we knew would recover within 4 years after onset were now evaluated as one group. Third, we did not compare these groups with normally fluent children because our interest was focused on observing differences in phonological progress between recovering and persistent stutterers. Moreover, evidence already was available in the literature concerning the typical ages of acquisition of phonological milestones by fluent children with which our groups could be compared (Hodson, 1997).

The longitudinal investigation we now undertook was unique in research on stuttering and phonology in several ways. Not only did it involve a much larger group of stuttering children than most previous studies of this issue, but it also examined their phonological development more thoroughly and over a longer period of time. Of more importance, it compared the phonological performance at three yearly visits of children who later proved to stutter persistently with others who would later recover without intervention.

Initial Observation of Expanded Groups

With the larger groups of children, it was possible to look for other ways in which the phonological performance of the two groups differed from or might resemble each other, when first assessed after stuttering onset.

Table 6.2

Mean and Age-weighted Mean Percentages of Error at Initial Visit
for 22 Children with Persistent and 62 with Transient Stuttering

Group	Mean Percentage of Error	Mean Age (in mos.)	Age Range (in mos.)	Age-weighted Mean Percentage of Error
Persistent	27.50	42.5	25–59	30.45*
Recovered	22.10	33.8	25–59	23.18

*$p = .002$.

Mean Percentage of Phonological Error. The first obvious difference between the two groups was in their mean percentage of phonological error.
In spite of their older age, the group whose stuttering would eventually
prove to be chronic had not progressed as far in phonological acquisition
as had the group who would recover from stuttering. The persistent group
was poorer (had a larger mean percentage of phonological error) than the
recovered, even when their scores were not age-weighted, but when age
was taken into account, the difference between the groups was significant,
as shown in Table 6.2.

There have been, as yet, no studies reporting children's rate of phonological acquisition before they begin to stutter.[1] We can safely assume,
however, that there will be wide differences in rate of phonological acquisition among these children, as there are in the population of children in
general. Our data suggest, however, that somehow the onset of stuttering
slows the rate of phonological acquisition for many children, and that the
slowdown will be greater for the group whose stuttering will become
chronic than for those who will later recover. Theorists may wish to offer
some explanation for why stuttering onset seems to have a more detrimental effect on phonological development of one group than the other.

Levels of Phonological Deficiency. Another way in which the persistent
and recovered groups differed was in how the children's individual mean

---

[1] Kloth, Janssen, Kraaimaat, and Brutten (1995), however, have checked the speaking rate of children at
risk for stuttering (i.e., children who came from families with histories of stuttering but who did not
presently stutter) and later found a difference in rate between those who developed stuttering and
those who remained fluent.

percentage of phonological error scores were distributed as to level of phonological deficiency. We used four levels to make this separation: *mild,* no more than 19% mean phonological error; *moderate,* 20% through 39% mean error; *severe,* 40% through 59% mean error; and *profound,* 60% mean error or more (Hodson, 1986). Looking at the distribution of the two groups in these levels (see Table 6.3), it can immediately be seen that no child in either group showed mean phonological error in the profound level of severity, even with the scores increased by age-weighting. In other words, none of these 84 children were virtually unintelligible due to phonological inadequacy. Thus, if stuttering is implicated as a cause of phonological impairment, in our large group its effects were limited.

Children who score in the mild level of phonological deficiency have already essentially mastered the early patterns, and there would be no concern about their future phonological progress. They are obviously uninhibited by stuttered speech as far as phonological development is concerned and are moving at a pace that would be comparable to that of most normally fluent children of their age. Almost half of the recovered group was at this level, but less than a quarter of the older persistent group showed similar ability. The moderate range, of course, indicates somewhat slower progress than the mild level. More of the persistent children than recovered fell in this range. For the younger children whose scores are in the lower half of the moderate range, this level may be considered acceptable, and many of the recovered children fell there. But for children who are 4 years old—and more of the persistent group were of that age—this progress is too slow.

Table 6.3

Approximate Percentages of Persistent and Recovered Groups
Scoring Within Each Level of Deficiency at Initial Visit
of 84 Children, Using Age-weighted Scores

Level of Deficiency	Percentage of Error	Percentage of Persistent Group	Percentage of Recovered Group
Mild	0%–19%	22	47
Moderate	20%–39%	50	40
Severe	40%–59%	28	13
Profound	60%+	0	0

The severe level indicates seriously delayed or possibly disordered phonological development. Again, more of our persistent children than recovered scored in the severe range. These children are probably at risk phonologically and should be closely analyzed and carefully monitored to check whether they progress appropriately. When Table 6.3 is examined with these levels in mind, it is impossible not to conclude that, overall, the younger recovered group showed better phonological ability than the persistent group.

Order of Pattern Acquisition. Another important factor to be checked in the phonological development of young children is the path they are following in acquiring Hodson's (1986) 10 basic patterns. When we checked, it was obvious that this was a way in which the groups did *not* differ, because the order in which both groups were acquiring new patterns was typical. (We say more about this later in the chapter.) However, at the time of their first visit, the persistent group was different from the recovered because it showed poorer ability on every pattern than the group that would spontaneously recover from stuttering. Again, the large number of older children in the persistent group should have resulted in better mastery by that group of all of the patterns.

Strategies for Patterns Not Acquired. Sometimes children who are not as advanced phonologically as others of their age use unusual or uncommon strategies when they are unable to produce the patterns they are attempting. When we examined inaccurate pronunciations of these children, however, we had difficulty finding examples of unusual strategies. Both groups of children relied almost entirely on the "natural simplification processes" (Stampe, 1973) that normally developing children most often use when patterns have not emerged—that is, for velars, the children used fronting (replacing velars with alveolar phonemes); for consonant clusters, they used cluster reduction (deleting one of the sounds in the cluster); and for liquids, they used gliding (replacing /l/ and /r/ with /w/ or /j/) or vowelization (replacing them with any vowel). In a very few cases, a child used an uncommon strategy that demonstrated his or her correct perception of the target pattern even though it was not correctly produced. A single phoneme used in place of a consonant cluster sometimes contained one feature from each of those in the cluster that was targeted (e.g., /f/ for the initial cluster in *smoke* includes the stridency of /s/ and the labial place of /m/). Only 3 children in the recovered group and 2 in the persistent group at this point in our testing used a strategy that was "unnatural" or in-appropriate when they attempted one of the more difficult patterns. In other words, we found virtually no instances among our participants to in-dicate that their stuttering was associated with abnormal or bizarre word productions.

Consonant Clusters: A Key to the Course of Stuttering? As mentioned earlier, Louko et al. (1990) analyzed the phonological abilities of a small group of children (28 males and 2 females) whose mean age was 4-4. They evaluated the children on the basis of the phonological processes being used, and reported that only one process, cluster reduction, was used by a significantly larger number of children who stuttered than by their nor-mally fluent paired group. Consequently, in evaluating our children, we paid specific attention to the amount of error they exhibited on consonant sequences (a pattern that is largely made up of consonant clusters). The re-sults showed that among the children ages 4 years or older, a large number of the persistent group, but not of the recovered, showed inadequacy on consonant sequences. It may be that reduction of consonant clusters among 4-year-olds who stutter is a strong indication that their stuttering will be persistent. This would lead us to guess that the stuttering of many of Louko et al.'s subjects would prove to be chronic unless therapy was provided. It should be noted that at our children's next assessment, when they were a year older, there was no longer an unusual number in either group who demonstrated poor performance on consonant sequences.

Strategies for Consonant Clusters. Because reports by other investigators (Louko et al., 1990; Wolk et al., 1993) suggested that children who stutter may have more difficulty acquiring consonant clusters than other patterns, Sambrookes (1999) examined all of our 84 participants to observe how those who were not yet able to produce clusters dealt with this pattern at their first visit. She found, as predicted, that by far the most common strat-egy used by all children was the deletion of one of the consonants in the cluster. The mean number of times this process was used per child was not significantly different between the persistent and recovered groups. How-ever, the children who were 36 months of age or older, and should be showing some progress toward mastery of this pattern, presented a differ-ent picture. With slight weighting added for each month of age over 36 months, the difference between the mean number of times the persistent group used cluster reduction was significantly larger than that of the recovered group. This finding added to the previous evidence that the persistent group was not progressing as well as the younger recovered group in acquiring consonant clusters.

Sambrookes (1999) also observed that these groups of children were alike in that they typically deleted from each cluster the same consonant that most fluent children do, this being the more difficult (therefore later developing) of the two sounds. Thus, stridents and liquids were the sounds deleted most often, whereas nasals and stops were deleted least often, but in virtually every 6-month age group, the recovered group deleted fewer of each of these sounds than did the persistent children. The small numbers of children in these 6-month age groups made it impossible to determine whether this difference was significant.

One further difference—and an interesting one—was noted between the two groups of children in their progress toward producing clusters. A few children in both groups occasionally used less common strategies for dealing with clusters they could not yet produce. These were epenthesis (inserting a vowel between the two consonants, e.g., /bəlu/ for /blu/), coalescence (combining features from the two sounds in a cluster into a single sound, e.g., /fok/ for /smok/), and metathesis (reversing the sounds, e.g., /mæks/ for /mæsk/). Using these strategies indicates that a child is aware of the presence of the two sounds, even though he or she has not yet mastered the ability to produce the two in proper sequence. Although the number of times these strategies were used was quite small, several children in the recovered group began using them between the ages of 24 and 42 months, whereas none of the persistent group used them until between the ages of 42 and 59 months. Thus, some children in the recovered group demonstrated awareness, without production, of the two sounds of a cluster much earlier than any members of the persistent group. Research with many more children, however, would be needed to determine whether this is a common difference between the two groups.

Summary. In every way we evaluated the two groups of children at their initial visit, we found that the mean performance of the group whose stuttering would persist lagged behind that of the group whose stuttering would disappear naturally. It is important to stress that the difference was rarely due to abnormal or unusual performance by the persistent group. For both groups, acquisition of the essential phonological characteristics of the language was following a normal course. If the persistent group continued to lag phonologically, it might later become a cause for concern.

This was one of the reasons that it was important to observe how our participants progressed after the first visit.

Phonological Development After 1 Year

By the 1-year assessment, we expected both groups to show less error than at their first visit, because most of the children were still within the ages when phonological ability improves rapidly. Indeed, that was the case in each of the ways we evaluated the two groups. Had we not assessed them soon after stuttering onset, however, we would have been unable to report the extent to which they had improved and a most unexpected difference we could now see between the two groups.

Mean Percentage of Phonological Error. At a mean age of a little over 4 years, the recovered group continued to show a lower age-adjusted mean percentage of phonological error than the persistent group, whose mean age was a little over 4½ years. The difference in mean phonological error between groups was now only 3.81%, less than half as large as at the first evaluation and, importantly, no longer statistically significant. What we had not anticipated was that the persistent group's mean error would improve (decrease) by almost twice as much as would the recovered group's. The children whose stuttering would persist clearly were beginning to catch up phonologically with the group whose stuttering would later disappear without intervention. In addition, the scores within the persistent group now were not as widely spread as were those of the recovered group.

Levels of Phonological Deficiency. The two groups had also made notable improvement in the levels of severity into which their mean percentages of error were now distributed. Not surprisingly, many of the children had moved into less severe levels than at their initial visit. In fact, all of the persistent group were now in the mild and moderate levels, as were 95% of the recovered group. The only children who still remained in the severe level were about 5% of the recovered group, who were the youngest and not yet old enough to be expected to score higher. Figure 6.1 graphically compares the distributions of the two groups at their initial and 1-year assessments, and shows the extent of their improvement. The recovered group's spread is the more "normal" of the two at both of these visits. Although the persistent group shows clear progress, its distribution still does not represent what would be expected of children whose mean age is ½ year older than the other group.

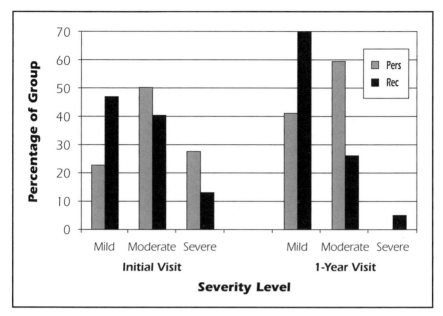

Figure 6.1. Severity levels of persistent and recovered groups. *Note.* From "Phonological Progress During the First Two Years of Stuttering," by E. P. Paden, N. G. Ambrose, and E. Yairi, 2002, *Journal of Speech, Language, and Hearing Research, 45,* p. 261. Copyright 2002 by American Speech-Language-Hearing Association. Reprinted with permission.

What cannot be seen in Figure 6.1 is that over half of the persistent group who fell in the moderate range of severity actually had mean percentages of error in the lowest one third (20%–26%) of that range, so that they were very close to being in the mild category. Thus, the improvement of the persistent group over 1 year is somewhat better than can be seen in the figure, even though they have not yet caught up with the younger group.

Differences in Pattern Acquisition. Both groups also improved on each of the 10 basic phonological patterns by the time of their second test. This improvement can be seen in Figure 6.2, where the new percentages of error (the shorter bars) are laid on top of those showing the children's initial percentages. The most obvious improvement is on the later acquired patterns, shown on the right-hand side of the figure. This would be expected because the children are a year older and many of them, especially in the persistent group, have achieved better mastery of the later acquired patterns.

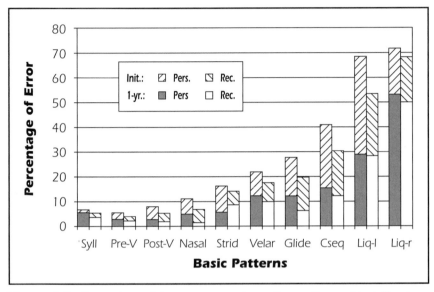

Figure 6.2. Comparison of the mean percentage of errors for persistent (Pers.) and recovered (Rec.) groups on 10 basic patterns (from left to right: syllables, prevocalic consonants, postvocalic consonants, nasals, stridents, velars, glides, consonant sequences, liquid /l/, and liquid /r/) at initial (init.) and 1-year visits. *Note.* From "Phonological Progress During the First Two Years of Stuttering," by E. P. Paden, N. G. Ambrose, and E. Yairi, 2002, *Journal of Speech, Language, and Hearing Research, 45,* p. 261. Copyright 2002 by American Speech-Language-Hearing Association. Reprinted with permission.

Many of the younger recovered group were not yet ready to acquire the liquids, for example. Even the liquid /r/ is beyond the capacities of most of the children in both groups, and the mean percentage of error for both groups is still about 50%. The recovered group still shows better average performance, however, than the persistent group on all of the patterns except stridents.

Overall, the recovered children once again present a profile on pattern acquisition that is close to what would be considered within the low normal range of phonological expectations for their age, with the persistent group noticeably catching up but still lagging somewhat on most patterns. The main question at this point seemed to be how long it would take for the older group to achieve the same level as the recovered group.

Strategies for Patterns Not Acquired. A review of the strategies the children in the two groups were now using produced the same results as when they were examined at the first visit. Both groups used the common ways of dealing with patterns they had not yet acquired (fronting for velars, deletion of one phoneme in consonant clusters, and gliding or vowelization for liquids). Unusual strategies were rare in either group.

Caution. We strongly reemphasize at this point that all of our evidence presented in this chapter so far has been for groups of children. In our exploratory study (Paden & Yairi, 1996), however, we reported a wide range of variation in percentage of phonological error among individuals, equally wide within all groups. Thus, our hope of identifying a way to predict the course of a child's stuttering solely on the basis of phonological achievement has not been fulfilled. It cannot be assumed that any 3-year-old who stutters and is obviously delayed in phonological acquisition will stutter persistently. At present, our data concerning the level of phonological ability indicate that this factor is less powerful in predicting the future course of a child's stuttering than was Van Riper's (1971) early Tracks of Development, in which his description of Track II (the only one of the four that includes "poor articulation") comes closer in accuracy of prediction.

Phonological Status at 2-Year Visit

At the time of their 2-year visit, more than half of the children were at least kindergarten age, when a normal level of phonological development can provide a highly desirable foundation for the academic challenges they are about to face in learning to read and spell. The mean age of the persistent group (5-9) and of the recovered group (5-4) now places them in the same range as the children who were studied in many of the early surveys and reports.

Because the children had now passed the years at which the most rapid phonological acquisition is usually seen, difference in age was no longer a critical factor to be considered in comparing the groups. Therefore, we looked at the true rather than age-weighted mean percentages of phonological error. It was interesting, and very surprising, that for the two groups these scores were now identical: only 7.91% mean phonological errors. The persistent group had indeed caught up with the recovered. Moreover, more than half of the children were within the "better" (lower) half of the mild level of severity of phonological impairment. Almost all of the children had mastered each of the 10 basic patterns, and the few errors some of them made were scattered ones, usually two or three errors on one or two patterns. Virtually all of these boys and girls, therefore, had the phonological ability that prepared them for formal schooling. Consequently, we were now primarily interested in analyzing the few who had *not* reached that level.

The broad criterion we used for satisfactory progress was no more than 40% error, or performance better than chance, on every pattern. Most of the children far exceeded this minimum goal. Failing to meet it were only 15 children, 3 in the persistent group and 12 in the recovered. All but 2 were 6 years old; one of them was 5, and the other was 7. Only 2 of the 15 were girls, 1 in each of the two groups. This provides more evidence not only that girls are less likely to stutter than boys, but that most girls who stutter will probably have mastered all of the basic phonological patterns by age 5.

It was especially important, however, that 14 of these 15 children were less than adequate only on liquids (/l/, /r/, or both). In that these are the last of the basic patterns expected to be acquired (/l/ and /r/ are usually mastered by 5 and 6 years of age, respectively), all 14 of these children were still progressing in the typical order of pattern emergence, as were both groups at the two earlier evaluations. If one wished to differentiate between terms, these 14 should more properly be said to be phonologically *delayed* rather than *disordered.*

The remaining child, who was in the recovered group, was the only participant who at the 2-year visit presented an unusual array of patterns acquired. Although he was almost 6 years old, he failed to meet criterion not only for both liquids, but also for velars and consonant sequences— patterns that are usually acquired before 4 years of age. Of more interest, he resorted to uncommon strategies for replacing velars, such as using /tʃ/ for /k/ (Paden, Ambrose, & Yairi, 2002). That this boy was the only one whose progress might be considered somewhat disordered, rather than simply delayed, emphasizes the normal path that virtually all of our participants were following.

Most of these 15 children were 6 years old, and although 14 of them performed with accuracy better than chance on all of the other basic patterns, all but 3 of the 15 showed 90% to 100% error on the liquids. Most speech–language pathologists probably would agree that phonological intervention should be provided for these children at this point and, in fact, 9 of them were receiving it. Although we did not offer this service within the research program, we always reported to parents after each phonological assessment whether the child's progress was within the expected range for his or her age. Children could be enrolled in such programs if their parents chose to do so. In fact, at this point we would have advised that therapy be sought for the other 6 children. (Remember that no child participated in fluency therapy.)

Because some phonological therapy had been received, our group now represents close to what would usually be seen in kindergarten children living in the many localities similar to ours. Recall that most of the early surveys for determining how many children who stutter also have articulation disorders were done at a time when articulation therapy was usually not provided by school systems before the first or even second grade; this may well account for the large numbers with articulation disorders among children who stutter reported by some of those investigators (see Nippold, 1990). At present, children with phonological problems are usually identified in preschool or before by school systems seeking to locate any children at risk in order to ready them for enrollment in kindergarten. Thus, surveys of children in school (kindergarten and up) would now probably report many fewer children who stutter and also are phonologically impaired than were found in the surveys completed in the 1950s to 1980s.

Two comments must be added about the children at their 2-year phonological assessment. First, it was interesting that 4 of the 12 children we identified in the recovered group as not having mastered all of the basic patterns were still stuttering at the time of this year's evaluation. Some might suggest that this was the reason they were behind phonologically, but recovery from stuttering had not resulted in phonological adequacy for the others. Second, the 6 who still stuttered and were also phonologically inadequate (3 in the persistent group and 3 in the recovered group) represented only 5% of our original group of 84 participants.

Observations with New Groups

By the time the series of studies just described had been completed, additional children in the University of Illinois Stuttering Research Program had finished their 2-year period of observation. It was possible to add more children and, of perhaps more importance, to make tighter restrictions on qualifications for each of the groups. For example, some children were removed because they were first evaluated more than 12 months past stuttering onset, and therefore stretched their qualification as beginning stutterers.

Table 6.4

Mean Phonological Errors (and Standard Deviations)
for the Persistent and Recovered Groups in the Original Study
(Paden, Ambrose, & Yairi, 2002) and in the New Study

	Persistent		Recovered	
Test	Original	New	Original	New
Initial	27.50 (12.6)	29.00 (12.1)	22.10 (12.9)	22.70 (12.1)
1-Year	13.99 (8.5)	14.63 (8.7)	12.08 (9.7)	10.76 (8.2)
2-Year	7.91 (6.7)	8.75 (6.9)	7.91 (8.3)	7.11 (7.8)

A few others were dropped because some question might be raised about whether they met the strict definitions of either group. Sixteen new children were added. The new persistent group consisted of 19 children, the new recovered group had 66, and the mean ages of the groups at onset differed by only about 3 months. The age ranges of the new groups at first testing were very similar (25–65 and 23–59 months for persistent and recovered, respectively), so that differences between the groups' mean phonological development could not be attributed to age differences. There were 4 girls in the new persistent group, and 20 in the new recovered group.

The mean phonological error and standard deviation at each of the 3-year tests for the groups in this new study were remarkably similar to those obtained for the original groups of participants. The difference between the mean phonological error for the two groups was never more than 1.5% at each of the three yearly evaluations (see Table 6.4). Likewise, the difference between the standard deviations was always less than 0.8%.

These results provided strong reinforcement for the conclusions drawn following the original study. In both instances, the older persistent group had a higher mean percentage of phonological error (poorer scores) when first evaluated than did the younger recovered group. A year later the persistent group had moved much faster than the recovered, so that the difference between the means of the groups was first reduced to less than 2 points, and a year later it was even smaller. Although the new means were still poorer for the persistent group, the persistent group essentially caught up to the recovered after 2 years. Still, we were reminded that the range of performance within each group was wide (see standard deviations in the table).

The course any one child's stuttering would take, therefore, could not be predicted by the amount of phonological error shown when first tested.

With the new groups, it was again possible to observe the strategies used when a basic pattern had not yet been mastered. Remember that we had examined consonant sequences in this way with the original groups. This time we looked closely at the liquid /r/ because this was the pattern on which there was apt to be the most overall improvement during the ages that we followed the children. Members of both groups almost invariably either omitted the /r/ when they were unable to articulate it accurately, or, in substituting for it, they almost always used the glide /w/. Thus, they were using the predicted natural strategy, gliding. In fact, it was almost impossible to find the use of any other strategy. Two children used the other liquid, /l/, once or twice as a substitute for /r/. In both groups, children usually progressed by reducing the number of omissions used on the previous test and substituting another consonant instead. This clearly showed progress toward their goal, especially because the substitutions demonstrated their awareness of what the phoneme should be. In other words, these children who stuttered were acquiring the phonological system of the language in exactly the same way as normally developing children. The fact that they stuttered did not alter this way of progressing.

Summary of the University of Illinois Stuttering Research Program Findings

Before the Illinois studies began, considerable evidence had been reported that children who stutter often show poorer phonological development than children who do not stutter. Our contributions to this issue result not only from knowing, when we analyzed their first performance data, what the course of their stuttering would be (persistent or transient), but also from our testing them annually over the crucial 2-year period when children's phonological development is especially rapid.

The important additions provided by the University of Illinois Stuttering Research Program to knowledge in this area are as follows:

1. Soon after onset, children who stutter indeed tend to be behind normally fluent children in phonological development.
2. Children who will eventually persist in stuttering are apt to be slower in phonological development than those who will eventually recover.

3. In spite of this delay, phonological skills alone are insufficient to predict the further course of stuttering.
4. The difference in level of phonological acquisition seen near stuttering onset between children whose stuttering will be persistent and those for whom it will be transient will probably have disappeared within 2 years.
5. The phonological delay that is associated with stuttering will be overcome much sooner than earlier research would have predicted.
6. The phonological development of children who stutter is similar in order of progression and strategies to those used by normally fluent children.

Our observations raise some questions about two current theories that seek to explain the relationship between stuttering and phonological impairment. The demands and capacity model proposed by Starkweather (1987) states that "fluency breaks down when environmental and/or self-imposed demands exceed the speaker's cognitive, linguistic, motoric and/ or emotional capacities for responding" (M. R. Adams, 1990, p. 136). The previously cited finding by Throneburg et al. (1994), later reaffirmed by Howell and Au-Yeung (1995), that, for all the groups of children they observed, about half of the words with stuttering-like disfluencies were ones with no phonological difficulty, raises doubt that these easy words would have so frequently overtaxed the children's linguistic or motoric capacities. Moreover, because the situations arranged for recording the children had been set up to be as nonstressful as possible, the demands of the situation would not seem to provide excessive challenge for most of the children's capacities. It must be remembered, of course, that other conditions besides these might challenge a child's capacities. As one example, N. E. Hall, Yamashita, and Aram (1993) observed that children whose vocabularies were not matched with adequately developed syntactic capacities exhibited high disfluency. This calls attention to the need for considering other factors in a child's current developmental status, in addition to phonological ability, that might limit that child's capacities. In the same vein, a child may have had experiences that would make some words that are not phonologically difficult extremely taxing emotionally for him or her. Likewise, situations that were considered by the experimenters to be nonstressful—and indeed *were* for most children—might cause traumatic distress for a few because of past experiences. Even allowing for the possibility of such factors, however, does not seem sufficient to account for as many as half of the disfluencies occurring on easy words by the children in both studies cited.

The Illinois study by Gregg and Yairi (2001) provides some support, as well as some contradiction, for the demands and capacity model. These researchers did find children who exhibited both poor phonology and severe stuttering, suggesting that inadequate phonological abilities may indeed have made these children unable to meet the demands for responding fluently in speaking situations. They also, however, found children who had poor phonology and mild stuttering. Thus, there was no consistent relationship between the two. Of course, these children may have had other deficiencies that were not observed within the protocol of Gregg and Yairi's study, but there were enough mismatches to raise some questions regarding the theory.

Paden and Yairi (1996) noted rather clear differences early on between *groups* of children whose stuttering would be transient or persistent. The group whose stuttering would persist showed poorer phonological development at first visit than did the group whose stuttering would later disappear, which might be interpreted as phonologic inadequacy *causing* chronic disfluency, whereas the better phonology of the recovering group resulted in only transient stuttering. These authors also stressed, however, that there were large differences in phonological ability among children in both groups, so that no certain relationship between the two disorders can be supported.

The covert repair hypothesis, proposed by Postma and Kolk (1993), suggests that adult speakers subconsciously monitor the formulation of their phonetic plan before actual utterance. If an error is detected, the utterance is subconsciously paused, and covert repairs are made prior to initiating production of a word. ("Error" was intended to include, but not be limited to, "phonemic slips.") Disfluencies, the hypothesis proposes, result from this detection and repair activity. Kolk, Conture, Postma, and Louko (1991) suggested that the covert repair hypothesis may also apply to children. Because children typically speak at a more rapid rate than adults, however, there may not be sufficient time for repairs.

Yaruss and Conture (1996) studied 3- to 6-year-old boys who stutter to investigate whether the covert repair hypothesis could account for their disfluencies. The researchers observed that when these 9 children, and also their pair group with normal phonology, produced systematic speech errors (i.e., used "natural processes") to replace the adult forms not yet acquired, they were less apt to be disfluent than when they made nonsystematic errors (omitted the sounds or used inappropriate replacements). This might be taken to mean that when a child used, for example, glides or vowels to replace liquids, and stops to replace stridents, both natural processes, he seemed to detect no error. Although both groups produced few words with nonsystematic errors (unusual processes or unnatural replacements), it is at this point that their within-word disfluencies were more apt to occur. The authors warned, however, that both their subjects and the number of within-word errors were too few to draw a positive conclusion from their findings about this apparent relationship.

Because it might be reasoned that the words most often in need of repair would be those that are phonologically most difficult for the child, studies by Throneburg et al. (1994) and Howell and Au-Yeung (1995) may also have some bearing on the covert repair hypothesis. The large proportion of non–phonologically difficult words that both of these groups of researchers found to be stuttered also seems to indicate that some rethinking of this theory is needed.

Questions That Invite
Theoretical Explanation

For decades, scholars have tried to explain why stuttering occurs. Our research may have added complexity to their task by providing evidence not only that stuttering is often accompanied by phonological delay, as has long been recognized, but also that there are two courses that phonological development may take in the presence of stuttering. This evidence causes further questions to emerge:

1. Why did our persistent group already exhibit a significantly poorer level of phonological development at the time of their first assessment, soon after stuttering onset, than did the recovered group? Is there a common genetic cause for both slow phonological development and stuttering, or did environmental factors result in this condition? This question is especially intriguing because the children in the persistent group averaged 5½ months older than the other group, and many of them were at the upper edge of the initial age range of our children (25–59 months). With this age advantage, when stuttering began, the children should have

been further along in phonological acquisition than the younger recovered group. However, when they were first assessed, the persistent group not only had a higher mean number of phonological errors, but also presented a poorer level of phonological acquisition on every one of the 10 basic patterns than did the younger recovered group.

2. Why did this slower phonological development continue for a few months in the persistent group? The children's within-group variation in mean phonological errors can, of course, be attributed to the diversity expected in young children's development in all areas, and this was equally wide in both of our groups. However, we have no explanation for the persistent group's poorer progress phonologically, compared with that of the recovered group, during the first months after stuttering onset. Obviously, the challenge of acquiring the phonological system of their language does not affect the two groups to the same extent. Why is this so?

3. Why was our persistent group then able to move faster through phonological development than the recovered group during the first year after stuttering onset? The phonological acquisition of the older children seemed to be more seriously affected by the advent of stuttering than that of those who later recovered, yet how were they able so quickly to increase their rate of development after previously being so slow, or perhaps having undergone an initial setback? We have suggested earlier in this chapter that it might be due to their being older, but are there other explanations?

Answers to these questions may require research in a previously untapped area concerning stuttering. Younger siblings of children who developed stuttering may need to be studied to observe factors that may have influenced stuttering to emerge and to become persistent.

At least two other questions result from our findings:

4. Can the larger proportion of girls, who often move faster in early speech acquisition than boys, account for the recovered group's showing fewer mean errors than the older persistent group at the initial and 1-year assessments? The percentage of girls in the recovered and persistent groups during the first two assessments was 39% and 18%, respectively, but at the time of their third assessment, only 1 girl remained in each group whom we determined required further monitoring and perhaps phonological intervention. This question requires study of a subgroup,

which we have not undertaken, but which might yield interesting information about the gender-related characteristics of stuttering.

    5. How can it be explained that some of the recovered group contin-
ued to be phonologically delayed after their stuttering had ceased? Is this
because they were more delayed at the outset, or was their progress slower
than most of the children, or were there other characteristics of subgroups that might affect the phonological progress of these children? Such
findings, as well as the wide range of phonological achievement within
each group, and the lack of a clear relationship between stuttering severity and level of phonological skills, would seem to indicate that the stuttering–phonology connection is not necessarily linear. Addressing this
question might yield interesting insights into the nature of the disorder.

Two observations were made clear on the basis of our study that might
be considered sidelights, but that have import too often ignored by researchers in this field. First, because the age at which young children are assessed makes an appreciable difference in what will be found about the
character and extent of disorders, results of investigations of young children at different ages should not be compared without keeping this fact in
mind. Second, and somewhat related, is that knowledge about speech pathology has gone through great changes in recent decades. For this reason,
surveys of the numbers of children in school who stutter that were done
even 10 and certainly 20 years ago may have produced very different findings from those that are more contemporary. As we mentioned earlier,
children typically are now receiving intervention for speech delay or disorders much earlier than they would have two or three decades ago. Consequently, in many localities the numbers of school-age children with
phonological impairments will be quite different from what was reported
in earlier decades. Therefore, surveys made, say, 20 years ago, which report
numbers quite different than our research suggests, are valuable only because of their historical importance. We hope that progress in research on
the phonological acquisition of young children close to the age of stuttering onset can be advanced even more during the next 10 or 20 years.

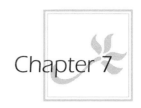

Chapter 7

Language Abilities of Young Children Who Stutter

Ruth V. Watkins

This chapter highlights key research findings from the University of Illinois Stuttering Research Program regarding language development and linguistic factors in young children who stutter. The primary goal of the chapter is to provide a summary and synthesis of the current status of knowledge regarding the interface of language and stuttering in young children, based on our empirical work. In addition, profitable areas for continued investigation of language are discussed, with the aim of stimulating research that is likely to yield better understanding of stuttering in young children and the role that language skills and linguistic variables play in the development of this disability.

Study Questions

1. *Summarize the central findings of the University of Illinois Stuttering Research Program in the area of the participants' expressive language abilities. How are these findings similar to and different from previous results? What factors might be related to divergence in research findings?*

2. *What is the evidence that linguistic variables (e.g., utterance length and complexity) influence the likelihood of stuttering.*

3. *Identify directions for future research into language and stuttering in young children that seem most promising. What research areas would you explore and what methods would you recommend?*

Case Example

The Henning family had never worried at all about their children's communication development. Their 2½-year-old son, Tommy, was incredibly talkative. Mrs. Henning noticed that Tommy used sophisticated vocabulary words, such as "bulldozer" and "curiosity," and that he tended to use very long and adultlike sentences when he talked. Tommy's child-care teacher had commented that he was one of the most "advanced talkers" in the class. Mr. and Mrs. Henning had observed that Tommy seemed to have a lot to say. As his parents, it was difficult for them to be objective, but he certainly appeared more mature in his language development than the majority of his young playmates. Then, sometime during the week after Thanksgiving, a bit before Tommy's third birthday in late January, the Hennings noticed that Tommy began stuttering. Quite suddenly, Tommy started to repeat sounds in words, as well as whole words in phrases and sentences. The Hennings also noticed that Tommy had started pausing silently at unusual times and for unusually long periods of time when he was attempting to talk. Worried, the Hennings contacted their pediatrician, who directed them to the University of Illinois Stuttering Research Program. In their initial visit to the Illinois project, the Hennings reported that their son seemed to have more to say than he was yet able to smoothly communicate, and that, in fact, "his brain seemed to be working faster and better than his mouth" could manage.

This example from the Henning family is actually a composite of a number of young children who have participated in the University of Illinois Stuttering Research Program or whose families have shared their children's stories and expressed interest in the project. Although the profile is clearly not applicable to every young child who stutters, the data summarized in this chapter suggest intriguing language strengths in many young children who stutter, particularly near the onset of the disability.

A connection between language and stuttering in young children is intuitive. As noted by Yairi (1983) and other scholars (e.g., Bernstein Ratner,

1997), stuttering onset coincides with a time of rapid expansion in expressive and receptive language ability in young children, given that stuttering most typically begins in young children between 2 and 4 years of age. Furthermore, it is in the process of using sounds to form words, and words to form phrases and sentences, that the repetitions and prolongations that characterize stuttering are observed. The apparent link between language and fluency has spawned theoretical accounts of stuttering that place emphasis on linguistic variables. For example, one working account of stuttering suggests that underlying difficulties with phonological encoding, difficulties that are self-corrected prior to actual language production but that slow language processing, yield disfluencies (Postma & Kolk, 1993). Linguistic factors are implicated in several other theoretical accounts of stuttering (Levina, 1966/1968; Perkins, Kent, & Curlee, 1991; Wingate, 1988).

Despite the intuitive appeal of connections between language and stuttering, many of the most fundamental questions in this area of inquiry continue to be debated. The language abilities of young children who stutter have been the focus of research and controversy for many years (see Yairi, Watkins, Ambrose, & Paden, 2001, and Wingate, 2001, for an example of the ongoing dialogue on this topic). Andrews et al. (1983) provided a detailed review of research in the area of stuttering. One conclusion they provided was that "stutterers performed more poorly than nonstutterers on some tests of language development" (p. 230; see also Andrews & Harris, 1964). As we discuss in this chapter, more recent work casts doubt on this early conclusion.

In addition to examinations of the language development status of young children who stutter, the connection between language and stuttering in young children has been studied in other ways, namely through evaluation of linguistic variables that appear to exert an influence on stuttering behavior. Relevant linguistic variables include grammatical complexity and location of stuttering events in the language planning or production process. In both the study of the developmental status of children who stutter and the study of linguistic influences on stuttering, there is a growing body of accumulated knowledge that speaks to the associations of language and stuttering in young children. This chapter highlights key research findings from the University of Illinois Stuttering Research Program regarding language development and linguistic factors in young children who stutter. The primary goal of the chapter is to provide a summary and synthesis of the current status of knowledge regarding the interface of language and stuttering in young children, based on our empirical work.

Language Ability and Stuttering in Young Children

The scholarly literature in the area of childhood stuttering reveals a relatively longstanding view of the child who stutters as more likely than typically developing peers to have language learning difficulties or impairments (for summaries, see Andrews et al., 1983; Bernstein Ratner, 1997). To some extent, current articles continue to propagate this view (Arndt & Healey, 2001; Wingate, 2001). Historically, standardized test measures have been used to compare the language abilities of children who stutter and those of nonstuttering peers. A number of older studies reported that children who stutter scored more poorly on a range of measures of language ability, most typically expressive language ability, than did matched, nonstuttering peers (e.g., Byrd & Cooper, 1989a; Murray & Reed, 1977). More recently, Ryan (1992) found that preschool children who stuttered scored lower than nonstuttering peers on the *Test of Language Development* (TOLD; Newcomer & Hammill, 1982), particularly on subtests that tapped expressive grammatical abilities. Anderson and Conture (2000) evaluated the language skills of preschoolers who stuttered and peers who did not stutter on several standardized measures, and reported that the children who stuttered (a) generally scored lower than nonstuttering controls and (b) displayed a greater discrepancy between receptive and expressive skills than did the nonstuttering controls. It is important to note that in these investigations the youngsters who stuttered generally performed within the average range of language abilities, but scored somewhat lower than typically developing cohorts in particular aspects of language ability. Also, although some differences in language ability were reported in selected studies (e.g., Ryan, 1992), the young children who stuttered did not differ from typically developing peers on other standardized measures of language within the same investigations (e.g., Ryan [1992] found no differences in scores on the *Peabody Picture Vocabulary Test–Revised* [Dunn & Dunn, 1981]).

Recent studies also have reported co-occurrence of language difficulties in young children who stutter. Arndt and Healey (2001), for example, asked speech–language pathologists to report whether the children they served for fluency disorders had concomitant language and/or phonological disabilities. Arndt and Healey reported that speech–language pathologists indicated that 44% of the school-age children on caseloads for fluency disabilities also had language and/or phonological limitations. There are a number of ambiguities in how speech–language pathologists may have determined or reported this co-occurrence of disability, but the 44% figure remains striking.

At the University of Illinois Stuttering Research Program, we used a different approach to evaluate the expressive language abilities of a large cohort of young children who stutter: the analysis of spontaneous language sample data (Watkins & Yairi, 1997; Watkins, Yairi, & Ambrose, 1999). As discussed in previous chapters, we prospectively tracked a group of young children who stutter, beginning as near stuttering onset as possible and continuing longitudinally for a number of years to monitor persistence in versus recovery from stuttering. To be able to contrast findings with previous investigations using standardized language measures, we obtained a global view of the language skills of our participants through analysis of performance on one standardized language test, the *Preschool Language Scale* (PLS; Zimmerman, Steiner, & Pond, 1979). Scores on both language comprehension ability, using the PLS Auditory Comprehension subtest, and expressive language skill, using the PLS Expressive Communication subtest, were calculated on all participants at the initial project visit. Table 7.1 reports basic demographic information and PLS subtest standard scores for the participants at the initial visit. As in previous chapters, participants are grouped according to later stuttering status, with recovered participants identified as those who recovered from stuttering within 36 months of onset and persistent participants identified as those who continued to stutter 48 months after stuttering onset.

As displayed in Table 7.1, the children's scores on both PLS subtests, Auditory Comprehension and Expressive Communication, were well above average at the time of entry into the study, near the onset of stuttering. Indeed, both persistent and recovered groups scored well above the test mean of 100 on both comprehension and expression components of the standardized measure. The high PLS scores of the recovered group are particularly striking. Figure 7.1 displays PLS scores over the first three visits of the project for both persistent and recovered groups. As illustrated in Figure 7.1, both persistent and recovered groups continue to score above the test mean of 100 throughout the three visits. At the third data collection visit, PLS scores for both groups have dropped to a level nearer the test

Table 7.1

Participant Performance on Standardized Language Measures
for the Persistent and Recovered Groups

| | Group | | | |
| | Persistent | | Recovered | |
Participant Information	*M*	*(SD)*	*M*	*(SD)*
N	19		70	
Age at onset	36.05	(7.93)	32.73	(6.70)
Age at initial visit	43.16	(9.52)	36.87	(7.66)
Initial visit PLS Scores				
Auditory Comprehension	114.96	(16.98)	129.37	(18.38)
Expressive Communication	110.10	(13.45)	122.78	(18.74)

Note. PLS = *Preschool Language Scale* (Zimmerman, Steiner, & Pond 1979); test *M* = 100, *SD* = 15.

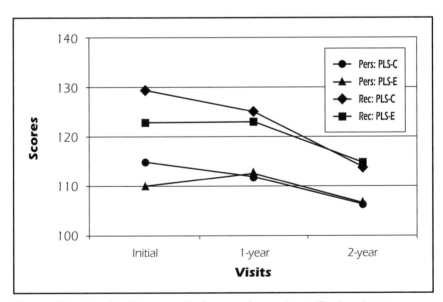

Figure 7.1. *Preschool Language Scale* scores for persistent (Pers) and recovered (Rec) groups at initial, 1-year, and 2-year visits. PLS-C = *Preschool Language Scale* Auditory Comprehension; PLS-E = *Preschool Language Scale* Expressive Communication.

average, and the scores of the recovered group are slightly higher than those of the persistent group. Although these results suggest advanced language abilities in both groups and a potential gap between persistent and recovered stutterers, the global nature of the PLS suggests only superficial information about the participants' language abilities, particularly abilities in handling the online demands of language use in context. Thus, the intriguing PLS results provided a wide-angle view from which we determined the next logical step in gaining understanding of the language skills of project participants.

In subsequent work, we shifted focus to the study of expressive language abilities through analysis of spontaneous language sample data. The availability of large (1,000-word) speech–language samples made this a particularly promising area of study. We compared the performance of young children who stutter to normative expectations on a range of language sample measures such as mean length of utterance (MLU, a general index of grammatical ability), number of different words (NDW, a general measure of vocabulary skills), and developmental sentence score (DSS, an index of grammatical skills). As a group, the children performed at or above normative expectations in their expressive language skills. More specifically, R. V. Watkins et al. (1999) reported findings from 83 preschoolers who stuttered. The children who entered the study between the ages of 2 and 3 years (i.e., exhibited stuttering onset between 2 and 3 years of age) scored about one standard deviation above normative expectations on a range of expressive language measures calculated from spontaneous samples, such as MLU and NDW. Children who entered the study between the ages of 3 and 4 years or 4 and 5 years performed at or near normative expectations. Interestingly, the children whose stuttering would ultimately persist (roughly 25% of the total sample) did not differ in expressive language skills from the children who would later recover from stuttering, when their language skills were compared near the time of stuttering onset. Figure 7.2 displays MLU for children who entered the longitudinal study at three different age groupings, relative to normative expectations. Figure 7.3 displays the mean NDW used in the language samples, again separated for children who entered the study at different ages, relative to normative expectations.

In this analysis, then, we found no evidence of pervasive expressive language difficulty in young children who stutter. On the contrary, as a group, these young children appear to be quite capable language users, based on frequently used metrics of linguistic development. The findings

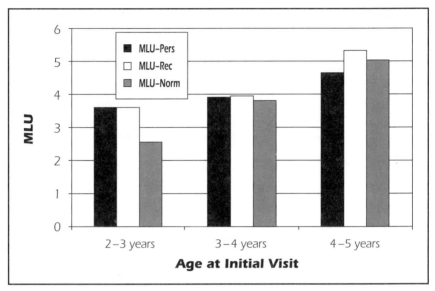

Figure 7.2. *Mean length of utterance (MLU) in persistent (Pers) and recovered (Rec) groups. Note. From "Early Childhood Stuttering III: Initial Status of Expressive Language Abilities," by R. V. Watkins, E. Yairi, and N. G. Ambrose, 1999, Journal of Speech, Language, and Hearing Research, 42, p. 1129. Copyright 1999 by American Speech-Language-Hearing Association. Reprinted with permission.*

of several other investigators lend support to these results regarding expressive language skills in young children who stutter. Over a decade ago, Nippold (1990) reported that there was no compelling evidence that children who stutter display language learning difficulties at a rate that exceeds the general population. More recently, Miles and Bernstein Ratner (2001) reported the language performance of a group of young children who stuttered on a range of expressive and receptive language measures; the children in their sample scored at or slightly above the average level of performance on every reported measure (i.e., the group scored at or above a percentile rank of 50 or at or above a standard score of 100 on the measures used). A group of German scholars (Häge, 2001; Rommel, Häge, Kalehne, & Johannsen, 2000), found that their preschool-age participants who stuttered demonstrated language skills at or above age expectations.

Thus, little empirical support can be found for a working hypothesis that language development and stuttering are linked to a common, underlying communication difficulty, at least in any significant number of young

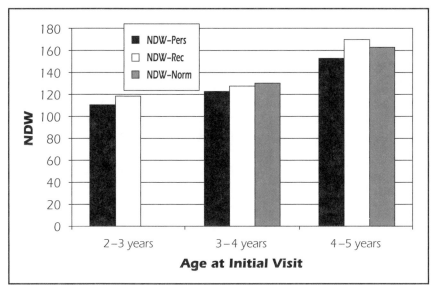

Figure 7.3. Mean number of different words (NDW) in persistent (Pers) and recovered (Rec) groups. *Note.* From "Early Childhood Stuttering III: Initial Status of Expressive Abilities," by R. V. Watkins, E. Yairi, and N. G. Ambrose, 1999, *Journal of Speech, Language, and Hearing Research, 42,* p. 1129. Copyright 1999 by American Speech-Language-Hearing Association. Reprinted with permission.

children. In closer examination of the research literature, methodological issues may account for the view that children who stutter frequently have concomitant language difficulties. Several early studies of language ability in young children who stutter did not consider socioeconomic status, potentially contrasting young children who stuttered and were from lower or middle-income backgrounds with typically developing youngsters from university-based families (see Bernstein Ratner, 1997). Furthermore, several past studies of language ability in young children who stutter did not evaluate skills in light of normative expectations (e.g., Byrd & Cooper, 1989a). Other studies have reported higher than expected rates of concomitant language disabilities in young children who stutter, but evaluated children long after stuttering onset or may have included children across very wide age ranges (e.g., Arndt & Healey, 2001). When the relationship between language ability and stuttering is examined long after stuttering onset, children may well have learned to adapt their expressive language in various ways to limit or reduce stuttering events. Although such studies are of interest, they are asking very different questions from investigations of language skills near stuttering onset. Any or all of these methodological choices would have considerable impact on findings pertaining to patterns and pathways of language acquisition in youngsters who stutter, and all could be in the direction that predicted a less favorable performance for the youngsters who stuttered in comparison to typically developing counterparts.

To better understand the expressive language abilities of young children who stutter, our next step was to longitudinally track language development in a subset of the participants from the large R. V. Watkins et al. (1999) investigation. R. V. Watkins et al. (2000) evaluated the expressive language development of 23 youngsters who stuttered over a 4-year period. Fifteen of these children recovered from stuttering within 3 years of onset; the remaining 8 children continued to stutter 4 years after onset. The 23 participants were selected from the larger study based on the following criteria: (a) the initial data collection visit was within 6 months of stuttering onset and (b) the child's age at that initial visit was less than 48 months. As in the larger R. V. Watkins et al. (1999) study, measures of expressive language were calculated, based on large (1,000-word) language samples that had been transcribed and coded using the *Systematic Analysis of Language Transcripts* (SALT; Miller & Chapman, 1997) software program. The primary measures analyzed were MLU, NDW, and number of total words used (NTW). Given that participants entered the study at somewhat different ages and were seen for follow-up visits at different ages, it was most informative to convert each participant's raw expressive language measure to a z-score, based on comparison with normative data. Calculating a z-score involves subtracting an individual's raw score from the normative mean and dividing the difference by the normative standard deviation. Thus, a z-score represents the group members' average difference in performance from the normative mean. For these analyses, the expected group average z-score is zero, if the population studied was performing at the level of normative expectations.

This longitudinal tracking revealed several noteworthy findings (see Figures 7.4 and 7.5 for results for MLU and NDW, respectively). First, this subset of youngsters displayed expressive language abilities at or above normative expectations across the 4-year period of development that was studied. This outcome was anticipated, based on the larger R. V. Watkins et al. (1999) investigation, but it is of interest that (a) the finding held for this subset of participants from the initial project and (b) expressive language skills were maintained near or above normative expectations over the

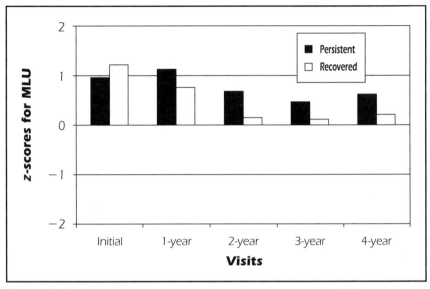

Figure 7.4. Longitudinal analysis of mean length of utterance (MLU) used by persistent and recovered groups.

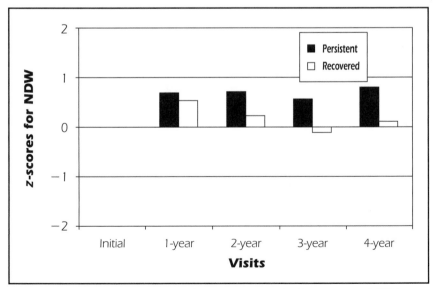

Figure 7.5. Longitudinal analysis of mean number of different words (NDW) used by children in persistent and recovered groups.

course of time and stuttering history. Second, the children in the recovered group appeared to decelerate in expressive language production over time. These youngsters did not begin to demonstrate language difficulties; they simply began to use sentences of average length, relative to developmental norms, and to use vocabulary with the level of diversity and richness that would be expected for their age. In contrast, the children whose stuttering persisted maintained somewhat higher than expected expressive language production across the time span of the study. Similar findings for children with persistent stuttering were reported by Häge (2001) in Germany.

These findings have piqued our interest regarding the extent to which the children who recover from stuttering do so about the same time that they decelerate their rate of expressive language production. If the development of stuttering involves some type of trade-off of linguistic resources (e.g., advanced language at the expense of motoric fluency), one would expect that those youngsters who recover from stuttering would do so as they slow a previously accelerated rate of expressive language development. At present, this possibility is just an intriguing hunch based on our data; findings to date do not allow full evaluation of this possibility. We are, however, pursuing this line of inquiry with a follow-up investigation. In this follow-up study, we are conducting a detailed analysis of the number and type of disfluencies produced by youngsters who recover from and who persist in stuttering, at the initial visit and at each of the subsequent four visits, in conjunction with specific expressive language skills analyses. Language and fluency patterns will be paired with information on the timing of recovery from stuttering, for those youngsters who do recover. Thus, through specific analysis of individual and group trends in both stuttering and language trajectories, we hope to better understand the nature of both language development and stuttering progression, and to gain insight into the possible link between these domains. We are approaching this analysis with the view that different subtypes of stuttering may be represented in our sample. Thus, it is important that we consider individual patterns as well as group trends.

Several summary points can be drawn from our findings in the area of children's language abilities. There is virtually no evidence that language development is vulnerable in any significant number of young children who stutter. On the contrary, there is some hint that early precocious expressive language abilities may be a risk factor for stuttering, or may simply be a by-product of some other operating risk factor. Results from the Illinois studies do suggest that continued and perhaps more detailed study of language strengths and challenges in conjunction with stuttering and other domains may be informative in revealing influential developmental asynchronies (e.g., perhaps accelerated language development in one domain, such as syntax or semantics, creates difficulties with fluency when proficiencies in other domains, such as motoric abilities, are less sophisticated). It appears that more complete understanding of the progression of stuttering in young children will require simultaneous consideration of multiple developmental domains, and an awareness that there may be varied pathways in the development of this disability (i.e., subtypes of stuttering, even in very young children). At present, our data do not support construction of a model of stuttering or explication of the relative role that language abilities would play in such a model. Our data do, however, reveal that (a) it is important to include language development in investigations of young children who stutter and (b) it will be crucial to consider the role that advanced expressive language abilities may play in early stuttering.

Linguistic Influences on Stuttering in Young Children

Beyond study of language development in children who stutter, there is ample evidence that stuttering events are influenced by linguistic variables. S. Brown (1945) was perhaps the first scholar to suggest linguistic influences on stuttering events with his groundbreaking report of apparent influences of a word's grammatical form class (i.e., content vs. function word) on stuttering loci in adults who stuttered. In brief, Brown found that adults who stuttered were significantly more likely to be disfluent on content words (e.g., nouns and verbs) than on function words (e.g., prepositions and pronouns).

Since S. Brown's (1945) seminal work, scholars have continually refined analyses in the study of linguistic influences on stuttering. Researchers have found, for example, that young children are generally more likely to stutter in sentences with greater degrees of grammatical complexity than in sentences with less grammatical complexity (Logan & Conture, 1995; Yaruss, 1999). Furthermore, several studies have revealed that the content–function variable is not the most relevant influence on stuttering loci. Instead, stuttering events are significantly more likely on either a content word or a phrase-initial function word that precedes a content word than in other phrasal locations (Au-Yeung, Howell, & Pilgrim, 1998; Howell, Au-Yeung,

& Sackin, 1999). The underlying influence is thought to be the planning unit in language formulation, such that disfluencies are significantly more likely to occur at the beginning of a language planning unit, when remaining components of the unit continue to be refined for production.

We have tentatively explored linguistic influences on young children's stuttering behavior in two investigations. B. Johnson, Humphreys, Watkins, Ambrose, and Yairi (2001) examined the influence that word frequency exerts on the likelihood of stuttering, based on analysis of the language samples gathered from young children near the onset of stuttering. A broad base of psycholinguistic research has revealed that word frequency has wide-spread effects on language production, including the findings that (a) frequent words are read more quickly than infrequent words and (b) speech errors are more likely on infrequent than frequent words (see Dell, 1990, for examples). Johnson et al. hypothesized that low-frequency words would more likely be stuttered than high-frequency words. To evaluate this prediction, they analyzed 1,000-word spontaneous language samples from the same subset of 23 young children who stuttered (15 who recovered within 36 months of onset, and 8 who continued to stutter 48 or more months after onset) as in the R. V. Watkins et al. (2000) longitudinal study described previously.

B. Johnson et al. (2001) found a complex relationship between word frequency and stuttering. When all words were included, the relationship between word frequency and stuttering was not significant. In contrast, when the corpus was limited to those words ever stuttered, the relationship between frequency and stuttering was significant, such that low-frequency words were stuttered significantly more often than high-frequency words. Johnson et al. interpreted this finding as general support for difficulties with phonological encoding posed by low-frequency words. In brief, once a word is stuttered, it becomes more likely that it will again be stuttered, particularly for low-frequency words. A single instance of disruption in phonological encoding for a low-frequency word is influential, whereas an instance of disruption for a high-frequency word is less influential, given the proportion of correct, fluent formulations of that word. This description of the frequency effect does not, however, provide an explanation for the factors that influence the initial likelihood of a stuttering event; future work will need to address this issue. Also, it is important to note that the influence of word frequency on stuttering held for both the persistent and the recovered groups. That is, the phonological encoding difficulty proposed to account for greater stuttering on low-frequency words was found in children whose stuttering would abate, as well as for those whose stuttering would persist.

A second investigation is currently under way. In this project, we are replicating the phrase-level analysis of stuttering loci implemented by Howell and his colleagues (Au-Yeung et al., 1998; Howell et al., 1999) with our population of young children who stutter, again using language samples gathered shortly after the onset of stuttering. The majority of previous investigations of stuttering loci have included very small numbers of children distributed across broad age ranges. We are particularly interested in whether a phrase-level analysis of stuttering loci will reveal the same trends found by Howell and his colleagues, in light of the fact that our population is younger and greater in number than those of previous studies. In addition, we are interested in whether we will find shifts, across developmental time, in stuttering loci for children as they progress from preschool to school age.

The preliminary findings of our own work, in combination with that of other scholars, reveal that aspects of language planning, formulation, and production exert an influence on stuttering for children and adults. These findings support the view that linguistic variables are relevant in characterizing stuttering events. It is noteworthy, however, that linguistic factors appear to influence disfluencies in a parallel way for stutterers and nonstutterers alike. That is, linguistic variables, such as grammatical complexity and the loci of stuttering, tend to influence individuals whose disfluencies occur at typical rates in language production, as well as individuals whose disfluencies are frequent enough that they are identified as stutterers. This working conclusion suggests that language formulation variables are likely to be more informative about the nature of language formulation and production, in general, than about stuttering, in particular.

Summary: Clinical Implications and Future Research

The domain of language is relevant in the study of early childhood stuttering. The empirical studies of the University of Illinois Stuttering Research Program have revealed that both persistent and recovered groups of young children who stutter display expressive language abilities at or above normative expectations, based on both standardized test data and analysis of spontaneous language samples. Analysis of patterns of recovery and persistence, in conjunction with language skills, are under way and are likely to be particularly informative. In addition, our own investigations reveal that linguistic variables, including word frequency and the position of words within phrasal units, exert an influence on the likelihood of a stuttering event. The influence of these linguistic variables is complex, and additional investigation is warranted to better delineate relevant influences.

Clinical Implications

From a clinical perspective, our findings regarding language abilities in young children who stutter do not yield clear guidance. Specifically, given that our data suggest that many young children who stutter have average or above average expressive language skills and that, as children recover from stuttering, their expressive language appears to reduce toward average, how would we advise parents like the Hennings, as introduced at the beginning of this chapter? We believe that our research agenda has not yet progressed sufficiently to offer absolute clinical implications in the area of language. However, there are several recommendations in the literature that we do not support. For example, Starkweather (1997) suggested that at least some young children who stutter may do so as a result of "language overstimulation" (p. 270), presumably meaning language input that is rich, complex, and frequent and that promotes children's language learning. On a related point, other scholars have recommended that adults simplify their language input in interactions with their young children who stutter. These recommendations seem flawed on several fronts. First, withholding language input or complexity from any child during the preschool years is a questionable practice; these years are crucial for full development of rich vocabulary that promotes later reading and academic achievement. Second, our own investigations suggest that children whose expressive language skills are at or above average levels ultimately develop as either recovered or persistent stutterers for reasons that, at least in our present analyses, seem to have little to do with language (see Chapter 9 for discussions of genetic contributions to stuttering). Instead, changes in expressive language production seem to be influenced by factors external to the language system, and the linguistic behavior we observe is merely a reflection of other developmental rearrangements. At present, then, the potential negative contributions of limiting or artificially manipulating language input to preschool-age children seem to far outweigh any possible positive influences. Clearly, more work is needed to better answer the clinical issues raised by the Henning family, as illustrated at the beginning of this chapter.

Future Research Directions

In terms of advancing our overall understanding of stuttering in young children, particularly the likelihood of whether a youngster who begins stuttering is likely to continue to stutter for a significant period of his or her life, several points are particularly relevant. First, to fully understand the nature and pathway of stuttering in young children, scholars need to use methods and measures that allow integration of findings of developmental strengths and limitations across varied developmental domains. Findings from the University of Illinois Stuttering Research Program suggest the possibility of linguistic strengths in the face of speech production challenges in many young children who stutter. Clearly, language ability alone cannot fully inform prediction of stuttering persistence or recovery; rather, it appears that language ability is just one component of an intricate puzzle. To date, most investigations have examined single puzzle pieces in isolation. Until findings are integrated across developmental domains, in the same children, our view of the puzzle will remain incomplete.

Second, future investigations need to look at old problems in new and complex ways. Considering language ability, for example, one of the most intriguing leads we have uncovered is the one expressed by the Henning family at the beginning of this chapter: Many young children who begin stuttering seem to have language abilities that exceed their capabilities for fluent production of speech. This idea has been circulating in clinical anecdotes for many years. Now, we have provided initial empirical validation of the concept. It is important that scholars develop creative methods to track this lead. The working hypothesis that sophistication in one developmental area, such as language, is gained at the expense of facility in another developmental area (e.g., motor control) must be fully and carefully evaluated. To be most meaningful and informative, the full range of potentially relevant areas (e.g., personality and temperament factors, genetic influences) must also be included in these analyses. It seems that the most promising future investigations for shedding light on language and stuttering in young children will move toward detailed and specific analyses of profiles of language strength, in parallel with evaluation of synchrony versus asynchrony both within and across multiple developmental domains.

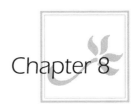

Chapter 8

Motor, Psychosocial, and Cognitive Aspects

Considerable study has been done of the involvement of motor, psychosocial, and cognitive skills in stuttering. Vocal fold function, speaking rate, and formant transition are some of the many aspects of speech motor functioning that have been investigated. Previous studies have shown mixed results, but overall pointed toward some aberrancies in all of these areas. The University of Illinois Stuttering Research Program studies indicated higher shimmer values, slower speaking rate in phones per second, and less frequency alteration in second formant transitions. In the psychosocial domain, our research into parent and child perceptions regarding anxiety and stress revealed higher levels for some children with persistent stuttering as opposed to those who recover, but few differences in the parents. Also, with regard to cognitive skills, children with persistent stuttering scored within normal range, but slightly lower than control or recovered children, on a measure of nonverbal intelligence. Awareness of stuttering has long been thought to be absent in young children who stutter, although a few studies have continued to report early awareness. Our work has shown that, for those children who continue to stutter, awareness enters the picture consistently after stuttering has continued for about 2 years, but some children give strong indications of awareness very early on. The interaction between stuttering and motor, psychosocial, and cognitive realms must be taken into account when planning evaluation and treatment, as well as research strategies.

Study Questions

1. *What have past and present studies shown about the motor control system in people who stutter? Briefly summarize.*
2. *Is there a consistent relationship between stress, anxiety levels and stuttering for both children who stutter and their parents? Discuss.*
3. *What role did awareness of disfluency play in the traditional view of onset and development of stuttering, and how has that idea changed?*
4. *How could knowledge of motor, psychosocial, and cognitive factors shape therapeutic strategies for children who stutter?*

he field of stuttering is rather uncommon in that it encompasses
myriad domains. When we work with people who stutter, we are
concerned not only about their speech, but also with their awareness of and reactions to their stuttering. And when we study stuttering, we
have found differences between people who stutter and those who are normally fluent in all of these areas. The overt disfluencies and secondary symptoms are the core of what we identify as stuttering, and clinicians can work
with these behaviorally. However, understanding what may underlie the
disfluencies, whether it be a direct cause or an additional factor, can help
speech–language clinicians and clients understand how and why treatment strategies work, as well as allow more specifically targeted treatment
strategies. For some who stutter, a program focusing on psychosocial concerns may be most productive, whereas others may benefit from treatment
with a strong motor component. Many, however, seem to benefit, or even
require, treatment that encompasses several or all aspects of the disorder.

There is a voluminous body of literature addressing motor speech, psychological constitution and reaction, and social concerns of people who
stutter, as well as parents of children who stutter. Past research also has
studied their intellectual abilities (IQ levels) and central processing. Cognition plays a role in the development of awareness of stuttering, as well
as in perceptions and abstractions that contribute to the development of
the disorder. The University of Illinois Stuttering Research Program has
addressed, to some degree, motor, psychosocial, and cognitive aspects of
stuttering.

Motor Speech

Regardless of its etiology, stuttering manifests itself as a breakdown in
speech motor control. The past 70 years of research in stuttering have been
replete with studies of the kinematic, electromyographic, and acoustic
characteristics of people who stutter and those associated specifically with
their disfluent and fluent speech. Dependent measures have included temporal parameters of speech, phonatory and respiratory aspects of speech
production, spatial dimensions of articulation, reaction time, and activation and tension of various oral, laryngeal, and nonspeech muscle groups.
The equivocal, sometimes conflicting, findings have been attributed to
either methodological differences, insensitive instrumentation, the wide

range of idiosyncratic motor processes used to produce both fluent and stuttered speech, and possible population heterogeneity (McClean, 1997). Furthermore, the great majority of studies have examined adults who stutter. When relevant research with adults is examined, on balance it would appear to suggest that the speech production processes of those who stutter are somewhat different from those of normally fluent individuals (Kent, 2000). Such a conclusion, however, is less likely to be reached in regard to young children who stutter. Past investigations, including those that examined spatial and temporal dimensions of young children's speech production, have concluded that if differences exist between stuttering and non-stuttering children, they are subtle (see review by Conture, 1991). Mostly, differences were observable in comparisons of temporal relationships between and among related events rather than for singular speech variables (Zebrowski, Conture, & Cudahy, 1985). One conclusion is that young children who stutter, as a group, do not exhibit pervasive deficits in speech motor function, but instead may exhibit different thresholds for perturbation. Stuttering occurs as a result of combined influences of increases in such factors as utterance rate and linguistic complexity, as well as communicative demand or pressure.

All of the information presented in Chapter 4 pertained to various analyses of disfluent speech of the child who stutters and normally fluent peers. It is, of course, quite apparent that much of the disfluent speech of the stuttering child is abnormal. This is why listeners perceive and react to it as "stuttering." It is the performance of stutterers when they speak *fluently*, however, that researchers have explored for evidence of possible underlying motor speech involvement. Such a focus is particularly valuable in helping us understand whether disturbances in the speech production system that are obvious during stuttering might be related to a generalized temporal discoordination between respiration, phonation, and articulation that affects all of the speaker's speech.

As stated previously, past research on the motor aspects of young children who stutter yielded few or no positive findings. Nevertheless, different opinions have been expressed. G. D. Riley and Riley (1985, 1999), for example, developed Speech Motor Training, a therapy program for preschool-age children who stutter, which was motivated by the assumption that these children suffer from reduced integration of the speech motor system. The University of Illinois Stuttering Research Program has made only a few contributions in this direction, which are summarized briefly in this chapter.

Vocal Fold Function

Several acoustic parameters, including fundamental frequency, jitter (cycle-to-cycle perturbation in fundamental frequency), and shimmer (cycle-to-cycle amplitude perturbation), have been traditionally used to make indirect evaluation of the underlying physiological functioning of the vocal mechanisms. Early studies by Bryngelson (1932) and Schilling and Goler (1961) reported reduced pitch range in adults who stutter. In the past 25 years, a good number of studies have examined the laryngeal dynamics of people who stutter, primarily adults, during both disfluent and fluent speech segments. Falck, Lawler, and Yonovitz (1985) and Sacco and Metz (1989) argued that adults who stutter exhibit greater fundamental frequency instability than those with normal fluency. One of the few studies investigating laryngeal behavior of young stuttering children's fluency (Conture, Rothenberg, & Molitor, 1986) used electroglottography to examine vocal fold movement patterns. The researchers reported small differences between children who stutter (mean age 4 years 7 months [4-7]) and their normally fluent controls in the amount of atypical laryngeal abduction. On the other hand, Conture, Colton, and Gleason (1988) failed to detect temporal asynchrony among respiratory, laryngeal, and articulatory functions in young stutterers (mean age 4-1) during repetition of a carrier phrase. Previous research in stuttering children, however, has not documented the acoustic measure of jitter or shimmer in fluent speech of young children close to stuttering onset, although these acoustic parameters have been used extensively to document developmental changes in normal speech (e.g., Glaze, Bless, Milenkovic, & Susser, 1988). It has been suggested that the decrease in the voice fundamental frequency, jitter, and shimmer observed in children between 1 and 3 years of age is related to their physical, linguistic, and cortical maturation, which results in greater control. In view of the rapidly expanding phonatory motor control in normally fluent children, data on acoustic measures that reflect the physiology of laryngeal function in children who stutter may shed more light on the disorder in the context of the developmental process of the speech system and speech motor control.

Our first study of fluent speech (K. D. Hall & Yairi, 1992) examined acoustic correlates of phonatory control in 10 preschool-age boys who had stuttered for less than 1 year and exhibited at least moderate severity of stuttering, and 10 normally fluent boys matched in age. For each child, 30 fluent utterances consisting of vowels and diphthongs in CV, VC, CVC, and

Table 8.1

Group Means (and Standard Deviations) for Fundamental
Frequency (F_0), F_0 Range, Jitter, and Shimmer Values

Group	F_0 (Hz)		F_0 Range (Hz)		Jitter (msec)		Shimmer (%)	
Experimental	278	(27)	236	(66)	.044	(.019)	6.61	(0.78)
Control	309	(35)	274	(130)	.031	(.019)	4.52	(1.25)

Note. Adapted from "Fundamental Frequency, Jitter, and Shimmer in Preschoolers Who Stutter,"
by K. D. Hall and E. Yairi, 1992, *Journal of Speech, Language, and Hearing Research, 35,* p. 1006.
Copyright 1999 by American Speech-Language-Hearing Association. Adapted with permission.

CCVC word shapes identified in recorded conversational speech were
selected for acoustic analysis using the Cspeech computer program
(Milenkovic, 1987). The program provided data for the fundamental frequency of the vocal folds, jitter, and shimmer. The mean value for each of
the three parameters is presented in Table 8.1 for the experimental and control groups. Unlike fundamental frequency, the jitter and shimmer values
were higher for the experimental group than for the control group. The statistical analysis, however, showed that only in the shimmer measure were
the groups' means significantly different. When a single outlier subject was
eliminated from each group, the difference in fundamental frequency also
became statistically significant, with the stutterers having a lower mean
value. Although the specific neuromuscular components of shimmer have
not been identified, compared with jitter, shimmer may reflect greater
difficulty with integrating respiratory, laryngeal, and cortical control. In
our opinion, these findings, suggesting the possibility of a slight instability
in laryngeal control in early stuttering, deserve additional research.

Speaking Rate

Our interest in uncovering factors that differentiate between those children who eventually recovered from and those who became persistent in
stuttering also has directed us to research the speed of their speech, or
speaking rate. Such knowledge may enrich our means of early prediction
of the course of stuttering. Both clinical interests and theoretical motivations in exploring stuttering as a disorder of speech motor control have led

to numerous investigations of speaking rate in people who stutter (see summary by K. D. Hall, Amir, & Yairi, 1999). Most have been conducted with adults and school-age groups, and studies of preschoolers were often clouded by inclusion of older children. No research has been conducted to answer questions about the possible developmental link between stuttering and the rate of speech, or about differences in speech rate development between preschool children who stutter and normally fluent children. The purpose of our team (K. D. Hall et al., 1999) was specifically to compare changes of what is known as articulatory rate, over time, of three groups: children who stuttered and later recovered without intervention (recovered group), children who stuttered and later became chronic stutterers (persistent group), and normally fluent controls. By articulatory rate, we refer to the number of speech units (e.g., syllables or phones) uttered per second, after excluding pauses and disfluent segments from the speech sample (i.e., only in fluent speech).

For our purposes, spontaneous speech samples were collected longitudinally over a 2-year period and analyzed acoustically, using the Cspeech computer program (Milenkovic, 1987), to determine the speaking rate at the initial visit, 1 year later, and 2 years later. As can be seen in Table 8.2, there were systematic differences among the groups when the phone metric was applied, with the recovered group tending to be the slowest talkers and the normally fluent (control) group always the fastest. Statistical tests showed significant differences among groups. Very close to stuttering onset, children who stutter tended to exhibit a somewhat slower articulatory rate

Table 8.2

Means (and Standard Deviations) of Articulation Rate
(phones per second) at the Initial Visit, 1-Year Visit,
and 2-Year Visit for Children Who Stutter and a Control Group

Visit	Recovered	Persistent	Control
Initial visit	7.68 (1.08)	9.56 (1.25)	11.42 (2.77)
1-year visit	9.78 (0.62)	9.66 (1.16)	12.17 (2.10)
2-year visit	9.38 (0.98)	10.22 (1.50)	11.88 (1.86)

Note. Adapted from "A Longitudinal Investigation of Speaking Rate in Preschool Children Who Stutter," by K. D. Hall, O. Amir, and E. Yairi, 1999, *Journal of Speech, Language, and Hearing Research, 42,* p. 1372. Copyright 1999 by American Speech-Language-Hearing Association. Adapted with permission.

than their normally fluent peers. The recovered children spoke significantly slower than the control group at all three visits but not statistically significantly slower than the persistent group. The persistent children spoke significantly slower than the control group only at the 1-year visit. All three groups demonstrated a significant increase in articulatory (phone) rates from the 1-year visit to the 2-year visit.

These findings are in harmony with theories that emphasize slower motor execution (Van Riper, 1982) as a contributing factor in early stuttering. They are also consistent with theories relating stuttering to slower central processing, which is then reflected in motor speech execution as slower speed of the articulators (Karniol, 1995; Postma & Kolk, 1993).

On the other hand, even though at the initial visit there was a tendency for children who later recovered to articulate speech at a slower rate than those whose stuttering persisted, the lack of a statistically significant difference prohibits the conclusion that articulatory rate can be used as a clinical prognostic indicator for the developmental paths of stuttering. Nevertheless, such a tendency should not be presently abandoned, especially in light of the very conservative statistics used. Further research is warranted. If this tendency reappears in future research, it could be hypothesized that oral motor or central planning deficiencies responsible for stuttering also contribute to the slowing of speech. As these deficiencies subside, both the fluency and articulatory rate improve. Alternatively, it might be hypothesized that the children who eventually recovered employed a strategy of slowing down their articulatory rate to cope with their stuttering.

Formant Transition

Another study of ours dealt with the dynamics of formants in the speech signal, particularly second formant (F2) transition. Although past literature did not provide a clear rationale for selecting F2 as a candidate predictor of the developmental patterns in stuttering, adults who stutter have been reported to exhibit appreciable aberrations in this formant (Harrington, 1987; Howell & Vause, 1986; Robb & Blomgren, 1997). Because variations in formant structure along the temporal and frequency domains reflect articulatory dynamics, such a line of exploration expresses the belief that stuttering involves difficulties with executing complex articulatory movements or maintaining spatial organization of the articulators (Kent, 1984).

Previous investigations that explored the usefulness of F2 transition in predicting persistent and recovered stuttering yielded contradictory results.

Stromsta (1965), the pioneer in this area, classified spectrograms of young children who stutter into those that display formant transitions and normal termination of phonation, and those that display lack of formant transitions and/or abnormal termination of phonation. Ten years later, parents' classifications of the children as either "stuttering" or "not stuttering" were checked against the initial spectrographic information. The great majority of children with F2 aberrations were those who later became persistent, whereas children exhibiting normal formant transitions later recovered. More recently, Yaruss and Conture (1993) studied F2 transitions in children classified as being at either high or low risk for developing persistent stuttering. Classification was based on the *Stuttering Prediction Instrument for Young Children* (G. D. Riley, 1981). The investigators concluded that the presence of abnormal F2 transitions during sound or syllable repetitions was not sufficient to differentiate the two groups.

In our opinion, however, methodological problems with the two studies invite additional research with children early in the course of stuttering, using adequate verification of their eventual stuttering status. Unlike the previous studies, which analyzed F2 in disfluent segments, our team (Subramanian, Yairi, & Amir, 2003) examined F2 transitions in the *fluent* speech of preschool children recorded soon after stuttering onset, long before they were distinguishable as persistent and recovered. More important, because the children were followed longitudinally, we were certain about their eventual status. Comparisons were made among 10 children who later persisted in stuttering, 10 who recovered, and 10 nonstuttering controls. All fluently repeated a standard set of sentences that contained CV target syllables (e.g., "She is peeking again"). The change in F2 frequency from onset to the offset of its transition from the consonant into the following vowel was measured, as was the time elapsed between these two points. The data showed that children who eventually persisted had significantly smaller frequency shifts than the recovered group. During the transition, the F2 frequency changed by 396 Hz for the persistent children, compared with 584 Hz for the recovered children and 502 Hz for the controls. A possible interpretation of the findings is that articulatory movements, reflected in the F2 transitions, are more restricted for children who later persisted in stuttering. Perhaps these children exhibit some problems in the fine coordination required for the control of normal speech production. The differences in the duration of the transition were not significant. The average transition lasted 59 msec for the persistent group, compared with 59 msec and 66 msec for the recovered and control groups, respectively. The relatively small number of children in this study and the great variability that they exhibited did not allow for strong conclusions. Nevertheless, in view of the few positive findings, we suggest that the F2 transitions should continue to be investigated as a possible predictor of stuttering pathways.

The encouragement to further pursue the motor domain in early childhood is supported by the work of other investigators who focused on kinematics. For example, Zebrowski, Moon, and Robin (1997) reported that children who stutter, compared with their nonstuttering peers, performed more poorly using their jaws to track sinusoidal frequencies and other signals. Sim (1996) experimented with a strain-gauge to transduce jaw and lower lip movements associated with speech of children who stutter. The kinematic measure differentiated the children's fluent speech prior to stuttering events as compared to their fluent speech at other times. Overall, it appears to us that the findings suggest a reasonable future research avenue for differences among subgroups or subtypes of stuttering.

Psychosocial Aspects

Exploration of genetic and physiological bases of stuttering and measurements of brain activation are rapidly growing research frontiers. Psychosocial factors have always been considered important, especially from the days of Freudian interpretations and behaviorism to the present. No one would contest the role of anxiety, family environment, personality, social pressures, and communication attitudes as critical in the development and maintenance of stuttering and the many behaviors surrounding it, especially in older children and adults. A number of current theoretical models assert that children's temperaments and self-perceptions, as well as parents' personalities, perceptions of their children, and child-raising practices, influence the developmental course of stuttering (e.g., Perkins, Kent, & Curlee, 1991; G. D. Riley & Riley, 2000; A. Smith & Kelly, 1995, 1997).

Furthermore, previous research has found heightened sensitivity, negative communication attitudes, and lower social competence in adolescents and adults who stutter (e.g., I. M. Blood, Wertz, Blood, Bennett, & Simpson, 1997; Janssen & Kraaimaat, 1980). School-age children who stutter, compared to normally fluent peers, have more negative attitudes about communication, and these attitudes become increasingly negative with age (DeNil & Brutten, 1990, 1991; Vanryckeghem & Brutten, 1997; Vanryckeghem,

Hylebos, Brutten, & Peleman, 2001). In addition, parents' perceptions of the social and communicative skills of their school-age children who stutter are even more negative than their children's self-perceptions (Vanryckeghem & Brutten, 1997). School-age children who stutter are perceived by their mothers as being more sensitive, more susceptible to stress, and more behaviorally inhibited than their nonstuttering peers (Glasner, 1949; Oyler & Ramig, 1995). Parents of children who stutter have been shown to be anxious and overprotective of their children and to raise them in environments that are less harmonious and more socially withdrawn than those observed in the families of nonstuttering children (see Yairi, 1997a).

There is similar preliminary evidence with regard to preschoolers who stutter. Conture (2001) reported that, compared with mothers of nonstutterers, mothers of preschool children who stutter perceive their children as more sensitive and inhibited. Vanryckeghem and Brutten (2002) also have presented preliminary data showing more negative attitudes about speaking among preschoolers who stutter.

Based on these various findings, investigators have hypothesized that children who stutter may be born with sensitive temperaments that persist over time and are heightened by the experience of chronic stuttering and by others' reactions to it (e.g., Conture, 2001; Guitar, 1998). It is difficult to discern whether these perceived characteristics of children who stutter and their parents are related to inherent temperament and personality differences, are a consequence of stuttering, or are a result of a combination of these influences. Exploration of such factors in young children just beginning to stutter, through their first years of stuttering, can shed light on this chicken-and-egg question. As part of the Illinois studies, we have investigated certain aspects of children's and parents' perceptions and behavior.

Parent Perceptions

Parent perceptions of their children's behavior were tapped both during the parent interview and in two formal questionnaires. This combination provided a more complete picture than would either method by itself.

Parent Interview

During the initial evaluation, parents were asked if, in their opinion, their child had any behavior problems, such as eating or sleeping difficulties, excessive crying or tantrums, unusual fears, shyness (enough to cause concern), excessive activity level, withdrawn behavior, and others. At the time of onset, 67% of the parents reported no behavior problems, 20% reported possible behavior problems, and only 13% indicated that their child clearly exhibited some types of behavior problems. Generally speaking, according to the great majority of parents, their stuttering children were not different in these behaviors from any ordinary group of children. Comparing parent reports of behavior for children who eventually persisted versus those who recovered, the spread is only slightly different; this is interesting in light of the fact that the reports were obtained shortly after the children began to stutter, long before they were determined to be persistent or recovered. Inborn temperament differences certainly may exist but, if so, were not seen to be reflected in the report of children's behavior, as a group. The presence of behavior problems in some children, however, may complicate an existing stuttering disorder.

Parents also reported their children's energy and maturity levels. At the time of stuttering onset, 70% of the children were described as having typical energy levels. None were thought to exhibit below average energy, and 30% were described as having higher than average levels. A comparison of persistent and recovered children yielded very little difference. The distribution of maturity levels among the children was skewed toward the higher end, with 5% below average, 69% average, and 26% above average maturity. Here, persistent and recovered children differed to some extent, although differences were not statistically significant ($p = .19$). For both groups, a majority were judged to have average maturity levels, but 14% of the persistent children were described as possessing less than average maturity, whereas only 4% of the recovered children were so judged. Overall, however, behavior problems, energy levels, and maturity levels of stuttering children close to onset did not appear remarkable in any way.

Parenting Stress Index

Parents were asked to complete the *Parenting Stress Index* (PSI; Abidin, 1986). Both mothers and fathers were asked to fill out forms independently. The PSI examines parents' attitudes and expectations with regard to their child. Scores for fathers and mothers of persistent and recovered children (status not yet determined for either group when the questionnaire was completed) and of control children fell well within the normal limits of the index (182–260), as can be seen in Table 8.3. Scores of mothers and fathers, or of parents of persistent, recovered, and control children, did not differ

Table 8.3

Mean Scores (and Standard Deviations) for *Parent Stress Index* (PSI) (raw scores) and *Walker Problem Behavior Identification Checklist* (*T*-scaled scores)

	PSI		Walker	
Group	Mothers	Fathers	Mothers	Fathers
Persistent	211.29 (39.77)	218.13 (24.32)	52.73 (10.34)	49.71 (7.81)
Recovered	211.39 (31.81)	213.19 (33.42)	53.67 (10.87)	51.75 (9.73)
Control	212.52 (34.04)	213.76 (36.86).	51.44 (7.49)	49.98 (9.19)

from one another. A small percentage of parents in all groups obtained scores above and below normal limits. As a whole, then, this measure did not distinguish any group of parents from norms or from each other.

Because stuttering runs in families, it is not unusual for a child who stutters to have a parent (most often the father) who stutters. The family environment for such a family may differ distinctly from that of a family with normally fluent parents. This important aspect of environment has frequently been ignored in stuttering research (Yairi, 1997a). In our sample of parents who completed the PSI, 14 fathers and 4 mothers stuttered. There were no cases in which both parents in a family actively stuttered. Looking at families in which either a father stutters, or a mother stutters, or neither parent stutters, scores were not significantly different. The highest (more stress) mean score was obtained for mothers in families where the father stutters; the second highest mean was obtained for fathers who themselves stutter.

Walker Problem Behavior Identification Checklist

Parents also completed the *Walker Problem Behavior Identification Checklist* (Walker, 1983); as with the PSI, both mothers and fathers were asked to fill out forms independently. This checklist assesses parents' perceptions of their child's potential behavior problems. It can indicate two things: (a) presence of behavior problems co-occurring with stuttering and (b) stress levels of parents who must cope with the perceived behaviors. Table 8.3 presents mean *T*-scaled scores ($M = 50$, $SD = 10$) for parents of persistent, recovered, and control children. All means and standard deviations are remarkably close to norms. We note, however, that the instrument contains some technical and outdated wording, and may therefore be unreliable. Additionally, it may be too gross a measure to detect possible differences, should they exist.

Child Perceptions

Previous literature, as well as common observation, has shown that people who stutter tend to have more negative attitudes and higher than average anxiety about their verbal communication skills, as discussed earlier in this chapter. For children of preschool age, it is not an easy task to discover their perceptions of themselves and their attitudes and feelings. A few children readily offer overt statements; others do not indicate whether they have such abstract constructs. Unfortunately for research, parent perceptions of their child's perceptions may not be accurate. By school age, most children can readily self-report and answer questions related to their self-perceptions and anxiety levels.

A primary question is, When does anxiety relating to communication develop? Does it evolve naturally out of reactions to stuttering? Or could it be part of a young child's temperament that is already established before stuttering begins? If the latter were the case, then children with higher anxiety levels would be expected to react more strongly toward their stuttering and their general communicative abilities. Most researchers would agree that a combination of the two, inherent personality traits and reactions to stuttering, shapes the perceptions of a person who stutters. The ability to adequately measure what anxiety-related traits a child has as he or she begins to stutter would be most beneficial in designing treatment to prevent loss of confidence, or increasing anxiety, as the child grows. It is possible that children who recover early and naturally from stuttering may be more outgoing, assertive, and self-confident, less apt to be ruffled. Perhaps the presence of higher anxiety is a factor in children who become persistent in their stuttering. Children enter the world with the genetic underpinnings of personality, which are shaped by environment. Therefore, a child with a low threshold for anxiety, who also begins to stutter, may experience more difficulty, and thus develop further anxiety, than a child who is naturally calm and content and begins to stutter. To explore this idea, we compared three anxiety measures in children who recovered from or became persistent in stuttering, and normally fluent control children.

We administered the *Child Anxiety Scale* (Gillis, 1980) to 4- and 5-year-old children. When these same children returned for a long-term follow-up visit at ages 10 to 14, they were asked to complete two scales: the *Revised*

Table 8.4
Range, Mean, and Standard Deviation (*SD*) for Age (in Months),
and Mean and *SD* for *Child Anxiety Scale* Raw Scores

	Age			Raw Score	
Group	Range	*M*	*(SD)*	*M*	*(SD)*
Persistent	50–83	59.81	(7.63)	11.79	(6.19)
Recovered	46–79	59.27	(7.65)	11.49	(5.46)
Control	47–83	59.98	(8.65)	10.45	(6.22)

Children's Manifest Anxiety Scale (Reynolds & Richmond, 1994) and The Communication Attitude Test (Brutten & Dunham, 1989).

Child Anxiety Scale

The *Child Anxiety Scale* (CAS; Gillis, 1980) can be given to children as young as 5 years old. It is designed for group administration but can be given to individuals also. Typically, for school-age children, the examiner reads the questions and instructs the children to draw a line through either a red or a blue circle, depending on which response they choose. We gave the test individually to children as young as 4 years of age, for whom we marked the responses. The younger children indicated understanding of the task by their responses, lending validity to the measure as we used it. Four-year-olds who did not appear to grasp the task were not administered the test. Although the results from 4-year-olds cannot be compared to the test norms, they can be compared within our own sample. The mean scores for the test are presented in Table 8.4. The raw scores are provided because test norms could not be used to convert scores for 4-year-olds into age-related percentiles.

The range, mean, and standard deviation for age at the time of testing are extremely close for the three groups of children. This makes comparisons between the groups meaningful. Each group contains a similar spread of 4-, 5-, and 6-year-olds. There is no significant difference between the means for persistent, recovered, and control groups [$F(2, 147) = .75$, $p = .47$], but it is nevertheless interesting to note that the persistent group has the highest mean (higher scores indicating higher anxiety) and the control group has the lowest. Although no firm conclusions can be

Table 8.5

Mean Scores (and Standard Deviations) for Total and Subscales
of the *Revised Children's Manifest Anxiety Scale* (RCMAS)

		RCMAS			
Group	Total	Physiological Anxiety	Worry/ Over- Sensitivity	Social Concern/ Concentration	Lying
Persistent	48.40 (5.94)	9.40 (3.05)	8.20 (3.11)	9.80 (1.64)	9.80 (1.30)
Recovered	45.12 (7.84)	9.00 (2.37)	7.69 (1.85)	7.81 (1.91)	8.94 (2.46)

made, further exploration of personality traits such as anxiety may prove enlightening.

Revised Children's Manifest Anxiety Scale

The *Revised Children's Manifest Anxiety Scale* (RCMAS; Reynolds & Richmond, 1994) yields a total anxiety score that consists of three subscales: Physiological Anxiety, Worry/Oversensitivity, and Social Concern/ Concentration. There is an additional subscale for Lying. For the total score, the norm is a *T*-scaled score of 50, with a standard deviation of 10. For each subscale, the norm is a scaled score of 10, with a standard deviation of 3. Higher scores reflect higher anxiety levels. Table 8.5 presents data for the persistent and recovered groups. Because 17 recovered children but only 5 persistent children completed the scale, the results must be viewed with caution. All mean total and subscale scores were within normal limits of one standard deviation above or below the normed mean. None of the individual scores for all subscales for all children exceeded norms; in other words, none of the children gave indications of higher than average anxiety. Although the recovered group tended to score lower (less anxiety) than the persistent group, especially on the Social Concern/Concentration subscale, no statistically significant differences were found.

Communication Attitude Test

The Communication Attitude Test (CAT; Brutten & Dunham, 1989) was developed to evaluate stuttering children's attitudes toward speech, as compared to normally fluent children's attitudes. It contains 35 statements, and children must circle "True" or "False" to indicate their agreement or disagreement with each item. The total number of negative responses (re-actions) is the score; thus, a higher score indicates that a child has a more negative attitude regarding his or her own speech. Vanryckeghem and Brutten (1997) tested stuttering and nonstuttering 6- to 13-year-olds, and reported a mean score of 17.44 ($SD = 6.81$) for stuttering children, and a mean of 7.05 ($SD = 4.69$) for normally fluent children. As part of the Illinois studies, the CAT was administered to persistent and recovered children in a similar age range, to determine whether children who continued to stutter and those who recovered developed, or continued to maintain, negative attitudes toward speaking. The mean score for persistent children was 10.80 ($SD = 6.80$), below the reported norm for stuttering children but above that for normally fluent children, reflecting, perhaps, the fact that a number of children who persisted in stuttering did so at a very mild level. Recovered children, however, yielded a mean score of only 4.12 ($SD = 3.28$), which is below the mean for normally fluent children. This is yet another indication that early recovery from stuttering appears to be complete. Not only do these children exhibit no speech symptoms of stuttering, but they also have positive speech attitudes.

Cognitive Skills

Past reports using a variety of cognitive measures, but primarily standardized intelligence (IQ) tests, have indicated lower overall mean scores for children who stutter as compared to their normally fluent peers, but only by a few points (Andrews & Harris, 1964; Okasha, Bishry, Kamel, & Hassan, 1974; Schindler, 1955). Otto and Yairi (1976) reported that incidence of stuttering and level of disfluency are higher in populations referred to as "mentally retarded," including in children with Down syndrome. Additionally, Andrews and Harris (1964) reported that mothers of children who stutter tended to have intellectual abilities below average. On the other hand, people who stutter, as a group, also have included many great minds and talents, such as Charles Darwin, Winston Churchill, Somerset Maugham, Demosthenes, Bob Love, and James Earl Jones. Except for the finding that the incidence of stuttering is higher among people with mental retardation, there are no indications of meaningful intellectual deficit in people who stutter, and no practicing clinician or researcher would associate intellectual deficit with stuttering. What, then, does the lower mean score on IQ tests mean? Clinically speaking, not a whole lot.

IQ tests are composed of many subscales and do not really indicate whatever overall intelligence might be, but the level of skill in a wide number of areas concerning intelligence. For example, someone might obtain extremely high scores in some areas and quite low in others, whereas a second person might perform similarly across all subscales, and their mean overall scores could be identical.

As we now know, numerous studies have pointed to differences in brain function between stuttering and normally fluent individuals, in that those who stutter tend to use the right hemisphere in language processing and production, and have slower reaction times, among other differences. None of these differences is perceptible to an observer, but can only be measured by sophisticated instrumentation. The different or poorer performance for people who stutter may simply represent skills at the lower end of the normal range, as a result of how their brains function due to stuttering (or to other disorders that may tend to co-occur with stuttering).

Arthur Adaptation of the Leiter Scale

In our project, the *Arthur Adaptation of the Leiter International Performance Scale* (Arthur, 1952) was given at initial evaluations simply to determine if each child's nonverbal skills were within normal limits, and comparable to the child's verbal skills. This test involves matching blocks with various colors, designs, and pictures, to a given set of drawings representing blocks. Skills tested involve recognition of basic color, shape, and number of items; analogies; functions; and patterns.

The scores shown in Table 8.6 for the stuttering children are overall above normal limits. The recovered group had a mean score above normal limits, and the lowest mean score, still within normal limits, was obtained by the persistent group. The ranges for both groups are similar, with the

Table 8.6

Range, Mean, and Standard Deviation (*SD*) for Leiter Scale (Arthur Adaptation)

Group	N	Range	M	SD
Persistent	26	78.17–151.05	113.67	16.84
Recovered	88	76.43–174.35	122.26	18.51
Combined	114	76.43–174.35	120.30	18.43

exception of two or three very high scores in the recovered group, which pulled the group's mean up. In sum, although some persistent children may have subtle processing differences, this is not apparent in the high average scores for this group. Perhaps the recovered children may be out of sync in their development, having precocious language or nonverbal skills, with motor speech systems that cannot keep up until the different domains catch up with each other. This theme is considered more fully in Chapter 7.

Awareness of Disfluency

Another aspect of childhood stuttering involving cognition is awareness of the disorder. *Awareness* has been defined in *A Dictionary of Psychology* (Drever, 1952) as "mere experience of an object or idea; sometimes equivalent to consciousness" (p. 26), but no adequate definition of awareness of stuttering, or lack of it, has been offered despite extensive usage of the term in the literature.

Awareness, in general, can occur at many levels. Awareness of stimulus change can be detected in infants by strength of sucking response or by head turning. School-age children can indicate awareness verbally or by body language and facial expression. As adults, we have a myriad of methods of indicating, or hiding, awareness. Children at 3 years of age, however, do not typically come up to their parents and announce that they seemed to have begun to stutter. Although, as indicated in Chapter 3, parents have reported that close to onset some children behaved in ways that, directly or indirectly, reflected awareness of their stuttering, more often children do not comment on difficulties with speaking. Does this mean that the majority of the children have no awareness of their stuttering? Traditionally, it was assumed that the brain of a newborn was a *tabula rasa*, and that a baby could not perceive or react much beyond his or her basic needs. We have come to realize how incorrect such beliefs were. Experts in child development now recommend providing optimal stimulation, visual and auditory, for infants' rapidly developing brains. Babies can respond to voices, music, shapes, and colors. They have personalities. However, babies cannot tell us that they love the sound of their father's voice, or that they prefer jazz to classical music. They do not have words yet. Therefore, when children begin stuttering, many continue on as before, giving little or no evidence of awareness of it.

Nevertheless, some children do project various levels of awareness. Some look a bit astonished at what their vocal tract has just done, some turn their heads and look down, and others frown or look unhappy. We have heard parents describe their children as saying, "I can't talk" or "I can't say it," or crying. One child was reported to throw himself on the floor, kicking and crying. Others have indicated overt awareness, but no concern, regarding their stuttering. These are 2-, 3-, and 4-year olds, close to the onset of their stuttering. Clearly, some children are aware of *and* bothered by their stuttering very early on, but do not have the words to describe it. Conscious awareness of self or others develops gradually through childhood. The timing and level of awareness are dependent on many factors, including sensitivity, experience, constitution, and environment. It is the marked situation, the extreme or unusual one, that is noticed first. Children take longer to become aware of characteristics that they share with people directly involved in their lives. Questions to consider include these: Is there a certain age at which children become aware of stuttering? Are there predictable features leading to awareness? Is awareness of stuttering "good" or "bad"?

Traditionally, awareness of stuttering has been considered an important milestone in the development of the disorder. As discussed in previous chapters, in Johnson et al.'s (1959) diagnosogenic view, awareness was the key element of the genesis of stuttering. Parents' awareness, or perhaps hyperawareness, of disfluency and their anxieties concerning it caused the child to become aware of his or her own normal disfluencies. Trying to stop or avoid the disfluencies allegedly caused stuttering. Following this highly questionable premise, it was only logical to advise parents and clinicians to avoid calling attention to disfluency or stuttering in the young child. Awareness also was deemed critical years prior to Johnson's work in that it was a necessary precursor for the appearance of anxiety, and presumably for "secondary stuttering" (Bluemel, 1932). It was a feature in Bloodstein's (1961) developmental scheme, especially in the transition from Stage I to Stage II, as well as in Van Riper's (1971) developmental tracks. In the most common track, awareness emerged gradually. Two of the other tracks were defined by presence of awareness at onset, and in the last track, awareness is not present initially or later in the course of the disorder.

Many researchers and clinicians of stuttering have anecdotally reported early awareness, and a few studies have documented some aspects of it. In a more systematic interview study, Yairi (1983) reported that parents of 18% of children who stuttered perceived indications of their child's awareness of stuttering close to the time of onset. Two additional investigations by members of our team assessed awareness of disfluency by testing children in a direct manner. In the first study to objectively measure correlates of awareness, Ambrose and Yairi (1994) found that 15% of pre-school children who stuttered indicated possible awareness of stuttering by indicating that they talk like disfluent puppets displayed on a TV screen significantly more often than like fluently speaking puppets. Nevertheless, because more than 5% of the normally fluent control children also chose stuttering puppets more frequently, it is difficult to interpret results at such young ages. As age progressed, the children's accuracy—the agreement between their own fluency status and a puppet with whom they identified—increased. Interestingly, the child's stuttering severity was not a significant factor. Ezrati-Vinacour, Platzky, and Yairi (2001) used a puppet task very similar to that of Ambrose and Yairi, but examined only normally fluent children ranging in age from 3 to 7 years. They showed consistent awareness of fluency by about age 5.

As time passes and children get older, the length of stuttering history increases. Undoubtedly, both factors contribute to awareness levels. At the same time, however, the fluctuating frequency and severity of stuttering present major difficulties in measuring awareness of its presence, especially in young children. Thus, they may be aware of their own speech patterns when stuttering is severe but have no idea of their fluency status a week or even a day later. In other words, awareness may be a fleeting phenomenon, which is to be expected at such young ages. Because fluency is the norm and stuttering varies from the norm, does awareness of stuttering arrive at an earlier age than does awareness of fluency? Plainly, as a majority of the children recover as they get older, their fluency awareness should increase. For children who continue to stutter, awareness of their own stuttering should become apparent as well. The clinical implications of this information are far reaching.

The Illinois Studies: Current Data on Awareness

As described in Ambrose and Yairi (1994), we developed an awareness test that uses a videotape portraying fluent and disfluent puppets as they utter different sentences presented as contrasting pairs of fluent versus stuttered speech. For example, the puppet at the right side of the screen says, "The ball is red," followed by an identical puppet at the left side that says, "The b-b-b-ball is r-red." The design controls for the side (left or right) and order (first or second) of the fluent and stuttered speech, so that a child who chooses, for example, all of the left puppets or all of the second presentations of the sentence, yield a score in the mid-range associated with randomness. The child is shown the video, one pair of sentences at a time, and is asked to point to the puppet that talks like him or her. A maximum score of 6 indicates choice of all stuttering puppets; a score of 0 results from choice of all fluent puppets.

Within our pool of participants, 110 children were seen within 12 months of onset and were given the awareness test for the initial through sixth visit, 3 years later. Not all children cooperated or completed the test on the various occasions. At the initial visit, these children ranged in age from 23 months to 56 months. There were 45 two-year-olds, 55 three-year-olds, and 10 four-year-olds. As explained earlier, a score of 0 represents identification with all and only fluent puppets, and 6 represents identification with all and only stuttering puppets. At the initial visit, of the 64 children who participated in the awareness task, 6 (almost 10%) indicated awareness of stuttering as measured by our procedure. This figure is comparable to the 12% of children reported by parents to be highly aware of their stuttering in the early months of the disorder, before their first evaluation.

Over all six visits, the percentage of children with each awareness score is shown in Figures 8.1a–f. At Visit 1, a normal distribution is clearly observed.

(*text continues on p. 276*)

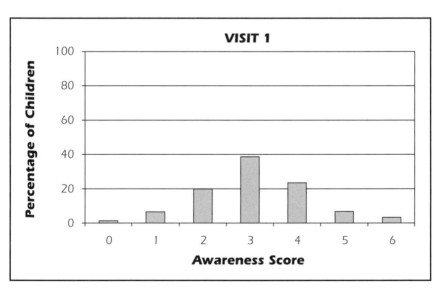

Figure 8.1a. Percentage of all children with each awareness score for each visit.

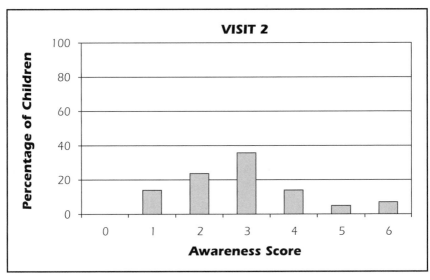

Figure 8.1b. *Continued.*

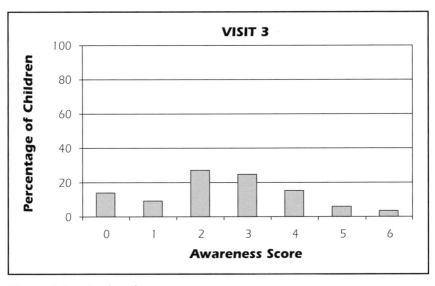

Figure 8.1c. *Continued.*

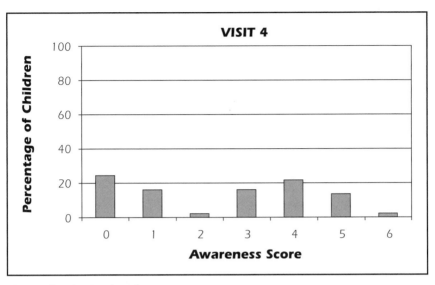

Figure 8.1d. *Continued.*

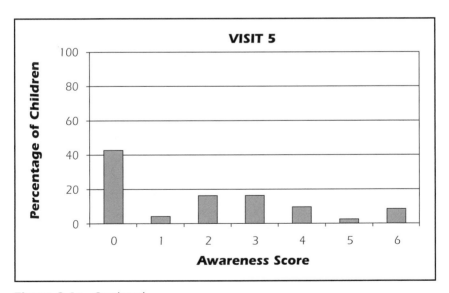

Figure 8.1e. *Continued.*

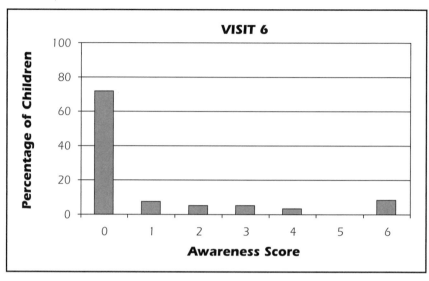

Figure 8.1f. *Continued.*

As the visits progress, children begin to make more choices indicating awareness of fluency. This converges nicely with the general decline in stuttering severity for a majority of children, with about 75% undergoing complete recovery over the span of the study. However, awareness of stuttering does not appear to increase over the visits. Does this mean that the children who continue stuttering do not become aware of their stuttering? One would think that by the time normally fluent children are aware of their fluency, stuttering children should already have become aware of their stuttering because of its "differentness." It is important to remember, however, that only 25% of the children continue stuttering throughout the study, so the lower percentage of children aware of stuttering is in large part due to the fact that there are many fewer of them as time progresses.

As noted, a complicating factor in measuring awareness of stuttering, especially at young ages, is that the severity, and even presence, of the disorder fluctuates in a good number of children. Thus, we may assume that awareness of very mild stuttering would lag behind awareness of severe stuttering. Perhaps the lack of identification with stuttering for some children is due in part to this fluctuation.

The naturally following question is, Does the level of awareness of fluency or stuttering correlate with stuttering severity at the time of testing?

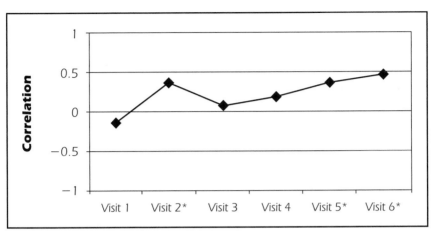

Figure 8.2. Correlation between awareness score and clinician severity score over the six visits. *Significant correlation.

In our early study (Ambrose & Yairi, 1994) in which only group means were examined, no such relationship was found. As time passes, however, does the match between severity and awareness grow, or do children at some point gain a self-image as "stutterer" or "normally fluent speaker" that overshadows fluency status on a given day? Figure 8.2 gives the correlation of awareness score and clinician severity score over the six visits. As can be seen, the correlation for Visits 1, 3, and 4 is relatively close to zero. At Visit 2, there is a significant correlation. At Visits 5 and 6, a significant correlation becomes consistent. In other words, it is only after 3 years or so of stuttering that the severity of the disorder should be taken into consideration in terms of its possible impact on the level of awareness.

To further examine the relationship between awareness and stuttering severity, we examined awareness scores for recovered and persistent groups separately. We included only those persistent children who exhibited at least moderate stuttering at the time of the awareness task. In this way, the development of awareness of both fluency and stuttering can be more closely followed, as can be seen in Figures 8.3a–f. Scores of 0 to 1 are interpreted as an indicator of awareness of fluency; scores of 2 to 4 may be broadly assumed to represent lack of awareness of either fluency or stuttering, or random choice; and scores of 5 to 6 indicate awareness of stuttering.

At the first visit (see Figure 8.3a), a majority of children in both groups appear unsure of their fluency status. At Visit 2 (see Figure 8.3b), persistent children tend to identify with stuttering. But at the third visit (see Figure 8.3c), 1 year following the initial visit, most of both groups again seem unsure. At this point, there is a slight increase in identification of fluency for the recovered group. At Visit 4 (see Figure 8.3d), the two groups are clearly delineated, with recovered children leaning toward awareness of fluency, and persistent children toward awareness of stuttering. This pattern continues at Visit 5 (see Figure 8.3e), which is 2 years following the first visit. At the final visit a year later (see Figure 8.3f), recovered children know they are fluent. At this point, there were only 3 persistent children who participated in the task and stuttered at least at a moderate level; 2 of them appeared aware of their stuttering, and 1 identified with fluency.

Awareness Conclusions

It can be assumed that many factors influence awareness of stuttering. These include age, severity, length of stuttering history, parental influences,

(*text continues on p. 281*)

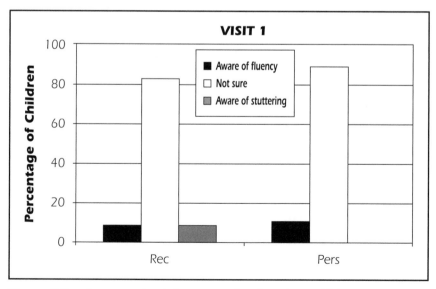

Figure 8.3a. Awareness levels for recovered and persistent children.

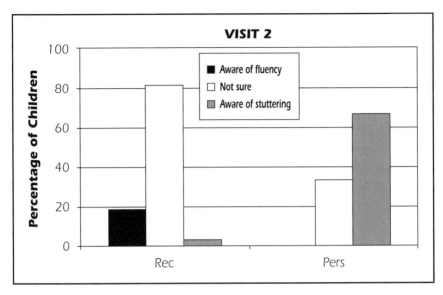

Figure 8.3b. *Continued.*

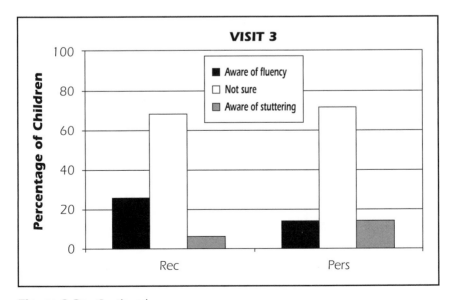

Figure 8.3c. *Continued.*

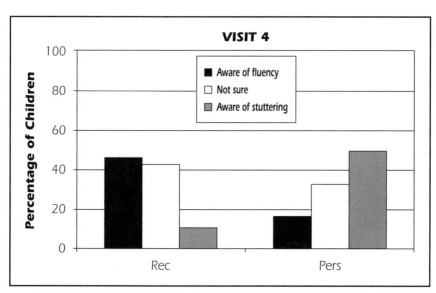

Figure 8.3d. *Continued.*

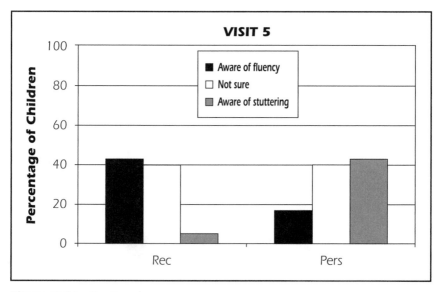

Figure 8.3e. *Continued.*

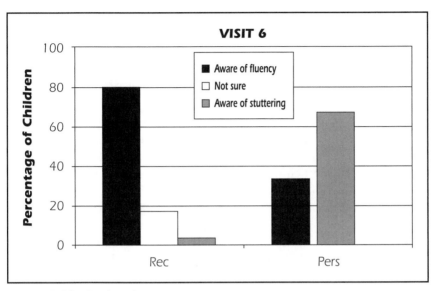

Figure 8.3f. *Continued.*

and treatment, as well as other forces, all of which combine with the child's own perceptive abilities. Thus, scientific assessment of awareness of stuttering in young children is a difficult challenge. Keeping in mind the additional limitations of the awareness task, it would appear that children who stop stuttering gradually gain awareness that their speech does not differ from the norm, and they know they do not talk like the puppet who stutters. Thus, awareness of stuttering in preschool children appears highly variable. As already mentioned, a number of the children we have seen, including 3-year-olds and even 2-year-olds, have had direct immediate negative reactions to their stuttering, whether or not they could choose stuttering puppets over fluent puppets as being most like themselves. Clearly, there should be no doubt that early awareness can and does occur.

The assumption of a lack of awareness and the focus on preventing awareness have left a heavy burden on speech pathologists, who, for many years, could not step in and modify behavior; on parents who were told to sit by and watch their child struggle; and, most of all, on the children themselves, some of whom were probably left wondering why Mommy and Daddy were ignoring them. Parents, after all, acknowledge and affirm, or at least notice and respond to, scrapes and bruises, or fights with siblings. Why should stuttering be treated differently?

Conclusions and Clinical Implications

In combination, motor, psychosocial, and cognitive data reveal an interesting picture. As a group, young children early in the course of stuttering do not appear to give strong indications of overt or obvious differences from normally fluent children, other than their disfluencies. Evidence indicates, however, that more subtle differences exist in laryngeal function (greater shimmer or amplitude variation), slower speaking rate (phone production), and a slightly more limited articulatory movement (second formant transition). Although the trends are not yet entirely clear, we are inclined to conclude that the motor speech systems of children who stutter are less stable and less flexible than those of normally fluent children. Similarly, a few possible early differences between children whose stuttering would eventually persist and those who would recover have been identified but need considerably more supporting evidence.

In the psychosocial domain, according to our findings, parents do not perceive their stuttering children appreciably differently than parents of children with normal fluency. This is yet more evidence against Wendell Johnson's diagnosogenic theory, discussed in more detail in Chapters 4 and 5. Early on, there are no clear indications of higher anxiety levels in young children who stutter, but as stuttering continues, anxiety related to communication increases for some children, as reported by previous investigators (Vanryckeghem & Brutten, 1997; Vanryckeghem et al., 2001). Recovered children do not show any presence of negative feelings associated with communication.

General cognitive skill levels for children who stutter are well within, or even above, normal limits. Children who recover from stuttering (early and naturally) may tend toward higher than average abilities, which could contribute to an uneven pattern of maturation, with language and cognition skills leading motor skills (more information in this regard is presented in Chapter 7). Although anxiety is not evident until children are older, some children do indicate awareness of stuttering very early. Whereas it is logical to assume that awareness of stuttering should precede anxiety about stuttering, anxiety is not a necessary outcome following awareness—and anxiety, of course, can develop for many reasons. Our studies have not shown any link between the development or presence of awareness and the instigation of anxiety. The awareness of listener reactions to stuttering, however, is quite different from self-awareness of stuttering. Negative reactions can cause awareness of stuttering and anxiety, but awareness of one's own stuttering is a natural and neutral aspect of development and maturation.

When a preschool child who stutters is seen for evaluation or treatment, responsible clinicians must consider all factors that might contribute in some way to the disorder of stuttering. Although present findings preclude the use of motor, psychosocial, or cognitive characteristics in isolation as predictors of persistence or recovery pathways, test scores or other relevant data for the individual child should be considered in conjunction with information derived from other domains, such as disfluency and familial history. The cumulative effect of diverse data can clarify the clinical picture. Similarly, although group data regarding motor, psychosocial, or cognitive function do not seem to make a significant contribution to the clinical differentiation between children who stutter and normally fluent peers, relevant information may play an important role in handling any individual case. Clinicians do not measure phones per second or second formant transition, but knowing that the motor speech system of children who stutter is more vulnerable leads clinicians to consider the effect of parent instructions or therapeutic method, particularly in regard to slowing of rate. Family environment, perceptions, and attitudes, including those of the parents or other caretakers and the child, must also be considered. As the child indicates awareness, with or without concern, parents can respond accordingly. It is also important for clinicians to understand, and to impart to parents, that *stuttering* is not a bad word.

Chapter 9

Genetics

The notion that genetics plays a significant role in the transmission of the susceptibility to stuttering has been discussed for many years and is widely accepted. Studies of family history, twins, and patterns of affected relatives have repeatedly illustrated genetic effects. Various genetic transmission models have been suggested, most converging upon the involvement of at least several genes, as well as environmental factors. More recent work has indicated a major locus in addition to polygenic factors, and the role of the environment appears to stem from nonshared (individually unique) factors in a family. Linkage studies to identify specific genes are currently under way. It is important for researchers and clinicians to be knowledgeable about the role of genetics in stuttering, in order to best tailor research design and treatment strategies, and it is equally important so that people who stutter can better understand their disorder.

Study Questions

1. *How do studies of family history, twins, and familial aggregation show that there is a genetic factor in stuttering?*

2. *What is the contribution of genetics to complex behavior disorders, such as stuttering? Is there one gene that causes stuttering? Are there other factors?*

3. *What is the best-fitting transmission model for stuttering? Explain how it directs further investigation of the etiology of stuttering and development of optimal treatment strategies.*

Background

The 20th and 21st centuries have seen intense interest and advancement in technology and science. The human genome project is a manifestation of scientific growth and progress, particularly in genetic research. Scientists at the project have, in fact, announced the number of genes in human DNA and found it surprisingly smaller than anticipated, at about 30,000. As the mapping and sequencing of the human genome progress, success for genetic research of common disorders becomes more likely. Progress in genetic studies has already been made in several areas related to speech and language, including apraxia with language disorders, where a specific gene (FOXP2) has been identified (Lai, Fisher, Hurst, Vargha-Khadem, & Monaco, 2001); specific language impairment (Tallal, Hirsch, Realpe-Bonilla, Miller, & Brzustowicz, 2001; Tomblin & Buckwalter, 1994); phonology (Felsenfeld, McGue, & Broen, 1995; B. Lewis, 1990; B. Lewis & Thompson, 1992); various syndromes involving speech, language, and hearing; and stuttering. Summaries and reviews of earlier genetic studies concerning stuttering may be found in Andrews et al. (1983), Yairi, Ambrose, and Cox (1996), and Yairi and Ambrose (2002).

But one might ask, What is inherited via genes? How much of a disorder is governed by genes? Why do scientists look for genes? It is important to realize that people do not inherit *behaviors* as complex as speech and language. People inherit *genes*, and these are the agents that affect behavior. How these genes are expressed is subject to environmental influences. For example, two neighbors may buy the same variety of strawberry plants, with genes for producing abundant large red tasty berries. One neighbor plants in a sunny area with rich soil and adequate moisture. The other neighbor plants in a drier, shady corner, in poor soil. The first condition allows the genes to be expressed, and the family enjoys a bountiful crop. The second condition results in a very poor harvest.

Any particular characteristic or behavior may be the result of the actions and interactions of many genes, as well as environmental contributions. The complex behavior that is defined as stuttering is its *phenotype*—the observable traits or characteristics of an individual that are genetically controlled. *Genotype* refers to the sum total of specific variants of genes that an individual possesses, with one copy of each gene inherited from the mother and one from the father. The underlying genes (genotype) transmit susceptibility to a wide variety of features that may play a role in speech–language–hearing disorders. Researchers continue to identify symptoms, or phenotypic characteristics, and attempt to relate them to particular variations of genes that can affect these phenotypes.

Genes interact with a host of environmental conditions or events that include more than the situations in which people are placed, such as economic status, family situation, lifestyle, political or religious beliefs, and air quality, to name a few. The environment includes all internal and external influences, some of which may be shared by a family and some of which are unique to an individual (e.g., birth order within the family, illness, trauma). Environmental factors may be specific, such as an event or condition that impacts expression of the gene, or may have purely random components that are difficult to identify or measure. It is also possible that the timing of exposure to environmental risks is critical, further complicating efforts to identify environmental factors. Some factors are difficult to classify as genetic or environmental because they reflect the influence of both. For example, cholesterol levels are considered to be an important influence on susceptibility to heart disease, but are influenced by both genetic (apolipoprotein structural genes and receptors) and environmental (diet and exercise) factors. Therefore, we are not looking for variation at a single gene that in and of itself causes stuttering, or controls any particular feature, such as the frequency of part-word repetitions.

Because the interaction of genes and environment is so complex, it becomes a daunting task to determine the necessary and sufficient factors resulting in stuttering. If the overall liability to stuttering is the summation of all the genetic and environmental agents that can affect this phenotype, then it is possible for an individual to have a number of factors and *not* stutter, but have parents, siblings, or children who do stutter. It may be that individuals in families with stuttering do not all have the same set of factors; there may be one or more primary genes that are involved in virtually all stuttering, but the remaining contributors probably vary at least to some extent.

Once a gene is identified as influencing a disorder, researchers still may not know what that specific gene actually does, and even if that information is known, researchers may not understand how it affects the phenotype. It can be difficult to identify the contribution of a single gene or of multiple genes because of their interactions with each other and with the environment. One or more genes may contribute to the underlying susceptibility to stuttering, and may have wider effects, affecting susceptibility to other disorders as well. These genes may also interact with other genes to cause a variety of phenotypic effects. Conditions that sometimes coexist with stuttering, such as phonological disorders, attention deficit, or even asthma, could possibly stem from this interaction.

The transmission of stuttering, then, is not a simple, straightforward process. The task before researchers is to identify genes that transmit the susceptibility to stuttering, and determine what combination of genes and environmental factors causes the overt onset and further development of stuttering. Successful identification of genes and characterization of their role in communication will enable further scientific endeavors, and make it possible to develop and customize new diagnostic, treatment, and counseling strategies for people with communication disorders.

Incidence and Prevalence

How common is stuttering? The *incidence* of a disorder is its rate of occurrence, or chance of occurring. The *prevalence* is an estimate of how many people have a disorder during a given time period, or at a given time. In a room of 100 people, the incidence of upper respiratory infection, the common cold, would probably be 100% because all 100 individuals likely have had a cold at some time in their life. However, the prevalence may be 5% or 13% or 27% or higher, depending on the season and area. This is how many people in the room have a cold at that particular time.

According to the more reliable studies of stuttering (Andrews & Harris, 1964; Mansson, 2000), the population estimates for the incidence of stuttering (how many have ever stuttered) are at about 5%, and the prevalence (how many stutter at any given point in time) is about 1%. Ambrose, Cox, and Yairi (1997) indicated that the difference leaves 4% as having stopped stuttering through recovery. In other words, on average, in a room of 100 people, 5 will have stuttered at some point but only 1 of them will currently be stuttering. Because stuttering tends to run in families, these figures would be expected to be considerably larger in a group of families in which at least 1 individual has ever stuttered.

Families for the Illinois Genetic Studies

The University of Illinois Stuttering Research Program data that we report in this chapter represent a majority of the children in the Ambrose et al. (1997) study, with additional families whose stuttering history has not been previously reported. Of the 163 children described in Chapter 2, those with identified first- and second-degree relatives (siblings, parents, uncles, aunts,

Table 9.1

Mean Age (and Standard Deviation) at Initial Evaluation
and Months Postonset of Stuttering by Gender

Gender	n	Age in Months		Months Postonset of Stuttering	
Males	84	39.93	(8.72)	6.48	(5.99)
Females	39	39.23	(9.29)	7.13	(7.74)
Total	123	39.71	(8.87)	6.68	(6.57)

cousins, grandparents) are included here. The families excluded were those
with no information for some relatives. A total of 123 stuttering children
met the criteria. Table 9.1 shows their age and months since stuttering onset. Of these children, 24 have been classified as persistent, 78 as recovered,
and the remaining 21 have not yet met criteria for persistent or recovered.

For each child's family, a pedigree was drawn, as described in Ambrose
et al. (1997). A pedigree is a schematic representation of related individuals,
indicating generational levels and degree of relatedness. In this family tree,
grandparents, parents, aunts, uncles, siblings, and cousins were included.
For each individual, stuttering status was noted as (a) never stuttered,
(b) stuttered and recovered by early school age, or (c) persistent (stuttering
duration of 4 or more years). Parents were given a definition and examples
of stuttering, and urged to check with family members. Individuals for
whom stuttering status was unknown were not included in counts of relatives. Pedigrees were verified repeatedly as children returned for their periodic visits over several years. Long-term contact with the families allowed
not only continued verification and updating, but also a chance to interact
directly with parents, siblings, and often grandparents of each child. Direct
observation of the speech of these individuals and confirmation of family
history of stuttering from several sources were thus possible.

Another unique and powerful aspect of the Illinois data is that pedigrees were ascertained through children who persisted in and who recovered from stuttering. Relatives reported to have recovered naturally and
early were also identified and included. No other genetic studies have included individuals who recovered from stuttering. Because other studies
have considered only persistent stuttering, they left out the large majority
of the stuttering population who recover while young. Our sample, then, is

representative of the stuttering population as a whole. Greater inclusion allows for consideration of possible subtypes of persistent and recovered stuttering, providing the means to explore possible underlying genotypes and their relation to phenotypes.

Exploration of Family Patterns in Stuttering

A majority of people who stutter can tell you that stuttering runs in their family. It has not taken any scientific studies or state-of-the-art technology to discover this. A question that does require research is why stuttering runs in families. Although some researchers have said that the disorder is purely learned, the past 40 years have seen a continuing exploration of the role of genetics in the transmission of stuttering. Several basic methods can be used to examine the role of genetics in complex behavioral disorders, including studies of the presence or absence of family history, twins, and familial aggregation (distribution pattern of affected versus unaffected relatives). When such studies point to a high possibility of genetic components for a phenotype, further investigations proceed into the biological sphere of genetic research aimed at identifying specific genes and their functions.

Presence of Family History

Adults often have childhood memories of their grandparents and even great-grandparents. In families with stuttering, some people have thus reported distinct recollections of stuttering grandparents or occasionally great-grandparents. Individuals interviewed in early stuttering studies no doubt gave similar reports. Published research on the topic began to appear in the 1930s, when Bryngelson and Rutherford (1937) reported that the incidence of stuttering among relatives of stuttering probands is higher than in the population at large. (The case through which the family is identified is referred to as the proband.) They examined familial incidence of stuttering for 74 children ages 4 to 16 with that of 74 normally fluent children matched for gender, age, socioeconomic status, and academic achievement. They found that 46% of those who stuttered had a family history of stuttering, compared with 18% of the control sample.

This general pattern has recurred in many subsequent studies that gathered data on familial stuttering, although the specific percentages have varied greatly. In our assessment (Yairi, Ambrose, & Cox, 1996) of the literature published between 1924 and 1983, we showed that the percentages of people who stutter who have a family history of stuttering ranged from 20% to 74%. The range among 12 nonstuttering comparison groups varied from 1.3% to 42%. The wide spread for both participant groups most likely reflects sampling biases. The majority of sample means for families of normally fluent individuals are below 10%, whereas the majority of means for families of people who stutter are from 30% to 60%. Three more recent studies focused on the familial incidence of stuttering. Goldberg and Culatta (1991) found that among 693 stuttering individuals (almost all adults), 46.5% reported a positive family history. Yairi (1983) and Ambrose, Yairi, & Cox (1993), using evidence from parents of preschool children shortly after the onset of stuttering, found stuttering in the immediate families of 42% to 45% of the children and in the extended families (grandparents, aunts, uncles, and cousins) of 64% to 71% of the children. No control groups were employed in these studies.

Looking at our own current data, a positive family history of stuttering was reported for 85 of the 123 families (or 69%), whereas 38 families (31%) indicated no identifiable family history. This figure is well in line with the previous estimates. However, because there is so much variation in family size, the percentage of families with multiple members who stutter is not a particularly meaningful number. For example, if a child's parents have only one sibling each, and those siblings have no children, and the child has only one sibling, the family has 10 members: 4 grandparents, 2 aunts or uncles, 2 parents, and 1 sibling, plus the child (proband). The small family size does not allow for much chance of expressing a complex behavioral trait such as stuttering, with an incidence of about 5%. On the other hand, if a child's parents have 4 siblings each, and each sibling has 3 children, and the child has 3 siblings, then the family has 42 members: 4 grandparents, 8 aunts or uncles, 24 cousins, 2 parents, and 3 siblings, plus the proband. If stuttering runs in this family, there is a much greater chance that it will be seen.

Given the small size of many families, it is interesting that the distribution of families with and without histories of stuttering, based on the eventual natural recovery status of the proband, was not equal. Of the 24 families of children with persistent stuttering, 21 (88%) had a positive history. Of the families of the 78 recovered children, 49 (63%) had a positive history. In other words, families of children who stuttered persistently were more likely to have at least one stuttering relative than families of children who recovered. Thus, the risk for familial stuttering among those who stutter varies. Statistics were not performed because of the variability of family size. This trend can be compared to the findings of Poulos and Webster (1991), who reported that negative family history was associated with probands who possibly had experienced brain damage early in life, whereas children without such a background were more likely to have stuttering relatives. They thus distinguished familial stuttering, due in part to genetic components, from idiosyncratic stuttering stemming from early brain damage, not genetics. In our study, we had only 2 children with serious medical complications, who were excluded from this database, so no comparison can be made. What lingers as a question, however, is whether more familiality versus no familiality is indeed a sign of different etiology.

Incidence in Twin Pairs

An obvious group to examine in the study of genetics of any complex disorder is twins. Because monozygotic (identical) twins share 100% of their genes, any differences in expression of a disorder must be due to environmental effects. In dizygotic (fraternal) twins, the genetic similarity is no different than in any set of siblings, but the shared environmental components are more similar than in other siblings. Variables such as family structure and events, locale, air quality, exposure to illness, and so forth, will be very similar for fraternal (and identical) twins, but may be quite different for siblings born years apart. It is important to note, however, that twins in general are more at risk for many disorders than are singletons. This fact can confound findings regarding incidence. Being a twin, then, can be a factor increasing susceptibility to stuttering.

The study of twinning in stuttering goes back seven decades. From the 1930s to 1970s, a number of investigations explored twinning and stuttering. Berry (1937, 1938) reported a connection between handedness and stuttering, whereas others reported the numbers of mono- and dizygotic twin pairs concordant for stuttering. Although Graf (1955) found only three concordant pairs, one monozygotic and two dizygotic, Godai, Tatarelli, and Bonanni (1976) and S. F. Nelson, Hunter, and Walter (1945) found many more concordant pairs of monozygotic than dizygotic twins, indicating a strong genetic factor. However, because the percentage of concordant monozygotic twins is considerably less than 100, which it would be if stuttering were *purely* genetic, there clearly are strong environmental factors. Howie (1981a, 1981b) continued to study twin pairs using a tighter sample of only same-sex twin pairs. She reported 63% concordance for monozygotic pairs (i.e., if one twin stuttered, so did the other) and 19% concordance for dizygotic pairs. These results affirm the assumption that both genetic and environmental factors contribute to stuttering.

Research on twins continues. In 1991, Andrews, Morris-Yates, Howie, and Martin used data from the Australian Twin Registry. Based on questionnaires, in same-sex pairs who reported stuttering, only 10 (20%) of the 50 monozygotic pairs were concordant, and only 2 (5.4%) of 37 were concordant in the dizygotic pairs. In opposite-sex twin pairs, only 1 of 48 pairs reported concordance. These data, however, were based on questionnaires and not verified by the researchers. Felsenfeld et al. (2000) also obtained data from the Australian Twin Registry, and directly interviewed 91 pairs of twins, of whom 38 were monozygotic (identical) and 53 were dizygotic (fraternal). Of the monozygotic twins, 45% were concordant for stuttering, and of the dizygotic pairs, 15% were concordant. These figures are intermediate between the findings of Howie (1981a, 1981b) and those of Andrews et al. (1991). In our own sample, we had only 5 sets of twins, 2 identical and 3 fraternal. In all sets both twins stuttered, but severity and duration varied.

Aggregation Studies

Although research concerning the presence or absence of a history of stuttering has verified clinical observations that stuttering tends to run in families, twin studies reinforce the interpretation that it is genetically based but with significant environmental effects. Neither of these two lines of research, however, takes into account the patterns of affected family members and family size. Aggregation studies allow us to identify the risk for both genders and for various classes of family relatives.

Aggregation studies are based on pedigrees, or family trees, of individuals who stutter. Pedigrees typically include first-degree relatives (immediate family of the proband) and second-degree relatives, such as cousins, aunts and uncles, and grandparents. Each individual is marked as having ever stuttered, never stuttered, or unknown. Many other details may also be included. In a pedigree, squares represent males, and circles represent females. A filled-in symbol indicates presence of the disorder. Children and parents are attached with vertical lines, and unions (e.g., marriage) with horizontal lines. The oldest generation drawn is the top row, the next generation the second row, and so on. In the sample pedigree shown in Figure 9.1, no stuttering has occurred on the father's side of the family.

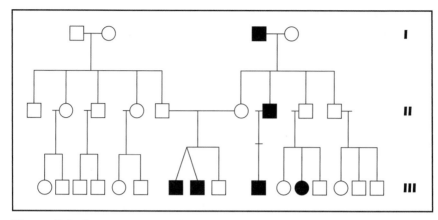

Figure 9.1. *Sample pedigree. Circles = females; squares = males; filled-in symbol = stuttering.*

In 1964 in Britain, Andrews and Harris published a unique (for its time) and remarkable aggregation study. Part of a larger research project concerning diseases and disorders in children, it was the first prospective investigation in stuttering, following children from birth to age 18. The longitudinal project followed the development of more than 1,000 children, of whom 43 were identified as having ever stuttered. An additional survey of over 7,000 children, ages 9 to 11 years, was conducted, and 80 of these were determined to stutter. Two investigators on their team, Kay and Garside, carried out a genetic analysis of these 80 children and two additional groups of stuttering individuals from the Speech Therapy Clinic, Newcastle upon Tyne: 83 children ages 2 to 14 years and 52 adolescents and adults. Among first-degree relatives, they found that the highest risk for stuttering was for fathers and brothers, at nearly 20%. This is not surprising in that many more males than females stutter. However, the risk differed for relatives of female and male probands: First-degree relatives of female probands had a significantly greater risk (20.2%) for stuttering than first-degree relatives of male probands (12.2%). The highest risk of all was for male relatives of female probands; the lowest risk was for female relatives of male probands.

In the United States during the 1970s, Kidd and his associates at Yale University performed the first large-scale investigation of genetics of stuttering. Their work was based on information obtained from first-degree relatives of 600 adults and adolescents who expressed persistent stuttering.

In a number of publications by Kidd and colleagues (Kidd, 1977, 1980, 1984; Kidd, Heimbuch, & Records, 1981; Kidd, Kidd, & Records, 1978; Kidd, Reich, & Kessler, 1973), the Yale group reported incidence and risk estimates. According to Kidd, in the families of the 600 probands, excluding the probands themselves, they found a 13% incidence of stuttering in immediate families (parents and siblings). As in the Andrews and Harris (1964) study, the risk for stuttering was significantly greater among male relatives (20%) than among female relatives (7%), and again, the risk for relatives of female probands was greater than that for relatives of male probands. Specifically, the highest risk was for male relatives of female probands (21.7%), followed by risk for male relatives of male probands (18.9%), female relatives of female probands (12.3%), and female relatives of male probands (4.2%). In their review of stuttering research and theories, Andrews et al. (1983) combined the findings of the British and U.S. studies just described and concluded that for males who have ever stuttered, the risk of stuttering is 22% for their sons and 9% for their daughters, whereas for females who have ever stuttered, it is 36% for sons and 17% for daughters.

In our project, Ambrose et al. (1993) provided data from a unique sample of 69 children who stuttered. Whereas the Yale studies included families of individuals with persistent stuttering, and Andrews and Harris (1964) studied families of children and adolescents who stuttered for variable durations and excluded from analyses 16 children who did not stutter for more than 6 months, Ambrose et al. (1993) used an unbiased sample drawn from families of children seen before persistence or recovery was determined. It was the first study to include analyses of families of children who recovered naturally from stuttering in the preschool years, without treatment.

For the 123 families reported in this chapter, familial patterns of expression of stuttering can be studied. The percentage of stuttering relatives for male and female probands is shown in Table 9.2. The first-degree relatives, or immediate families of probands, include siblings and parents. The second-degree relatives include cousins, aunts, uncles, and grandparents. Inspecting the percentages for the total immediate families, it is most obvious that the expected incidence of 5% is vastly exceeded. This simply confirms that stuttering does tend to run in families. It is also clear that the incidence among males is two to four times as great as that for females, as would be expected. The rates of occurrence drop off sharply for the second-degree relatives. This pattern is typical for traits with significant polygenic or environmental components. Also note that the rates of

Table 9.2

Percentage of Relatives Who Ever Stuttered in Families of Male and Female Probands

Probands	N	Brothers, Fathers	Sisters, Mothers	Total First-Degree Relatives	Male Cousins, Uncles, Grand-fathers	Female Cousins, Aunts, Grand-mothers	Total Second-Degree Relatives
Male	84	23.7	8.1	16.2	5.1	2.3	3.7
Female	39	25.0	9.3	17.3	4.2	2.8	3.5
Total	123	24.1	8.4	16.5	4.8	2.4	3.7

occurrence of stuttering are comparable for immediate families of both male and female probands. The highest risk is for male relatives of female probands, and the lowest is for female relatives of male probands, similar to the previous findings of the previously cited Andrews and Harris and Kidd studies. The differences between relatives of male versus female probands in our study, however, are not statistically significant. Because the Illinois studies used a considerably more representative sample in that it included individuals who recovered from stuttering early without formal intervention, there are reasons to believe that our findings reflect accurately the overall population of people who stutter.

Genetics and Subtyping

Although everyone can recognize stuttering, is all stuttering the same disorder? Researchers do not really know. It is becoming increasingly clear that stuttering, as a complex behavior disorder, stems from a variety of genetic and environmental components, and cannot be considered a uniform or homogeneous disorder. Upon what basis can subtypes be determined? Characteristics of people who stutter, such as gender, language skills, age at onset, and brain activation, or characteristics of stuttering, such as disfluency types and frequencies or presence of accessory physical behaviors, could provide a basis. Certain features of stuttering remain relatively consistent, such as age at onset, or presence of short repetitions, but wide variations in expression of symptoms and in severity are the rule, rather than the exception. The question to ask is whether stuttering is one disorder spread over a wide continuum, or whether there are specific discrete subtypes.

As discussed in Chapter 5, the idea of subtypes of stuttering is not new; a number of typologies have been suggested over a long period of time (for reviews, see Preus, 1981; Yairi, 1990). Some of the work of Kidd and his associates at Yale University concerned subtyping. Kidd, Heimbuch, Records, Oehlert, and Webster (1980) analyzed data from 184 stuttering adults and determined that severity of stuttering was not related to genetic risk for stuttering; in other words, individuals genetically at higher risk for stuttering did not exhibit more severe stuttering. Gladstien, Seider, and Kidd (1981) examined birth order and age difference between siblings, and found no relationship to frequency of stuttering.

The Illinois studies are not the first to examine genetic influences in recovery from stuttering. Cox and Kidd (1983) asked whether recovery could be a genetically milder subtype of stuttering, an independent disorder, or even nongenetic. They were unable to identify any meaningful patterns. It is important to remember that the families they studied were all identified through adults with persistent stuttering, and the authors stated that their negative findings were not definitive because of the nature of their sample. Seider, Gladstien, and Kidd (1983) also investigated recovery from stuttering as a possible subtype of stuttering, using data from families of adults who stuttered. They determined that recovered and persistent stuttering were not two independent disorders, and that handedness, birth order, and duration of stuttering did not differentiate the two groups. Females tended to recover more often and earlier than males.

More recently, Janssen, Kraaimaat, and Brutten (1990) found that people who stuttered and had histories of stuttering in their families differed significantly from those without such a history in frequency of sound prolongations and in speech motor skills. Poulos and Webster (1991) also examined family history of stuttering to identify possible subtypes. They found that adults and adolescents who stuttered and had a history of birth or developmental trauma or illness tended to have a negative family history of stuttering. They proposed two subtypes of stuttering, one that is familial, and another that is induced by trauma or illness.

The most extensive treatment of possible subtypes of stuttering has come out of the Illinois studies. We have focused on persistent stuttering, which continues beyond early childhood, and recovered stuttering, which remits of its own accord (naturally) during the preschool years.

Table 9.3

Incidence of Risk for Persistent and Recovered Stuttering by Gender

Group	Persistent	Recovered	All Stuttering
Males	1.5%	5.3%	6.8%
Females	0.5%	2.7%	3.2%
All children	1.0%	4.0%	5.0%

To compare the incidence of persistent and of recovered stuttering, it is necessary to understand how the overall stuttering incidence figure of 5% can be broken down. We have shown that up to 80% of children who ever stutter recover. This means that the incidence of recovered stuttering is about 4%, and the incidence of persistent stuttering is 1%. The last figure equals the prevalence, usually measured by looking at persistent adults. Furthermore, it has long been established that more males than females stutter. Bloodstein (1995) summarized a number of studies and found that a ratio of about 3:1 was relatively consistent. These studies, however, used children from kindergarten through adulthood, and many included no young children at all, missing most cases of early natural recovery. This number, then, can be taken as our best estimate of the gender ratio for *persistent* stuttering. In *recovered* stuttering, which occurs only in young children (by our definition of recovered stuttering), the male-to-female ratio is about 2:1. Accordingly, it is possible to break down the incidence figures more accurately, as shown in Table 9.3. Given that a child is a boy, we can say that the risk of persistent stuttering is 1.5% and the chance for recovered stuttering is 5.3%, with a total risk of 6.8%. Given a girl, the risk is about 0.5% for persistent stuttering and 2.7% for recovered stuttering, with a total risk of 3.2%. These figures apply to the population at large, and as discussed previously, we expect the percentages to be considerably higher in families with one or more people who have ever stuttered.

Persistent stuttering and recovered stuttering can be examined independently, as reported in Ambrose et al. (1997). Analysis of only persistent stuttering relatives of persistent probands would most closely approximate the samples used by previous researchers, who did not include cases of early recovery. Indeed, our current data, in Table 9.4, show that this is the case. The highest risk for stuttering occurs in male relatives of female

Table 9.4
Percentage of Persistent Stuttering Relatives in Families
of Persistent Male and Female Probands

Group	N	Persistent Brothers and Fathers	Persistent Sisters and Mothers	Total Immediate Families
Persistent male probands	17	24.2	7.4	16.7
Persistent female probands	7	33.0	12.5	23.5
All persistent probands	24	26.2	8.6	18.2

probands, and the lowest risk in female relatives of male probands, although the difference is not statistically significant. With such a limited number of persistent female probands, however, the statistics must be viewed with caution. The percentages are consistent with the findings of Andrews and Harris (1964) and Kidd (1980). This pattern of higher incidence in relatives of females who stutter has been explained by Kidd et al. (1981), who made the supposition that females have higher thresholds, requiring more genetic factors in order to express stuttering. Therefore, they have more factors to transmit to males, who appear to have a greater vulnerability or greater but not complete penetrance. In genetics, *penetrance* refers to the degree of expression of a disorder, given the susceptibility genes. Because not every person with susceptibility genes stutters, penetrance is incomplete; penetrance is somewhat reduced for males, and considerably reduced for females.

What, on the other hand, does an analysis of only recovered stuttering yield? The picture is quite different, as Table 9.5 indicates. Again, the incidence of recovered stuttering in the families of recovered probands is much greater than the expected 4% for the general population, except for female relatives of male probands, for whom the risk is only slightly greater than expected. In contrast to persistent stuttering, however, the highest risk is for male relatives of both male and female probands, with a much lower risk for female relatives of female probands. As in persistent stuttering, the lowest risk is for female relatives of male probands.

A comparison of the patterns of affected relatives for persistent and recovered stuttering shows clear differences between the two possible subtypes of stuttering. Males appear to have greater penetrance than females in

Table 9.5

Percentage of Recovered Stuttering Relatives in Families
of Recovered Male and Female Probands

Group	N	Recovered Brothers and Fathers	Recovered Sisters and Mothers	Total Immediate Families
Recovered male probands	54	15.3	3.8	9.8
Recovered female probands	24	15.2	5.4	10.0
All recovered probands	78	15.3	4.3	9.9

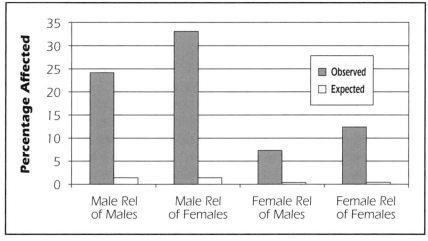

Figure 9.2. Persistent stuttering: Observed versus expected incidence in male
and female relatives (Rel) in immediate families.

both types, but the difference is not as extreme in recovered stuttering. This
can also be seen in the male-to-female ratios: approximately 4:1 for persistent stuttering and about 2:1 for recovered stuttering. The percentages of
risk in Tables 9.4 and 9.5 do not, however, indicate how these figures compare to the risk expected for the population as a whole. When we make such
comparisons, it becomes very clear that, although the observed incidence is
greater for both genders for both types of stuttering, it is not uniformly
greater across the board. Figure 9.2 illustrates the difference in the observed
versus expected incidence of persistent stuttering for male and female rela-

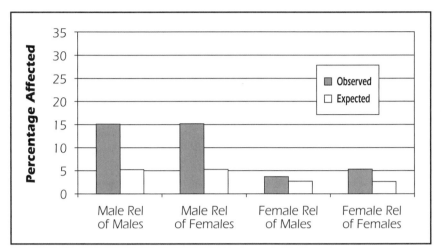

Figure 9.3. Recovered stuttering: Observed versus expected incidence in male and female relatives (Rel) in immediate families.

tives of male and female probands. The observed values are extremely high compared to the expected values; in fact, they are 15 to 25 times greater. This comparison indicates that persistent stuttering is very familial and likely to have a strong genetic factor. The picture for recovered stuttering, shown in Figure 9.3, is different. The observed incidence of recovered stuttering is greater than in the general population, but only 2 to 3 times greater. Recovered stuttering, then, is less familial than persistent stuttering, and may have a greater environmental component.

In many families, cases of both persistent and recovered stuttering are reported, so in actual families, we cannot look at only persistent or recovered stuttering. A count of the proportions of persistent and recovered stuttering in actual families of persistent and recovered probands reveals a startling pattern, first reported by Ambrose et al. (1997) and illustrated in Figure 9.4. Using a considerably larger sample of probands, our current data confirm that persistent stuttering tends to run in some families, and recovered stuttering tends to run in others. In families of persistent probands, there is a vastly higher proportion of persistent stuttering than in the population. The proportion of recovered stuttering is also somewhat higher than expected. In the families of recovered probands, just the opposite is seen. The proportion of recovered stuttering is much greater than in the population, and the proportion of persistent stuttering is greater

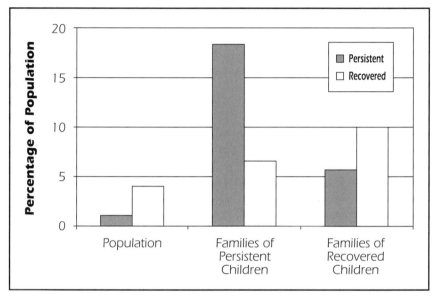

Figure 9.4. Proportion of persistent and recovered stuttering in immediate families.

than in the population but to a lesser degree. This finding, as we discuss in Chapter 10, has important prognostic implications.

What Is Transmitted?

It has become clear that susceptibility to stuttering is transmitted genetically. What is not at all clear, though, is what those genes actually do: What is the nature of the defect that prompts stuttering? Do the genes involved underlie a motor speech problem? A fine motor problem? A deficit in motor planning? A language deficit? Unusual pattern of cerebral dominance? The literature shows that people who stutter tend to have some subtle abnormalities in these areas, but these traits might be a result of stuttering, or associated with but unrelated to stuttering, or the primary defect itself. To explore this question, we have collected additional data (a) from people who stutter, (b) from relatives of people who stutter who are at high risk for stuttering (i.e., people who appear to have transmitted genetic components of stuttering to their offspring, but they themselves do not stutter), and (c) from normally fluent individuals without family histories of stuttering. In this study, several traits known to be associated with stuttering were examined—specifically, cerebral dominance and skill in motor sequencing tasks as shown in finger tapping, word retrieval, and interference as indicated by the Stroop test (Stroop, 1935), and sequencing of nonwords through the nonword repetition task developed by Dollaghan and Campbell (1998). It would be expected that people who stutter would do more poorly on all of these. If only the stuttering group exhibited poor performance, the trait might be one that is transmitted independently of stuttering (otherwise the high-risk group would also exhibit the trait). If the stuttering and high-risk group behaved in a similar fashion and differed from the control group, then that trait might be transmitted as part of, or along with, stuttering. The study (a doctoral dissertation project by Subramanian, 2001) found that the stuttering group performed more poorly than the high-risk and control groups on the tapping task, and the stuttering and high-risk groups performed more poorly than the control group on portions of the Stroop test. There were no differences on the nonword repetition task. These interesting findings must be confirmed in further studies.

How Is Stuttering Transmitted?

Both persistent and recovered stuttering are often present in the same families and, as discussed in Chapter 5, share many indistinguishable features, especially closer to onset. There is no rationale for considering them to be independent disorders, although they have certain clear-cut differences. To further explore this relationship, it is necessary to discuss genetic transmission models.

When susceptibility to a disorder is genetic, the genes involved are passed from parent to child. Genes are located in chromosomes that come in pairs. Humans possess 46 chromosomes, or 23 pairs; half are inherited from the mother and half from the father. Genes are represented on both chromosomes of a pair, so genes also come in pairs. When there is variation at a gene, the different forms are called alleles, or variants. In the case of disease controlled by a single gene (a Mendelian disorder), only one of the alleles can affect susceptibility to disease. Each individual has two alleles for the gene (one on each chromosome), but they may have two disease alleles (they are homozygous at that gene), two normal alleles (homozygous), or one of each (heterozygous at that gene). Each parent passes down one of his or her two alleles to each offspring; in other words, for each gene, a child receives one allele from the mother and one from the father.

When a disease allele is *dominant,* it requires only one of the two alleles in an individual to be the type that increases risk for the disorder; the second allele can be either a disease or a normal allele. When the disease allele is *recessive,* then an individual must have two disease alleles, one from each parent, in order to express the disease. Thus, recessive traits or disorders can be rare, unless the overall frequency of the allele is very high in the population. Therefore, for a dominant trait, either parent must have at least one disease allele, but for a recessive trait, each parent must have one. The chances for expression of a disorder due to a single dominant or recessive allele, without additional environmental factors, can be easily calculated. For example, if both parents are heterozygous for a dominant trait (both have one disease and one normal allele), then the following are likely:

> 25% of the children will have normal allele from mother, normal allele from father.
> 25% will have normal allele from mother, disease allele from father.
> 25% will have disease allele from mother, normal allele from father.
> 25% will have disease allele from mother, disease allele from father.

The only case here without the dominant disease allele is the first of the four, so 25% of the children would be normal for that trait, and 75% would express that trait. If only one parent has one disease allele, then 50% of the children would express the disorder. Of course, these figures reflect probability, not reality. A family with 100 children might approximate this distribution, or 100 families with several children, but for an individual family with 2, 3, or 4 children, we can only say that each child has a 75% (in the first case) or 50% (in the second case) chance of exhibiting the disorder. However, this easily discernible pattern occurs only for disease controlled by a single gene.

There is little doubt about the contribution of genetic risk factors in the transmission of the susceptibility to stutter, but the model of transmission has not been entirely clear. In a complex behavioral trait, such as stuttering, several models are possible. First, a trait may be controlled by a single dominant or recessive gene, that is, a single major locus. This is most unlikely. If stuttering were to be controlled solely by a single major locus (by a dominant allele of a gene), then if only one parent had that allele, that parent would be affected, and on average, 50% of the children would be affected. If a recessive allele were solely responsible, a child would stutter only if he or she received one of these alleles from *each* parent. The pattern of stuttering in families lends no support to either scenario.

Second, a trait may be multifactorial polygenic, or controlled by a number of genes in an additive fashion. The genes establish a potential range of expression of the trait, which is further controlled by environmental factors. Multifactorial polygenic traits are continuously distributed, as in height, weight, and intelligence. If environmental factors are optimal, the trait expresses variation only due to its genetic factors, but if environmental factors are less than optimal, variation increases. The amount of phenotypic variance attributable to the additive effects of the polygenic component is referred to as *heritability*. To complicate matters further, a trait may involve a single major locus *and* multifactorial polygenic components (mixed model).

A number of studies have estimated the best-fitting model of inheritance for stuttering. In 1964, Andrews and Harris determined that single-gene transmission was highly unlikely. They concluded that stuttering was most likely accounted for either by polygenic inheritance or by a dominant gene in conjunction with multifactorial polygenic components.

Scientists on the Yale University genetics of stuttering study headed by Kidd performed more sophisticated statistical analyses. The study was based on data obtained from almost 400 people who stuttered and their first-degree relatives. In 1978, Kidd et al. reported that the best statistical fits for the data were for either multifactorial polygenic or single major locus. Cox, Kramer, and Kidd (1984) performed a segregation analysis and obtained different results, ruling out a model of a single major locus. Their calculations were consistent with either a multifactorial polygenic model, or a multifactorial polygenic plus major locus model. The major locus appeared to be non-Mendelian; in other words, it did not follow the pattern of strict Mendelian transmission.

Andrews et al. (1991) studied stuttering in twins identified through the Australian Twin Registry, obtaining their data through responses to questionnaires. They assessed the contribution of genetic and environmental components to stuttering liability by testing various transmission models. Remember that environmental factors can be either shared by a family or unique to an individual, as described earlier in this chapter. Because Andrews et al. were examining the contribution of environmental factors, they did not consider a transmission model of a single major locus.

Rather, they limited testing to four models: (a) shared environmental effects only, (b) additive genetic effects (polygenic), (c) additive genetic effects and shared environmental effects, and (d) additive genetic effects with unique environmental effects. Whereas models a and c were rejected, models b and d both fit the data well, providing estimates of about 70% of the transmission due to additive genetic effects and about 30% due to unique environmental factors. This work provided an important lead for research on contributing environmental factors.

In another study that drew on the Australian Twin Registry, Felsenfeld et al. (2000), using telephone interview-based data, reached virtually identical conclusions to those of Andrews et al. (1991): 70% additive genetic effect and 30% nonshared environmental effect. Their data were considerably more accurate than in the Andrews et al. study, in that direct interviewing enabled confirmation of stuttering status. Whereas in the past, some potential shared environmental effects, such as perfectionistic parents, were explored as causes of stuttering, these studies provide support for nonshared, or unique, factors. It is not known what those unique factors are, but future exploration must move in this general direction.

The Illinois studies have employed a quite different approach in testing genetic models for best fit. Because all of the studies discussed above were based almost exclusively on adults with persistent stuttering, the findings are generalizable only to that group, which is a small minority in the population of those ever studied. As pointed out many times before, children in the Illinois studies constituted a unique sample in that it is truly representative of stuttering in general, and is not confined to one specific subgroup. In 1993, members of our team (Ambrose, Yairi, and Cox) published results of segregation analyses for families of 69 stuttering children, a sample that included both children who recovered from and those who persisted in stuttering. At that time, we shared particularly exciting findings, as we were the first ever to report statistically significant evidence for the presence of a Mendelian major locus component. Still, the data indicated that other genes were also involved. The reason for the excitement is quite obvious: If there is a major gene, the chance to locate it is good.

A follow-up study (Ambrose et al., 1997) on families of 66 stuttering children, some of whom were children included in the previous study, focused on possible subtypes of stuttering. Segregation analyses were performed separately for the families of children who recovered from stuttering (excluding persistent stuttering relatives) and families of children who persisted in stuttering (excluding recovered stuttering relatives). In both analyses, the findings confirmed our previous conclusions regarding the presence of a major gene component, but indicated that the likelihood of the mixed model for the entire sample was significantly greater than that of other models. Here, too, in contrast to the Yale studies, the single major locus component conformed to Mendelian expectations.

Two additional findings were remarkable. First, the parameters for the single major locus were almost identical in each analysis, indicating that this component involves (at least) one major gene that is present in both forms of stuttering, persistent and recovered. Second, for the multifactorial polygenic parameters, the heritability component (phenotypic variation attributed to a polygenic, additive effect) differed. Thus, the Ambrose et al. (1997) study advanced knowledge about the role of genetics a step further. The results showed that not only does the initial expression of stuttering have strong genetic components but also that its developmental course is influenced by genetics. Specifically, the researchers showed that children who stutter and have a familial history of chronic stuttering would tend to follow that pattern, and that children who stutter but have a familial history of recovered stuttering would tend to follow that pattern. Therefore, the type of family history (predominance of persistence or recovery) appears to be a strong basis for early prediction of a child's recovery from or persistent stuttering.

In summary, we suggest that both forms of stuttering share a common major gene, but that persistent stuttering varies more due to additional genetic components, whereas recovered stuttering may be less genetically controlled, with evident but less prominent family history, governed perhaps equally by genetic and environmental factors. Many factors must be considered as possible components of subtypes, but persistent and recovered stuttering appear to be the best lead, at this time, in identification of subtypes of stuttering. Their power as prognostic indicators has immediate consequences for diagnosis, counseling, and treatment of stuttering.

Linkage Analysis

As we have discussed, ample evidence supports a genetic factor in the transmission of susceptibility to stuttering. To date, however, no specific genes have been identified. Linkage analysis can be performed as an initial step to identify the genes that underlie a disorder, and it has proceeded with good results for several disorders, including Alzheimer's disease, diabetes, and attention-deficit/hyperactivity disorder. Linkage analysis works by identifying alleles for certain known marker genes on each chromosome that are coinherited with the disorder in question. When a marker gene is coinherited with stuttering, it means that the gene contributing to stuttering is on the same chromosome as the marker gene and, in fact, very close to it. These regions can then be further studied to identify specific genes involved in the transmission of stuttering.

There are currently three investigations utilizing linkage analysis. One is directed by Drayna (1997) at the National Institutes of Health and involves saliva samples from individuals with persistent stuttering. Weak evidence for linkage has been reported by this group (Shugart et al., 2003). A second investigation is being completed by a team from the University of Chicago, which includes one of our research team members. The group has been conducting a linkage study on the Hutterites, a population isolate in North Dakota. The first full-genome scan (386 markers) of families with stuttering has already been conducted on 750 individuals, as part of a larger genealogy being studied for a variety of genotypes. Within this group is a 127-member pedigree, in which 31 individuals have ever stuttered. Preliminary analyses have proceeded successfully, and several chromosomes have been identified as possible loci. This information has been reported (Cox et al., 2000) but not yet published in a scientific journal.

A third investigation, currently in progress and funded by the National Institutes of Health, is conducted by the University of Illinois Stuttering Research Program along with Drs. Nancy Cox and Edwin Cook from the University of Chicago; Dr. Ruth Ezrati from Tel Aviv University, Israel; and Cecilia Lundstrom and Marie Garsten from Sweden. This study holds great promise. We have been drawing blood samples from a unique population, all people who have ever stuttered, rather than only people exhibiting persistent stuttering. Our approach will allow for a more complete picture of genetic involvement, and may also clarify potential genetic factors differentiating persistent and recovered stuttering. The study is expected to be completed in 2004.

The information provided by linkage analysis could prove to be an enormous step forward in the understanding of the basic nature of stuttering, and could have a profound impact on clinical practice and research. It may become possible to tailor treatment to specific genetically transmitted defects and eventually to achieve early prediction of persistence or recovery for an individual child who begins stuttering.

Clinical Applications

Several of the exciting recent findings on the role of genetics in stuttering can be clinically applied. A speech–language clinician can apply information about genetics and stuttering to diagnosis, prognosis, treatment, and counseling. Evaluation and diagnosis should be performed for any person reporting possible stuttering in him- or herself or a child. When a strong family history of stuttering exists, the clinician should be alerted to the fact that individuals in such a family are at greater risk for stuttering than the general population. Although new treatment strategies have not yet been devised, prognosis and the question of whether to treat may be considered in light of genetic factors. For young children beginning to stutter, there is a greater likelihood that they will follow the predominant stuttering pattern of their family: If there are several people who stuttered into adulthood, then there is a greater chance that the child might also; if there are relatives who stuttered, but recovered, apparently completely, at a young age, then there is a greater chance that the child will follow this pattern. This history is, at present, the single most reliable predictor of persistence when it comes to prognosis of children just beginning to stutter. If history does indicate persistence in stuttering, then treatment for a young child who has just begun to stutter should be considered much sooner than for a child with indications of tendencies for recovery. This point and its implication to treatment will be discussed further in Chapter 10.

Although it is likely that in the long run better understanding of the genetic component of stuttering and its interaction with environmental factors will have profound implications for treatment of stuttering, specific predictions are limited as long as no reasonably clear clues about what is being transmitted are available. Still, inasmuch as some of the genes may not only be responsible for the underlying susceptibility to stuttering but may have wider effects in interacting with different genes affecting susceptibility to other disorders, such as phonological and language deficits, our understanding may become more comprehensive.

Assuming that genes underlying stuttering are discovered, one should realize that the probability of quickly developing more effective treatment is not high (Yairi, 1998). Once specific genes are identified, their function must be identified. Then, we will need to discover how that function ultimately affects fluency. However, there are still some more immediate implications for speech therapy. For example, identification of genes might help sort out the heterogeneity of stuttering, such as persistent and recovered forms, and it might eventually be found that certain forms of stuttering are more amenable to a certain speech therapy than others.

As knowledge of specific genes becomes increasingly applied therapeutically, ethical considerations arise, especially the issue of privacy. As Yairi (1998) pointed out, genetic analysis may produce information that may be quite significant for the person who stutters, as well as for current or future family members. Currently, the decision regarding whether to share results or provide no information regarding genetic analyses is decided as a whole for a project before anyone participates in it. If such information is found, however, what should be done with it? Should it be written in the participant's file? Discarded? Another potential problem may occur when obtaining genetic information for one part of the family requires participation from others who may not want to participate. Is there a proper ethical principle to persuade their participation? Another rather sensitive issue is counseling: As information about the genetic component to stuttering increases, some parents may wish to be more reliably advised about the chances of having a stuttering child. Or, an infant might be diagnosed as high risk for stuttering even before the onset of speech. Who is qualified to provide the counseling?

There are also possible thorny issues involving the interaction between pharmacology and young age at stuttering onset. Imagine that there is ultimately a pharmacological treatment for stuttering that requires taking the drug with some risk of negative side effects. There would undoubtedly be some parents who would want their child to take the drug even though stuttering is not a life-threatening condition. How does one weigh any risks against the benefits of fluency? How can a parent, especially one who has never stuttered, make decisions about the benefits of fluency?

Putting ethical issues aside and returning to the more positive side, knowledge of the role of genetics in stuttering may be of great assistance in therapeutic choices. For children with an inherited tendency toward natural recovery, treatment may not be necessary, but it may very well hasten the recovery process. For some individuals for whom therapy has not been successful, whose stuttering appears to continue unabated regardless of treatment, it may be helpful to understand the possible role of genetic factors contributing to persistence in stuttering. Caution must be exercised because stuttering is complex and typically many factors are involved at any stage, but at times a "hopeless" case may be better viewed as a case of relatively "permanent" stuttering. In such cases, the fault may not lie with the person's or therapist's failures, but with the nature of the stuttering.

This is not to say that further treatment cannot help, but that it might refocus on adjustment and coping strategies, in conjunction with one of various instruments that facilitate fluency. Ultimately, it is the parents' or individual's choice. In the future, however, genetic information may aid in development of treatment strategies that are based on data and targeted at specific deficits, and it may also lead to the use of pharmaceuticals as part of the treatment regime. Overall, treatment will become more effective by targeting those who need it most (e.g., those children with the genotype of persistent stuttering) and by being better tailored to the individual's stuttering and other relevant characteristics. Lastly, understanding what ultimately causes stuttering will be a great boon to people who stutter and those who treat them.

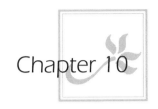

Chapter 10

Assessment of Early Stuttering

Typically, parents of young children who stutter correctly diagnose the problem, making the professional evaluation a task of describing and quantifying the disorder rather than differentiating it from other disorders. Further differentiation within the disorder is not currently possible because there is no accepted clinical system for distinguishing subtypes of stuttering. The initial evaluation, as described in this chapter, begins with an extensive case history through parent interviews that emphasize various aspects of the child's onset of stuttering. The chapter includes specific practical suggestions for obtaining adequate speech samples, procedures for comprehensive disfluency analyses, and methods for obtaining other data such as secondary characteristics and speaking rate. We provide a four-dimensional scale to assess overall stuttering severity, as well as minimal criteria for differentiating early stuttering from normal disfluency. After completion of the description and quantification of stuttering, the next task is that of prognosis. We list and discuss primary and secondary criteria for estimating a child's chances for natural recovery versus persistent stuttering. Using specific examples, we illustrate the rationale for arriving at clinical recommendations.

Study Questions

1. *What specific questions concerning the onset of stuttering are suggested for the initial evaluation of preschool children who stutter? Briefly explain each.*

2. *What are the four dimensions used to rate the overall stuttering severity? Explain the procedure for deriving the final score.*

3. *What are the minimal disfluent speech characteristics associated with clinician perception of mild or very mild stuttering?*

4. *What are the primary criteria for assessing a child's chance for natural recovery or persistent stuttering?*

The Objectives of Assessment

The term *diagnosis* means the conclusion or findings following analysis of a condition or disease. At times, an extensive analysis is required when the nature of the disease or condition is not clear. Such a process is frequently required in relation to various everyday situations, including automobile problems, computer failure, and human ailments of physical or emotional nature. The professional, being a mechanic, electrician, physician, or speech–language clinician, faces the challenge of identifying the specific nature of the condition or disease through analyses of its presenting signs (objective indications) or symptoms (subjective indications). Whereas in some cases a single indicator may be sufficient, in others the search is for a pattern of signs or symptoms. The overall motivation for diagnosis is to facilitate intelligent decisions concerning the best course of action to correct an undesirable condition or for dealing with a disease.

When it comes to stuttering, however, the majority of persons who seek help already have a correct diagnosis. Without hesitation, callers state the diagnosis of stuttering when they first talk to a clinician or consult with a pediatrician. We never have disagreed with self-referred adults who diagnosed their speech difficulties as stuttering or with referrals made by other speech–language clinicians. Rarely have we questioned parents' diagnoses of their child's speech as stuttering. Occasionally, parents have mislabeled other communication disorders as stuttering. In one referred case, the parents complained about their child's so-called stuttering, but our examination revealed that the actual problem was hypernasality that diminished the child's speech intelligibility. In only rare instances is there a question of whether a child exhibits stuttering or normal disfluency; these situations indeed require diagnoses in the classic sense.

Differentiation Between Stuttering and Normal Disfluency

Our impression that parents usually are reliable in diagnosing stuttering in their child was formed early on in studies of the onset of stuttering (Yairi, 1983) and has been repeatedly confirmed over the years (Ambrose & Yairi, 1999). In our experience, the identification of early stuttering in clinical settings is seldom difficult. We wonder why several authors (e.g., M. R. Adams, 1977; Conture, 2001; Gordon & Luper, 1992; Manning, 2001; Pindzola, 1987) have expressed a different opinion, emphasizing the great overlap and possible confusion between early stuttering and normal disfluency, and cautioning clinicians of the difficult task. Gordon and Luper (1992) stated that "speech–language pathologists often struggle with the differentiation of stuttering from normal disfluencies in young children" (p. 43). Perhaps this thinking results from a combination of the remaining influence of Wendell Johnson's theory about parents' mistaking normal disfluency for stuttering and his disfluency data that led him and others to emphasize overlap between children regarded as stutterers and those regarded as normally fluent, overlooking certain critical differences. As stated, our experience has shown no evidence that many parents confuse normal disfluency with stuttering. The data demonstrate that our clinical judgment that a child stutters and our overall severity rating of the stuttering are close to those of the parents (Ambrose & Yairi, 1999; Yairi, 1983; Yairi & Ambrose, 1999a). A similar conclusion was reached by Curlee (1999b, p. 3), who wrote, "I can recall only a handful of parental misdiagnoses of stuttering in over 25 years of clinical practice." Regardless of the degree of ease of identification, comprehensive diagnostic data are helpful in facilitating the next step: the decision regarding treatment of the young stuttering child (Yaruss, LaSalle, & Conture, 1998).

One of the reasons for the general ease in diagnosing is that clinicians typically do not examine large random samples of the entire population of preschool children ages 2 to 5. They do not face the task of dealing with the full range of the fluency–disfluency continuum in children who do and do not stutter. When the full disfluency range of the population is plotted, one may expect a gray area. The typical clinical caseload, however, is a selective subset of the population at large, consisting of children suspected by concerned parents or others to exhibit behaviors or characteristics that are beyond normal. Furthermore, when stuttering begins mildly, parents typically wait until their concern grows before seeking help. Therefore, it is very likely that these children are above the gray area for the population at large. In fact, only 24% of parents in our studies rated their children's stuttering as mild and, for the most part, those were also clear cases.

Occasionally in clinical settings, a child suspected of stuttering falls within a zone of uncertainty in terms of disfluency characteristics. As discussed in Chapter 4, however, when disfluency data are analyzed properly, possible overlap can be greatly reduced. Several disfluency measures (Ambrose & Yairi, 1995, 1999) may be applied to make reasonably clear differentiation between unambiguous stuttering (Onslow & Packman, 2001) and those few who are, by inference, ambiguous cases or normally fluent.

Additionally, perceptual data such as severity ratings from clinicians and parents can add significantly to diagnostic decisions. On the other hand, there is also a question in principle of whether the concept of ambiguous stuttering is clinically meaningful. If a case is so unclear as to be difficult to determine whether it is very mild stuttering or normal disfluency, a stuttering problem does not exist at that time. This is the key issue for the practicing clinician. Borderline disfluency–stuttering is *not* a phase through which all children who stutter must pass; it is not a gate to stuttering that can be shut. Finally, although the confusion between normal and abnormal disfluency in the clinical setting has been exaggerated in the literature, this does not mean that a distinction is always clear-cut at the time when parents notice, for the *first* time, something different in the child's speech. At that time, the child is not yet a part of the more selective group eventually seen in clinical settings. Nevertheless, as we have conceded, if the speech sample of a very large number of randomly selected children in the general population were to be examined, a few would fall into a gray area and be difficult to classify as either normally fluent or stuttering (Ambrose & Yairi, 2001).

Stuttering Subtypes Differentiation

Whereas the differentiation of early childhood stuttering from other communication disorders is typically a straightforward matter, further differential diagnosis *within* the disorder of stuttering is limited at present. The idea that people who stutter can be classified according to types or subgroups can be traced back several hundreds of years (Preus, 1981). Hypothetical *etiologies* have been used as the bases of several classifications. For example, Luchsinger and Arnold (1965) proposed six types of stuttering: organic (inherited), symptomatic (of organic lesions), developmental, traumatic, physiological, and hysterical. In 1963, St. Onge suggested three types: organic, psychogenic, and speech phobic. Brill's (1923) psychologically based classification and Canter's (1971) neurogenic types of stuttering provide additional examples.

A second frame of reference for subtyping has been prominent *characteristics of stuttering* or behaviors of the stutterer. Froeschels (1943) suggested clonic or tonic stuttering, whereas Douglass and Quarrington (1952) proposed the interiorized versus exteriorized stuttering distinction. A third approach to classification was based on *characteristics of the stutterer,* such as familial history (Seider, Gladstien, & Kidd, 1982, 1983) or ear preference in dichotic listening (Hinkle, 1971). Still others used grouping of variables into *factors* pertaining to the characteristics of stutterers and/or stuttering (Andrews & Harris, 1964; G. D. Riley, 1981; G. D. Riley & Riley, 2000; Van Riper, 1971). Within this approach, H. D. Schwartz and Conture (1988) used objective measures of speech and nonspeech characteristics, such as disfluency type ratios, to derive subgrouping factors.

In spite of the apparent diversity in stuttering manifestations and a good number of references to typology in the literature, overwhelmingly, experts have dealt with stuttering as a single disorder. In countless studies and clinical programs, adults and children who stutter participated under the assumption that all exhibit the same disorder. To date, despite the long list of proposed typologies, there have been no indications either in the literature or among professional circles, such as the International Fluency Association or the Fluency Specialty Division of the American Speech-Language-Hearing Association, of any progress toward either identification or agreement on subtypes or subgroups of stuttering. Currently, whatever differentiation is made appears to be limited to statements regarding the general developmental stage of the disorder, such as early or advanced stuttering, or its overall severity as mild, moderate, or severe. Recent years, however, have seen encouraging progress in the prognostic aspects of the initial evaluation of early childhood stuttering, especially in assessing risks for persistent stuttering. Such advancements enhance clinicians' ability to recommend further action and provide more individualized parent counseling.

Describing and Quantifying the Disorder

Given the limited diagnostic opportunities and differential diagnostic alternatives, the clinician's typical task when first meeting a child who stutters is that of characterization and quantification of the stuttering. In other words, it is more a matter of confirming the parents' diagnosis and of describing the disorder and related factors than of actually diagnosing something that was not apparent right from the beginning. Actual diagnostic work still may be required, considering the risk for concomitant disorders, communication or otherwise, that tend to occur more frequently in children who stutter than in children who do not stutter (G. W. Blood & Seider, 1981). Therefore, the initial evaluation of a young child who stutters also includes comprehensive testing of hearing, language, phonology, motor, and cognitive skills that constitute an integral part of standard speech, language, and hearing evaluations of children. Hence, the clinician has to (a) obtain the pertinent background and history of the disorder, (b) describe and quantify the various aspects of the child's disfluency and other features of stuttering, (c) identify other factors relevant to the stuttering, (d) assess the current stuttering in light of its history and the potential risk factors in order to reach prognosis, (e) assess other communication skills and related conditions, and (f) provide feedback and suggest a course of action. With these considerations in mind, it becomes clear that parents are extremely important participants in the evaluation process of preschool-age children who stutter. They are the case history source; they take part in the data collection from the child, receive the counseling, and ultimately make the decision about the course of action.

In Chapters 2 through 9, detailed information was provided concerning our research procedures for recording and testing young children who stutter, as well as updated data about disfluencies, onset and development, phonology, language, motor, awareness, genetics, and other aspects and issues pertaining to early childhood stuttering, and upon which clinical interpretations and decisions should be based. At the risk of some duplication, the present chapter addresses all of these with an orientation toward the practicality of clinical situations. Whereas comprehensive initial evaluation protocols with detailed discussions of their components can be found in other sources (e.g., Conture, 2001), our purpose here is to present our point of view on selected issues.

Background and Case History

Assuming that standard items, such as personal identity, family background, health, and physical and speech–language development, are covered in the case history taking, the clinician should ask additional questions aimed at tapping the event of onset and the course of stuttering up to the present. Such questioning is important because the disorder's progress is one of the key components in its overall assessment. Several lead questions and the rationale behind them follow.

🔘 **When did the child begin stuttering?** This question is worthy of patient investigation because information on the time since onset is critical to reaching conclusions regarding the present stuttering status, especially for considering the need for intervention. The reason is simple: Short postonset intervals weigh in favor of a waiting period. As the postonset interval increases, the chance for natural recovery becomes smaller, and intervention may be sought more aggressively. Obviously, the length of post-onset interval depends on accurate determination of the onset date. Because few parents keep documentation about this event, they need to be guided to identify that time period through questions that follow a systematically reduced bracketing pattern that narrows the possible time range. Encouraging the parents to recall the onset in reference to other events, such as birthdays, holidays, trips, illnesses, and so forth, can be quite helpful. For example, if the parents estimate that the child began stuttering in March or April, asking if he was already stuttering during the Easter holiday might help their recollection. If onset is estimated to have occurred in early summer, then these questions are appropriate: Did he already stutter before school let out? Was he stuttering on the 4th of July? We take our time on this single question, revisiting it later in the interview and in subsequent meetings, asking parents to search their memory and consult with other family members. Examples of exchanges with parents in an attempt to pinpoint the date of onset were presented in Chapter 3. Interestingly, a study in Britain (Buck & Lees, 2000) found a trend for children who had early onset to also recover, whereas those reported with late onset had a greater tendency to persist. Our data confirm such a trend, bordering on statistical significance, but more data and detailed analyses are needed.

Ⓠ **What were the initial signs or characteristics?** We ask parents to describe in their own words, as well as imitate, the earliest possible indications of stuttering—that is, how the child spoke and what she did that was thought to be stuttering. It is best to obtain a variety of examples. Next, we seek more structured input by verbally presenting parents with a list of common disfluencies, secondary characteristics, and emotional reactions, one at a time, accompanied with vivid examples and clinician demonstration. The checklist is used because many parents are unable to express in words all the details of the stuttering and because their passive memory, triggered by the list, is often better than their active memory. For each item, they are to indicate whether the characteristic was present *at onset*, and if so, to what degree (see Figure 10.1). Throughout this procedure, it is important to continuously remind the parents to focus on the onset, *not* on the current stuttering.

The resultant checklist and additional description constitute the baseline symptomatology. Although Van Riper (1971) used initial symptomatology for his subgroup classification, so far our research has discerned only a few possible trends in this regard. In any event, we conclude this

EARLY STUTTERING: SPEECH, SECONDARY CHARACTERISTICS, AND COGNITIVE AND EMOTIONAL REACTIONS

Directions: Indicate whether the following characteristics were observed at onset.

Characteristic/Reaction	Never	Sometimes	Frequently
Speech			
1. Repeating syllables (ba-ba-baby)	1	2	3
2. Repeating words (and-and)	1	2	3
3. Repeating phrases (let me-let me)	1	2	3
4. Prolonging vowels (a→a)	1	2	3
5. Prolonging consonants (s→s, m→m)	1	2	3
6. Broken words (Ba——by)	1	2	3
7. Incomplete words (ba-)	1	2	3
8. Silent blocks (→b←aby)	1	2	3
9. Interjecting (ah, um)	1	2	3
10. Upward swings in pitch	1	2	3
11. Loudness during disfluencies	1	2	3
12. Others _____	1	2	3
_____	1	2	3
Secondary Characteristics			
13. Facial grimaces	1	2	3
14. Eye closing/blink	1	2	3
15. Tense lips	1	2	3
16. Tense tongue	1	2	3
17. Wide-open mouth	1	2	3
18. Tension in throat	1	2	3
19. Respiratory irregularities	1	2	3
20. Head tilt	1	2	3
21. Tense movement of arms and legs	1	2	3
22. Others _____	1	2	3
_____	1	2	3
Cognitive and Emotional Reactions			
23. Awareness (describe) _____	1	2	3
24. Emotional reaction (describe) _____	1	2	3

©2004 by PRO-ED, Inc.

Figure 10.1. Inventory for initial signs and characteristics of stuttering.

part of the case history by having parents respond to the Parent Stuttering Severity Scale (see more details in Chapter 2) by judging the stuttering at the time of onset. It requests overall stuttering severity judgments using an 8-point rating scale from 0 to 7. Zero is defined as *normally fluent*, 1 as *borderline*, 2 as *mild*, 3 as *mild to moderate*, 4 as *moderate*, 5 as *moderate to severe*, 6 as *severe*, and 7 as *very severe*. Parents are allowed to choose points halfway between intervals. After obtaining this severity baseline, the clinician can compare the parents' judgment with the clinician's own rating.

In this part of the interview, the objectives are to verify the parents' judgment that indeed it was stuttering that they recognized at the identified time of onset, help them focus on the details of the problem, and derive onset baselines. The importance of baseline data becomes apparent as the evaluation progresses because the current stuttering can be compared to that at onset. Also, the parents' task of analyzing the child's stuttering and its background might produce secondary therapeutic values, helping them take a good look at and reassess their home environment and family style. Johnson et al. (1959) were convinced that the lengthy parent interviews they conducted for their study of stuttering onset were instrumental in the eventual improvement reported for many of the children.

⊚ **How did it happen?** This question pertains to the manner of onset. Did the stuttering begin gradually or suddenly? How long did it take the parents to realize that the child was stuttering? Was it over several weeks or a few days, or was it an abrupt, overnight change? Again, although at present, the state of knowledge about the manner of onset does not provide definite clues for either differential diagnosis or prognosis, the details are revealing and can turn the parents' or the clinician's attention to various possible contributing events or conditions. (These are pursued in considering the next question.) Our data show that stuttering associated with sudden onsets tends to be perceived as more severe; perhaps it is the severity that calls parents' immediate attention.

⊚ **What were the circumstances surrounding onset?** The general issue of circumstances surrounding onset invites several related questions regarding the child's physical and emotional health at the time of or a few weeks prior to onset, with attention to conditions and events in the child's personal life or in the family that could have triggered or complicated the stuttering. Was the child sick or exceedingly tired? Was a new sibling born? Was there a death in the family? Was there a job loss in the household? Was there a problem in the day care center? Was there a change in sitters or day care personnel? In essence, we pursue leads for possible stressors that may have facilitated or complicated the onset. At the least, these questions shed light on the child's home environment and the parents' evaluation of and reaction to the events discussed. Information gathered about the manner of onset may prompt us to discuss additional specific circumstances more intensely. For example, sharp recollections of a sudden onset would tend to increase our interest in either emotional or physical events. On the other hand, an apparent noneventful, gradual onset would prompt us to look for more subtle events or processes that parents may have overlooked. This possibility leads us to the next question.

◎ **What other factors might have been involved?** This broad question invites parents to look at parameters that have not been among their or the clinician's prime suspects. Conditions, processes, and behaviors, such as accelerated or delayed language development, nutrition, and apparently unrelated medical issues, might surface.

◎ **Who might be a contributor?** Attention is focused on specific people the parents suspect to have directly or indirectly contributed to or influenced the child's stuttering but who have not been brought up earlier in the interview. Negative influences assumed by the parents, such as models provided by relatives who stutter or by other children who stutter at the sitter's home or day care center, as well as actions or expressed attitudes by parents, siblings, and others, should be explored. In several cases, an uncle's tickling the child under the armpit has been seriously stated as a plausible cause of the child's stuttering. Although many of these explanations are typically rejected by most scientists, they should be evaluated on their merit in each case. What appear to be "fantastic" stories may contain elements of truth.

The main line of inquiry related to this question is the history of stuttering in the families of both parents. Currently, it appears that a general positive or negative familial history of stuttering has little diagnostic value. Inasmuch as history is positive, however, what is important is the specific type of history. The objective is to identify trends for either persistent or recovered familial stuttering, because such trends do have diagnostic value, as discussed later in this chapter. Toward this end, drawing a complete pedigree that comprises the families of both parents, including the child's grandparents, uncles, aunts, cousins, parents, and siblings, serves to keep

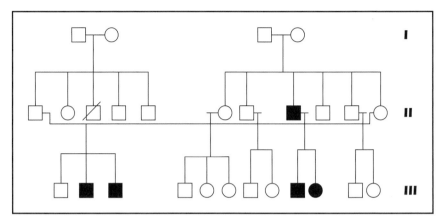

Figure 10.2. Sample pedigree. Circles = females; squares = males; filled-in symbol = stuttering; line through symbol = deceased.

reasonably accurate records of all members. Each family member is added to the picture using conventional genetic symbols. Past or present stuttering is indicated, as well as the time period when the person stuttered and the severity of the stuttering, if known. Other relatives in the extended family, such as a grandparent's sister, can be added if stuttering history was indicated. Of course, the source of information and all possible verifications are sought. Parents are always encouraged, and repeatedly reminded in future contacts, to investigate stuttering history with all living relatives and in the family's record. Telephone calls to these relatives may add significantly to the reliability of claims. Figure 10.2 provides a sample pedigree. The top row represents the grandparents; the second row, the parents, aunts, and uncles; the third row, the child, siblings, and cousins. A horizontal line represents union, and a vertical line links parents with their offspring.

ⓠ **How has the stuttering progressed?** This is a good point in the interview to pursue an examination of the developmental course of the stuttering. Alterations in overt and covert characteristics from onset to present are brought into focus, keeping in mind that this information is likely to have important practical implications. Neither the description of the initial stuttering nor the present stuttering, each in and of itself, is as meaningful as the comparison of the amount and direction of the differences that have taken place over time. Such an understanding of the course of the child's stuttering places the clinician in a good position to assess the problem in perspective. For example, a current severity rating of 5 (on our 0-to-7 scale) should be alarming if the case history reveals that the initial stuttering was rated by the parent as 2. A rating of 5 would be viewed as a positive sign, however, if the initial stuttering were rated as 7. Knowing that the disorder has diminished in severity would have a significant impact on the outlook for the child's prognosis and on the counseling given to parents concerning intervention.

In answer to the question about progression, parents are to describe in their own words the general course of stuttering and changes they have observed in the overt stuttering characteristics and in the child's reactions. We encourage parents to provide several imitations that are as accurate as possible. Next, we proceed with a more structured input concerning the course of stuttering by asking parents to respond again to the list of characteristics presented previously (Figure 10.1) but applied to current stuttering. The clinician provides examples and vivid demonstrations. For each item the parents indicate whether it has been recently present and, if so, at what frequency. The questioning proceeds into details such as the number of iterations per instance of repetition, the estimated length of sound prolongations, and the level of tension; all are factors that contribute to the assessed direction of the change. Moving through the list this time, however, the clinician needs to continuously remind the parents to describe the *current* stuttering, not the status at onset. Finally, we ask the parents to rate the child's current overall stuttering severity using our 8-point scale. When parents report substantial changes in severity between onset and the present, we ask them to give additional ratings to indicate peaks or valleys in severity during that period.

In summary, parent input regarding stuttering at onset and its current status, including general description, responses to checklists, and severity ratings, provides excellent information to be used in the final assessment of the case.

Speech Data

Having obtained a comprehensive case history and the parents' subjective descriptions, judgment, and rating of the child's stuttering, or, in the rare situation, upon learning that they are uncertain of whether the child truly stutters, the clinician shifts the focus of the evaluation to his or her own observations and subjective impressions, as well as more quantitative analyses of the child's speech. Typically, prior to any formal procedures, clinicians have several opportunities to hear the child talking as they accompany the family in the hallways, elevator, waiting room, and so on. The child may talk to the parents, respond to the clinician's greetings, or speak in another context. These are important encounters that contribute to forming initial impressions of stuttering. For this reason, we advise keeping a small hand-held tape recorder with a small, but sensitive cord microphone. It might provide useful segments of the child's spontaneous speech to add to the recordings obtained in the formal session. Nevertheless, now is the time for an in-depth analysis using a sufficiently long recorded speech sample of a reasonably good quality. This sample constitutes part of the hard data for the child's disfluency, as well as other speech and language parameters.

Recording Settings and Materials

Desirable conversational speech can be obtained in one of several alternative physical settings, such as a testing room with the child sitting at a small table or on a playroom floor while interacting with a parent or clinician. The evaluation also can be performed at home. For achieving a more accurate as well as complete analysis, a video recording of the conversation is preferable to audio only. Unclear, complex instances of disfluency that are difficult to discern from audio recording often can be resolved by observing the visual image of the child. Secondary characteristics or affective reactions during stuttering also can be better documented upon reviewing the videotape. To be effective for all of these purposes, the camera should be focused on the child's face. Occasionally this is difficult, if not impossible, to achieve if the child is allowed to move about the room while the camera remains stationary. Some clinicians prefer the unrestrictive play situation, assuming that it elicits more natural verbal expression. This kind of setting, however, significantly diminishes the usefulness of video recording for the purposes of stuttering analyses. We have had excellent experience obtaining speech samples with the child seated, quite happily, at a chair–table setting in a small test room (e.g., sound-treated booth), yielding both good speech output and high-quality video and audio recordings.

A cord-connected microphone rather than a built-in microphone is recommended because it yields considerably cleaner-sounding speech. A small tie-tack microphone attached to the child's shirt or a high-quality desk microphone may be used. If the latter is used, the microphone should be positioned several inches above the table (on a separate wall-mounted shelf or suspended from above) to protect it from the child's banging on the table, movement of toys and paper, and so on. Along these lines, quiet play material, such as clay and several interesting action pictures are preferable. Plastic and wooden toys generate noise that interferes with the quality of the recording. Additionally, the clinician should consider removing the child's shoes, because restless children sometimes repeatedly bang the chair or the floor with their shoes, creating interfering noise. In less restricted settings, when the child is allowed to move about the room, the tie-tack microphone is superior to other types. We also have obtained good results with sensitive, inexpensive, omnidirectional microphones.

In some situations, audio recording alone can provide sufficient information for clinical purposes. Even when video is used, simultaneously obtaining audio recording as a backup is desirable. The audio recording also serves as the working copy when transcribing the sample and relistening for disfluencies. The ease of transcription depends on the type of equipment available. Recently, computer programs have become available that allow speech analysis from compact discs (CDs).

The Speech Sample

As stated in Chapter 4, a minimum of 30 minutes of verbal interaction, obtained over two sessions separated by several days, is recommended. Approximately half of the speech sample should be between the child and a parent and half between the child and the clinician. Although a sufficiently long sample can be obtained within a shorter time, depending on the talkativeness of the child, and although there are no data showing that 30 minutes is the minimum, time is needed to observe the child's behavior, reaction, and interaction. We record 40 minutes total over 2 different days to obtain a long speech sample, as well as to minimize the effects of any known or unknown factors that influence the child's speech on a given day. Long speech samples also are desired for the sake of valid and reliable speech data. The longer the sample, the better the opportunity to observe the child's full potential for stuttering. In particular, we are interested in observing what the child does when he or she stutters, which may be during only part of the sample, especially in very mild or borderline cases. Although we have settled on 600 syllables as the minimum, to obtain solid disfluency data, speech samples should approximate 1,000 syllables or even more. Data by Sawyer and Yairi (2003), as discussed in Chapter 4, show that in four consecutive 300-syllable segments taken from continuous 1,200-syllable speech samples of 20 children who stutter, the greatest amount of disfluency tended to occur in the last two segments, especially the fourth one. Therefore, had we used only the first 300 syllables, some or much of the children's disfluency would not have been reflected in the data.

Given that there are several measures of clinical interest, including disfluency, language, and phonology, quality speech samples yield quality data. Several scholars (e.g., Lund & Duchan, 1993) have suggested that reliability and validity are significantly enhanced through the use of longer samples. In regard to our focus, several disfluency types, such as sound prolongations or blocks, and complex disfluent events (e.g., those containing four or more repetition units) might occur in low frequency and simply cannot be adequately assessed if only one or two specimens occur in a short sample, if at all. The validity of the data would then be questionable and the reliability at risk. Therefore, we take a skeptical view of the typical 300-syllable samples often reported in disfluency studies (Conture & Kelly, 1991; Meyers, 1986; Yaruss, 1997) or the fewer than 100-utterance length used in many past investigations involving language analyses. Although 300 syllables or words may be sufficient for a good number of children, subject variability is large, making it impossible to trust that a short sample would be sufficient. As we have reported, longer samples appear to be particularly desirable for children who initially exhibit mild stuttering. Although Conture (2001) opined that clinical situations are not always ideal and shorter samples are, at times, inevitable, this argument does not explain why short, clinically obtained speech samples have been used in many basic and clinical studies. Unfortunately, it appears that short samples have become the standard rather than the exception. Clinicians should be encouraged to conduct a thorough evaluation. If the speech sample is short, it should be supplemented with additional recording time either at the clinic or at home.

For recording purposes, having clay on the table is very helpful in getting a conversation started and keeping the child busy and in place. After starting with a conversation about what the child is making, we switch to open-ended questions and prompts regarding the child's favorite toys, TV shows, or movies to stimulate longer responses. Questions that invite yes–no or other one-word responses should be minimized; not only can they be conversation stoppers, but also single words typically are not stuttered as often as words in phrases and sentences. Unless the child is significantly delayed in language skills, too many single words in a speech sample will bias, in a downward direction, his or her apparent level of stuttering. Single words are also less desirable for language analysis purposes.

To elicit more than single-word responses, the clinician should ask, for example, "So what happened next in the show?" rather than "Did the good guys win?" or "Why do you fight with your sister?" instead of "Do you fight with your sister?" In discussion of a TV show or movie, it is often helpful for the clinician to mention something specific about it, to bring the child's mind into the story. Remarks such as "Did you see the movie *Shrek*? I thought it was really gross when he put bugs on his toothbrush" often draw much more conversation than "Did you see *Shrek*? What was it about?" The clinician should ask the parents about topics that particularly excite the child, including recent family events or mishaps, particular pets, toys, TV shows, and so on. With the younger child, age 2 or so, the clinician needs to focus on the present, on what is happening right at the moment. Skills in abstraction often limit the ability of a child this age to explain a plot or report what he or she did over the summer. It is important to follow the child's lead. If the clinician asks, "What movie do you like?" and the child responds "Make a bigger monster," then the clinician should make the monster and pursue that topic. On the other hand, it is important for the clinician to minimize his or her own talking to leave the child space for expression.

Using these techniques will elicit more complex and longer utterances from the child, and this is where stuttering tends to be exhibited. Typically, however, stuttering also increases with heightening emotion, such as excitement or frustration. The conversational partner can fairly easily control these (e.g., by feigning ignorance of a topic, asking the obvious, or acting and sounding excited). We have found all of these strategies to be excellent for stimulating ongoing verbal output and for revealing more of the child's stuttering. It is a most enjoyable goal to discover what triggers increased speech output for each child.

Overall Stuttering Severity

While recording, the clinician makes online subjective estimates of four aspects of the child's disfluencies to derive an overall stuttering severity rating. If a videotape is available, rating can be done at a later time. As discussed in Chapter 2, in our Clinician Stuttering Severity Scale (see Figure 2.1), scoring is broken down into four components: Stuttering-Like Disfluencies (SLD), duration, and tension of disfluency, as well as the extent of secondary characteristics. The first three are rated from 0 (*normally fluent speech*) to 6 (*severe stuttering*) and their mean is calculated. Secondary characteristics are then rated separately, on a scale from 0 to 1, and this number is added to the mean of the first three items. A maximum score of 7 (*very severe stuttering*) could thus be obtained if frequency, duration, and tension are rated as 6 and secondary characteristics as 1.

Disfluency Analyses and Counts

Type and Frequency

After securing a tape-recorded speech sample, the clinician's next task is to identify and quantify stuttering or disfluency. Some clinicians prefer making categorical judgments of each word or syllable as either stuttered or not. The number of stuttered words per 100 spoken words (or the percentage of words stuttered) in the speech sample is then determined. For example, in a 583-word sample, a clinician judged 28 words as stuttered. To calculate the percentage of words stuttered, the clinician multiplies the number of stuttered words by 100, then divides the outcome by the total number of words in the sample. Applying this formula to the sample specified above looks as follows: $28 \times 100/583 = 4.8\%$. The same calculations can be performed with the metric of percentage of stuttered syllables.

In some respects, this is the easiest, least time-consuming method of quantifying stuttering, and does provide basic information. As suggested in Chapter 4, however, in addition to difficulties arising from differences in listeners' identification of stuttering, the percentage of stuttered words or syllables metric provides virtually no information about the specific characteristics of an individual child's stuttering. Does the stuttering consist primarily of repetitions? Are sound prolongations included in the repertoire? Such information is missing when clinicians report 4.8% stuttered words. Furthermore, the report does not indicate whether words that contained repetitions were repeated once or eight times. Because there is a growing body of information showing the significance of specific disfluency types in differential diagnosis and prognosis (e.g., H. D. Schwartz & Conture, 1988; Throneburg & Yairi, 2001), we much prefer a complete analysis of frequency, type, and length of disfluencies. Furthermore, inasmuch as the child's progress is monitored over time, whether the child is in therapy or not, changes in the specific disfluent types and their extent or length, rather than simply the total number of stuttering events, are of great interest.

Toward this end, after carefully transcribing the child's speech, we replay the tape, sentence by sentence, phrase by phrase, or word by word.

Using symbols for the six disfluency types that we use (see Chapter 4 for detailed descriptions), we mark all disfluent speech events on the transcript. The total of each disfluency type in the sample and per 100 syllables is calculated. Next, we add the numbers of those types that constitute SLD and those that constitute Other Disfluencies. We then add these two figures to yield Total Disfluencies. The resultant data for a sample of 1,238 syllables is shown as an example in Table 10.1. These disfluency data are well within the typical range for the early stage of stuttering, reflecting a level between high-mild and low-moderate stuttering. The largest number of disfluencies are of the repetitive type (part-word and monosyllabic-word repetition). Furthermore, the SLD constitute 67% of the total number of disfluencies. Yairi (1997a) has shown this to be an important group characteristic of early childhood stuttering. It should be recognized, however, that individual children vary in this respect.

Length: Extent and Duration

In addition to type and frequency determinations, the disfluency analysis also should include calculation of the *extent* of SLD types that are of repetitive character. For each instance of part-word and single-syllable word rep-

Table 10.1

Example of Disfluency Data Collected on a Sample of 1,238 Syllables

Disfluency Type	Number in Sample	Per 100 Syllables
Stuttering-Like Disfluencies (SLD)		
Part-word repetition	31	2.50
Monosyllabic-word repetition	22	1.78
Disrhythmic phonation	19	1.53
Total SLD	72	5.81
Other Disfluencies		
Interjection	16	1.29
Revision	11	0.89
Phrase repetition	9	0.73
Total Other Disfluencies	36	2.91
Total Disfluencies	108	8.72

etition, the clinician counts the number of *extra* productions. For example, in "bu-but," the number of repetition units is one. In "bu-bu-but," the number of repetition units is two. In "bu-bu-bu-bu-but," the number of repetition units is four. Part-word and whole-word repetitions are combined for this purpose. Several measures can be obtained. The data can be used to calculate the range and the mean number of repetition units. Additionally, it is important to keep track of the number of disfluency instances that contain various numbers of repetition units (i.e., 1, 2, 3, or 4 units). This information can yield a very useful measure: the number of disfluency instances per 100 syllables that contained two or more repetition units. In fact, this measure is perhaps the most powerful diagnostic information for differentiating early stuttering from normal disfluency (Ambrose & Yairi, 1995, 1999). From our own current data, as described in Chapter 4, very early stuttering contains an average of 8.72 part-word and single-syllable word repetitions per 100 syllables. Of these, 5.60 are single-unit repetitions, and 3.12 are repetitions with 2 or more units. In contrast, normally fluent speech in children the same age has only 1.34 instances of repetitions per 100 syllables, of which 1.15 are single-unit repetitions and 0.19 are multiple-unit repetitions. In other words, over 35% of the repetitions of children who stutter are multiple-unit repetitions, whereas about 14% of the repetitions of normally fluent children contain 2 or more repetition units.

If a child exhibits many instances of sound prolongation, estimates of the mean *duration* of the three or five longest instances are informative. Because a large percentage of sound prolongations fall within the 1-second range (Bloodstein, 1995), the mean duration of all prolongations is not particularly meaningful. However, information concerning the high end of the range can be revealing. A few prolongations of 2 seconds or longer are sufficient to critically increase the overall perceived degree of stuttering severity. Thus, the clinician is encouraged to identify and measure or estimate the length of the longest prolongations. Those above 1 second are strong indications of stuttering (Zebrowski & Conture, 1989).

Another parameter to consider in evaluating length of disfluencies is the *intervals* between repetition units. These deserve special attention as they may reveal information that is more important than the total duration of the disfluent event. We showed in Chapter 4 (see Table 4.8) that, compared with normally fluent children, children who stutter tend to exhibit considerably shorter silent intervals between syllables or words that they repeat. In other words, children who stutter repeat faster, whereas normally fluent children repeat slower (Throneburg & Yairi, 1994; Yairi & Hall,

1993). This behavior appears to be true from the very early stage of stuttering. In children who stutter, the interval constitutes the smallest portion of the total disfluency; it is the biggest portion in disfluencies of normally fluent children. Our analyses revealed that interval duration alone was sufficient to differentiate stuttering from nonstuttering children with 72% to 87% accuracy, depending on disfluency type. In short, clinicians should pay attention to the tempo of repetitions.

Metric

A few additional comments regarding the merit of employing the disfluencies-per-100-syllables metric are of special relevance to the clinician. Its general advantages over the disfluencies-per-100-word metric were discussed in Chapter 4 (see also Yairi, 1997a). In brief, because the length of young children's words increases as the children grow older, 10 disfluencies per 100 words at age 2 may not be the same as 10 disfluencies per 100 words at age 4. Because at age 4, children tend to use longer words in greater frequency, their speech samples contain more speech. Thus, 10 disfluencies affect a smaller proportion of the speech output than at age 2 years: Whereas the number of disfluencies (10) is the same, there appears to be a reduction in the 4-year-old's disfluency relative to the amount of speech. That is, the child seems to have improved.

Recently, however, Conture (2001) questioned our position, arguing that there have been no data to support our argument about the advantage of the syllable metric and that, in any event, it would make no difference in making the distinction between a normally fluent child and a child who stutters. Conture perhaps has overlooked the essence, as well as the specific implications, of our position. First, because children during the preschool years increasingly use longer words and show a wide range of language skills, the syllable measure provides a constant common denominator for comparing frequency of disfluency among children of different ages and of different language skills. Being based on smaller units, it is undoubtedly a more precise measure than the word metric. If clinical decisions are to be scientifically sound, why advocate a less precise measure purely for the sake of convenience? We should strive to match proclaimed clinical ideals with actual clinical routine. Second, the objective of the initial evaluation is not limited to the determination of whether or not the child stutters. There are additional goals, such as providing sound baseline data for future comparisons of the same child (e.g., in monitoring progress in therapy or without therapy). For this purpose and in the stated age range, the syllable metric has a clear advantage.

Secondary Characteristics
As discussed in previous chapters, secondary characteristics have received little attention in research of early stuttering, perhaps because traditionally they have been regarded as late developing, occurring with more "advanced" stuttering. More recently, frame-by-frame videotape analyses of disfluent events in the speech of young children who stutter have demonstrated the presence of head and neck movements in children near the onset of stuttering (Conture & Kelly, 1991; Throneburg, 1997; Yairi, Ambrose, & Niermann, 1993). Present data on the actual number of movements during disfluencies are rather sparse and inconclusive; as Throneburg has shown, quite a few movements also appear in matched fluent segments.

In Chapter 4 we also provided perceptual rating data, estimating that almost 75% of the children had some physical behaviors during stuttering that were observed without the aid of slow-motion video. These behaviors ranged from lip pursing and eye blinking to foot stomping, head turning, and so on. Our strong impression is that these movements were part of the stuttering, without the children's conscious thought of coping or adapting mechanisms.

Diagnosing and
Differentiating Stuttering

As previously stated, the risk for a "false alarm" (inappropriately identifying a child as a stutterer) or a "miss" (incorrectly judging a child who begins to stutter as being normally fluent) is rather small, especially in conventional clinical settings or schools. In most cases, clinicians' judgments based on overall impressions, with particular attention to the presence of Stuttering-Like Disfluencies, confirm parental diagnoses. Subjective perceptual judgments of the presence of stuttering, which also serve as the basis for severity ratings by clinician and parent, require substantiation with descriptive speech data obtained from the child. These individual data are matched against current population data on the average percentage of stuttered words or syllables, type or frequency of disfluency, extent or duration of disfluency, level of tension, and secondary characteristics. We have preferred employing detailed disfluency analyses rather than straight "stuttering counts" because they provide much more information about the characteristics of the stuttering and other disfluent speech behavior.

Average Disfluency Data for Stuttering Preschoolers

Practically speaking, what should a speech–language clinician look for in the disfluency data derived from the speech sample for either the initial diagnostic evaluation of a young beginning stutterer or in subsequent evaluations of the child's progress? Primarily, it is important to have a good idea about stuttering preschool children's average data for various dimensions of disfluency. For the majority of children for whom diagnosis based on perceptual judgment and analyses of speech features is clear cut, clinicians would probably wish to compare the child's speech characteristics with such averages. Searching past and more recent literature, including our own findings (see Chapter 4), we have identified several disfluency indices for early stuttering that are of special interest because of their strength. Those that are of more immediate practical value to the practicing clinician are listed in Table 10.2 in Group 1. Others that are important but more difficult to assess in conventional clinical settings are presented in Group 2. (See Yairi, 1997a, for a comprehensive review.) Hopefully, with improved skills and availability of technology, measures listed under Group 2 also will become part of the routine protocol.

The disfluency data in Table 10.2 indicate wide ranges. They can be used, however, as a guideline for meaningful, comprehensive descriptions of a child's speech relative to that of other children who stutter. Future, perhaps computerized diagnostic instruments may become more sophisticated by incorporating many of these features. In order to judge severity, the clinician needs to consider combined measures.

Table 10.3 gives ranges for both the clinician stuttering severity rating (based on the frequency, length, and tension of disfluencies, plus the rating for secondary characteristics, as calculated using the scale shown in Figure 2.1), which is a more subjective measure, and weighted SLD (frequency, type, and length of disfluencies), which is more objective. Children usually, but not always, fall into the same or a similar severity level for both measures.

Table 10.2

Disfluency Data for Early Stuttering: Mean, Range, and Percentage

Measure (Frequency per 100 Syllables)	M	Range	Percentage
Group 1			
Part-word repetitions (PW)	5.5	1.5–9.5	
Single-syllable word repetitions (SS)	3	1–25	
Disrhythmic phonation	2.5	0.5–12	
Repetition units	1.5	1–5	
Stuttering-Like Disfluencies (SLD)	11	3–40	67% of Total Disfluencies
Weighted SLD	20	4–100	
Repetitions (PW + SS) with 2 or more *extra* units	3	1–20	30% of repetitions
Other disfluencies	6	1.5–16	36% of Total Disfluencies
Total disfluencies	17	5–50	
Group 2			
Disfluencies in clusters	3 per cluster		50% of Total Disfluencies
Face and head movements per disfluency		1.5–3	
Duration of disfluencies	750 msec		
Duration of interval between repetition units	200 msec		
Proportion of silent interval to total duration for repetitions (PW + SS) with 1 *extra* unit		0.25–0.33	

Table 10.3

Severity Levels of Stuttering and Corresponding Clinician Severity Ratings and Weighted Stuttering-Like Disfluency (SLD) Scores

Severity Level	Clinician Severity Rating	Weighted SLD Score
Mild	1.00–2.99	4.00–9.99
Moderate	3.00–4.99	10.00–24.99
Severe	5.00–7.00	≥25.00

Differential Criteria

For "borderline" children—that is, those perceived to present a challenge in terms of determining their fluency status as stuttering—consulting with group means is not very helpful for differential diagnosis decisions. In these cases, the clinician needs data that define a cardinal rule for what are indictors of stuttering: the minimal requirements of overt disfluent characteristics needed to classify a person as exhibiting stuttering or, in other words, data that show points of no, or minimal, overlap between children who stutter and normally speaking children. These are combined with descriptive information and the perceptual rating to facilitate conclusions.

Several previous diagnostic protocols (see review by Gordon & Luper, 1992) have offered criteria for speech and nonspeech characteristics of stuttering that, for the most part, seem to fit the typical range of cases, but do not provide clear grounds for discrimination at the very low end of the range where the difficulty may lie. In 1977, M. R. Adams suggested five criteria for differentiating stuttering from normal disfluency. Children who stutter are likely to exhibit (a) at least 10 disfluencies per 100 words, (b) high frequency of part-word repetitions and sound prolongations, (c) repetitions and prolongations marked with abnormal termination of voice and airflow, (d) repetitions consisting of at least three iterations, and (e) vowels in repetitions that are perceived as schwa. In contrast, normally fluent children have no more than 5 disfluencies per 100 words, only a few of which are part-word repetitions. These part-word repetitions do not involve abrupt stoppages of voice and airflow, do not include more than three iterations, and do not involve inappropriate inclusion of schwa. Adams assigned equal significance to each of the five parameters.

Unfortunately, the scientific basis of Adams's (1977) scheme is questionable. He relied on information that was outdated at the time, while overlooking the large body of disfluency data published by Johnson et al. (1959). It is not clear why 10 disfluencies were set as the minimum, what kinds of disfluencies were included, and what a "high frequency" of part-word repetitions and sound prolongation means. He suggested that repetitions containing *at least* three iterations should be taken as a sign of stuttering; however, this number is greatly exaggerated and does not reflect the relevant data. His statement that Stromsta's (1965) findings indicate abrupt termination of phonation as a differential sign between normally fluent children and those who stutter is in error. Actually, Stromsta differentiated between children who persisted in and those who recovered from stuttering. Finally, Adam's claim regarding the schwa characteristic of repeated vowels has not received experimental support. Our overriding concern, however, is that these criteria serve to characterize stuttering that can be easily diagnosed, not those cases that may present diagnostic challenges.

This last concern also applies to the differentiating protocol by Pindzola and White (1986), which reorganizes many of the suggestions made by M. R. Adams (1977) and Van Riper (1982) but considers more updated data reported by Yairi and Lewis (1984). Furthermore, it also extends to differentiating persistent from episodic stuttering. An important feature, however, is the inclusion of observations of secondary characteristics: facial grimaces, head movement, and body involvement. We agree that the early presence of observable secondary characteristics associated with instances of disfluencies is a helpful diagnostic sign of stuttering. Yaruss et al. (1998) reported diagnostic data that influenced decisions concerning recommendations for treatment, but their report did not offer differential diagnostic criteria.

A well-known clinical attempt to set up minimal differential guidelines was made by Van Riper (1971), who grouped 26 items under seven classes of behaviors: syllable repetitions, prolongations, gaps, phonation, articulating postures, reaction to stress, and awareness. Most of the list's 26 items, however, rely on qualitative judgment. Among the few quantitative items, one requires at least 2 syllable repetitions per 100 words, and another requires a single 1-second sound prolongation per 100 words. Combining these two, it would appear that 3 SLD per 100 words reflect Van Riper's concept of minimum stuttering. Interestingly, however, scientific data gathered by Johnson et al. (1959) for 68 boys and presented according to deciles show that the lowest decile—that is, the 10% of the participants who were least disfluent—exhibited fewer than 3 SLD per 100 words in their speech samples. Only the second decile, those between 11% and 20%, reached that criterion. As described in Chapter 4, however, we have reservations about the composition of that particular sample of children.

To focus attention on the borderline cases that may show signs of stuttering but at low frequency and perceived severity level, we reexamined our past data, as well as those reported in Chapter 4, carefully searching for any indication of minimal group overlap. For stuttering and normally fluent children, group means for frequency of SLD types and repetition units are highly significantly different. This observation, however, is difficult to apply to any single case because of some overlap at low frequencies. For borderline cases (i.e., those with a lower frequency of SLD), two specific features can be helpful in determining stuttering status. The first is presence of clear disrhythmic phonation (i.e., blocks and prolongations) of at least 1 second in duration with physical tension. Even a single instance is a strong indication of stuttering. Normally fluent speakers may exhibit very occasional relaxed sound prolongations, and these are not perceived as abnormal. The second discriminating feature, reported by Ambrose and Yairi (1995), involves long instances of repetitions, those containing three or more units. Therefore, we reemphasize that clinicians should pay careful attention to the number of times a child repeats a syllable or word. Even a few instances of "bu-bu-bu-but," "a-a-a-and," and "on-on-on-on" may literally seal the diagnosis.

The more challenging cases for differential diagnosis are those that are mild. What are the minimal disfluent speech characteristics associated with clinician perception of mild or very mild stuttering? What are the upper limits for normal? Our analysis of data obtained from speech of children perceived as stuttering and those perceived to be normally fluent yielded the differential criteria scheme shown in Table 10.4. At least three of these criteria must be met to consider a child as exhibiting observable stuttering. A few normally fluent children may meet one or two of the criteria.

Although these criteria are somewhat solid, we caution that none has been established as an absolute differential diagnostic sign. Individual dif-

Table 10.4

Disfluency Criteria To Diagnose Mild Stuttering

Measure (Frequency per 100 Syllables)	Minimum Criteria for Stuttering
Part-word repetitions (PW)	≥1.5
Single-syllable word repetitions (SS)	≥2.5
Disrhythmic phonation	≥0.5
Repetition units	≥1.5
Stuttering-Like Disfluency (SLD)	≥3.0
Weighted SLD	≥4.0
Repetitions (PW + SS) with 2 or more *extra* units	≥1.0

Note. The child must meet three criteria to be diagnosed with stuttering.

ferences present strange cases at times. Therefore, we again emphasize that the key to diagnosis lies in multiple measures and indicators. Parents' detailed descriptions and imitations of the child's stuttering at home can provide useful hints. When parents designate the severity of the child's current stuttering as 1.5, clearly describe the stuttering they refer to as occasional "a-a-a-and" or "a-a-a-ai," and by "occasional" they mean daily occurrence, the case should not be dismissed even if the speech sample recorded in the clinic contained only isolated disfluency events that could have been perceived as stuttering. Additional speech samples should be elicited and the child should be closely monitored. In the reverse situation, if parents are unsure but the clinician perceives stuttering at a rating above 1, and the disfluency analysis yields three of the six critical signs, the child should be regarded as exhibiting stuttering. Thus, it is important to integrate the parents' rating, the clinician's rating, and the objective disfluency data. Currently, we are developing a structured, step-by-step differential diagnostic guide for borderline cases.

Other Diagnostic Work

The initial evaluation of children who stutter, like that of other children, should include comprehensive testing of the speech mechanism, phonology, language, and motor skills, as well as a hearing screening. Standard tests or tape-recorded conversational speech samples can be used for phonological and language analyses. Because deficits in these domains may have implications as to whether therapy is initiated, and, if so, what approach should be pursued (e.g., Conture, Louko, & Edwards, 1993), careful assessment must be pursued in addition to the original focus on the stuttering. These aspects of the evaluation, however, are not discussed in this book. Other factors of relevance can be included in an evaluation. Two very different but informative aspects are speaking rate and affective reactions.

Speaking Rate

The overall speaking rate—the number of words or syllables, whether fluent or disfluent, spoken per minute or second—is negatively correlated with stuttering severity. Therefore, rate information is clinically useful in describing and assessing the speech of children who stutter, as well as in monitoring the progress of their stuttering. Reasonable estimates of overall speaking rate can be obtained by measuring several minutes of conversational speech using a stopwatch. As reported in Chapter 8, we employed the more sophisticated measure of articulatory rate derived from fluent speech only. Our data showed that close to stuttering onset, children who stutter tend to exhibit a somewhat slower articulatory rate than their normally fluent peers. Whereas the mean for the stuttering subgroups was 8.43 phones per second ($SD = 1.16$), the mean for the normally fluent group was 11.42 phones per second ($SD = 2.77$). At present, however, the sophisticated instruments and computer software needed for such analyses are not available to the great majority of practicing speech–language clinicians.

Awareness and Affective Reactions

A unique part of the initial evaluation of preschool-age children who stutter pertains to their awareness of stuttering and their possible affective reactions to it. Although previous chapters reported that some children project various levels of awareness and that our experimental studies have supported such clinical observations and parental reports, current assessment methods are quite crude. Nevertheless, useful information may be obtained for some children seen by clinicians using multiple diagnostic avenues.

The first approach involves the parent report. Parents are asked if they know or suspect that the child is (a) not at all aware, (b) slightly aware, (c) highly aware, or (d) if aware, not bothered. Positive responses are further pursued: What is the reason for the parent's answer? Did the child make a verbal statement (e.g., "I cannot talk")? Did the child display an affective nonverbal response to the stuttering (e.g., clear indications of frustration) or a physical response (e.g., hitting his or her head)? Have the parents been openly reacting to the child's stuttering, thus making the child aware?

A second approach is for the clinician to engage the child directly in brief questioning, such as, "Do you like to talk? Are you a good talker? Do you ever make mistakes when you talk?" The clinician might stutter on several words and ask the child, "Do you know anybody else who talks like me? Do *you* talk like me?" Some children respond positively to these questions; in our experience, some smiled, and one laughed outright in response to the clinician's stuttering.

Third, the clinician can use a systematic test of self-identification as employed in our experiments (see Chapter 8). The clinician holds two identical puppets, one on each hand. In turn, each puppet says an identical sentence, with one puppet speaking fluently and the second one stuttering. The child must decide which one talks the way he or she talks. The clinician repeats this procedure several times, changing the order of the fluent and disfluent puppets. Look for correct identification of greater than 50%. The cumulative information on awareness and emotional reactions gathered through the three approaches could be clinically quite useful and, at times, rather critical for making recommendations to parents.

Prognosis

Growing evidence for a large natural recovery factor was presented in Chapter 5. As a result of this evidence, attempts have been made to identify early prognostic indicators for either recovery or persistent (chronic) stuttering. The ability to predict the course of any disorder in a given case could be a tremendous asset and would provide added flexibility to practitioners in a position of making clinical recommendations and decisions about the course of action. Would we recommend treatment knowing that the disorder will disappear or substantially improve within 3 months? Would we recommend waiting, knowing that the disorder may disappear 6 months from now? Within a year? These are critical questions in terms of treatment philosophy. If the answer is positive, then how long of a waiting period is too long? How sure must we be of the accuracy of our predictions: 100% or 95%? Would 80% do? In addition to philosophies and principles, various practical issues need to be considered.

With increasing frequency, speech–language clinicians must focus treatment on those who most need it because there are not resources to treat everyone at the same time. Selective treatment policies have begun to force speech–language pathologists into making more knowledgeable treatment decisions. Information about risk factors can assist clinicians in making reasonable risk assessments concerning young preschool children who have begun stuttering. Past work in this area falls into categories of informal clinical guidelines, structured instruments, and acoustical studies.

Clinical Impressions

Initial ideas for differentiating children likely to recover from those who are candidates for persistent stuttering are reflected in various general guidelines, based primarily on clinical impressions, that were not incorporated into systematic procedures or dedicated clinical instruments. One such attempt is seen in Van Riper's (1971) developmental tracks that linked natural recovery with various characteristics of stuttering. Van Riper suggested that children who had very early stuttering onset, exhibited repetitions as the primary symptom, and demonstrated up-and-down stuttering cycles were inclined to either recover naturally or show quick positive response to therapy. Children who began stuttering concurrently with late speech development, produced few sound prolongations, and showed little fear were more likely to eventually evidence only mild stuttering or cluttering. In contrast, children with a higher chance of becoming severe and chronic stutterers were those who abruptly began stuttering at a somewhat older age, after a period of normally fluent speech; exhibited blocks as the primary early symptom; and developed fears of speech.

Curlee (1980) took a backtracking approach to determining isolated risk factors. He first identified characteristics of chronic stutterers that he viewed as barriers to recovery, including effortful vocal and articulatory attacks, fear of stuttering, and the sense of being handicapped. In his opinion, these should be the target of early remediation in order to facilitate remission of stuttering. Thus, young children should be observed for specific signs of these characteristics expressed in (a) part-word repetitions of two or more units on 2% or more of words spoken, (b) prolongations longer than 1 second, (c) involuntary blocks longer than 2 seconds, (d) secondary characteristics, (e) noticeable emotional reactions, (f) complaints of not being able to function satisfactorily, and (g) marked variations in frequency and severity of stuttering.

Another clinically based prognostic scheme was suggested by Conture (1990). According to Conture, young stuttering children displaying two or more of the following characteristics are at risk for developing chronic stuttering: (a) sound prolongations or blocks that constitute more than 25% of the total disfluencies produced by the child; (b) lack of eye contact during more than 50% of conversations; (c) frequent or unusual use of phonological processes; (d) prolongations, blocks, or part-word repetitions on the first production of diadochokinesis tasks; and (e) oral motor scores or neurological screening scores that indicate delayed neuromotor development. Interestingly, the criteria listed at the top of Conture's and Curlee's lists emphasize the type or ratios of disfluency. Conture also believed that the use of fast speaking rate or complex vocabulary by the parents might aggravate the child's stuttering, making it more difficult for the child to become fluent. Again, some of his suggestions were not backed by hard data, and it is not clear for what age or for how early in the stuttering history they apply. This is an important reservation that will be discussed later in the chapter.

Structured Tools

The past two decades have seen some effort directed toward developing structured assessment tools to help clinicians determine in advance which young children are most likely to persist in or recover from stuttering. To a considerable extent, however, these instruments have been based on clinical impressions. A pioneering and influential contribution in this area of differential prognosis was the work of Glyndon Riley, seen especially in his *Stuttering Prediction Instrument for Young Children* (1981). To assess persistence risks, this tool uses information gathered from parent interviews and characteristics of the children's speech. The items that are considered predictive of chronicity include: (a) secondary characteristics, (b) child's frustration with disfluencies, (c) parents' reactions to disfluencies, (d) more than three repeated units in part-word repetitions, (e) part-word repetitions repeated "abnormally," (f) presence of prolongations and blocks, and (g) frequency of disfluencies per 100 words. Each item can be scored on a range of possible points, which varies across items. Thus, reactions to stuttering can receive a score from 0 to 12. In the repetition section, target vowels perceived as "hurried," "abruptly separated," or "abnormally tense" can increase the score from 0 to 7. As blocks and prolongations increase in duration from 0 to 4 seconds or longer, the score for this item may rise from 0 to 12. The instrument also requires the analysis of a 100-word speech sample. As the percentage of part-word repetitions, prolongations, and blocks increase from 0% to more than 28%, the score on this section rises from 0 to 9. The total score from all the sections combined ranges from 0 to 40. A score of 10 or greater suggests that the child will continue to stutter.

G. D. Riley (1981) commented that the predictive usefulness of the instrument is unclear. The subjects upon whom it is based are defined rather vaguely as 85 children between 3.0 and 8.9 years who received therapy for stuttering in various settings, versus 11 children who were monitored for 1 to 3 years by the author but in whom "abnormal disfluency had not developed" (p. 20). It appears that receiving therapy was the only criterion for judging chronicity because the instrument does not mention a specific duration of stuttering history that defines "chronic." The instrument also does not reveal the criteria for selecting the 11 recovered children who were monitored.

Several years later, Cooper and Cooper (1985) published their Chronicity Prediction Checklist (CPC), based on data reported by McLelland and Cooper (1978) and on clinical observations, not on longitudinal data. The CPC includes 13 indicators for chronicity: (a) family history of stuttering, (b) increased severity of disfluencies, (c) presence of persistent rather than episodic disfluencies, (d) disfluent for more than 2 years, (e) child's frustration and negative perception of speech, (f) presence of sound prolongations, (g) part-word repetition with more than three units, (h) faster than normal tempo of repetition, (i) uneven or interrupted prolongations longer than 1 second, (j) schwa inserted in repetition, (k) presence of blocks, (l) restricted inflection, and (m) presence of secondary characteristics. The checklist comprises 27 yes–no questions. If the total number of "yes" answers varies from 0 to 6, the score is taken as predictive of recovery; a score from 7 to 15 indicates that the child requires vigilant observation; and a score from 16 to 27 is predictive of chronic stuttering. The authors listed six items considered key clues for stuttering chronicity:

1. Disfluencies are produced on 5% or more of words uttered, for over 6 months.
2. The average duration of disfluencies is greater than 2 seconds.
3. Struggling articulatory gestures or blocks accompany disfluencies.
4. Secondary characteristics are present.
5. Child has negative feelings about disfluencies.
6. Parents have negative feelings about disfluencies that may be detrimental to the child.

As can be seen, the prominent and common elements in the Riley and the Cooper instruments emphasize frequency of disfluency, long disfluencies, the blockage character of disfluency, presence of secondary characteristics, and the child's affective reactions to stuttering. Overall, the main focus is on the severity of overt stuttering with some consideration of the emotional reaction to it.

Critique of Current Prediction Schemes and Instruments

Undoubtedly, the authors of both the informal prognostic guidelines and the more structured instruments just described are to be credited for the impetus they provided to promote the concept of prognosis in early childhood stuttering and the beginning of research in this domain. We are sincerely grateful for their inspiration. It is also clear, however, that their specific ideas and procedures for making prognoses fall short of the type and quality of data required to establish predictive criteria. There are two fundamental requirements. First, early prediction criteria must be derived from longitudinal data obtained from a large *unbiased* sample of stuttering children. Second, follow-up must begin from *close* to stuttering onset. This is the only way to establish and verify early predictions.

In regard to the issue of bias, a reasonably unselected sample is needed. However, in G. D. Riley's (1981) sample, upon which the SPI is based, the proportion of persistent (75%) and recovered (25%) children is the reverse of what is expected for the population. A more balanced distribution could have changed the conclusions about differences. In regard to the issue of being close to onset, it is apparent from descriptions of the subjects who were observed or tested, as well as from the characteristics of several items on informal clinical checklists (e.g., Conture, 1990) and formal instruments (e.g., Cooper & Cooper, 1985), that the guidelines and instruments are not intended for use in the very early stages of stuttering when prediction is most needed and presents the real challenge. For example, the age of the children used extended to almost 9 years. By that age, most children who stutter are already persistent, and prognosis at this stage comes more than a bit too late. Some items on Cooper and Cooper's Chronicity Prediction Checklist assume 2 years of stuttering history or refer to negative emotional reactions. Although some children present clear expressions of frustration from near onset, negative emotions are more likely to be found in older children who have stuttered for some time. It is not known at what time in relation to stuttering onset the information presented in the instruments was gathered. This information is critical to the clinical value of any set of suggested criteria.

The expression "early stuttering" has been used too often without clear definition. How long can the disorder's history last and still be "early"? A major point that must be reemphasized is that 1 or 2 years after onset may not be "early." Certain characteristics of stuttering that may have prognostic significance 1 or 2 years after onset could be totally insignificant during the first few months of the disorder. A good example is the frequency or severity of stuttering. Whereas during the first few months postonset, this parameter is not useful for signaling danger, 2 years later, after many children have already recovered, those exhibiting severe stuttering have a better chance to continue stuttering. It goes without saying that the longer the stuttering history is at the point when data are collected, the less applicable they are to predicting the course of very early stuttering, when prognosis is needed the most. When prognosis is made after the child is far into the course of stuttering, the less it is needed and the easier is the "prediction." We simply know that chances for recovery become increasingly smaller because, by then, the many children who would recover have already done so. In other words, even if the information in those instruments is valid, they seem to be oriented to prediction of persistent stuttering for children, many of whom have already persisted in the disorder and are statistically more inclined to continue in this course. Additionally, since the time when these instruments were published, a significant amount of new information has been gathered. For example, the assumption that secondary characteristics are late to appear and are a sign of advanced stuttering has been questioned. Quite a few parents report the presence of such symptoms from the very beginning of the disorder (Yairi, 1983). Furthermore, in the past decade, Conture and Kelly (1991) and Yairi, Ambrose, Paden, and Throneburg (1996), using frame-by-frame video data, have dispelled the belief that secondary characteristics are late symptoms, showing their presence in many children close to onset.

Speech Acoustics Clues

In addition to clinical hunches, valid as they may prove to be, and the early instruments, there have been isolated research activities aimed at discovering attributes that could be used for early identification of children at risk for developing chronic stuttering. One of the first and a rather intriguing endeavor was carried out by Stromsta (1965), who searched for acoustic cues in the speech sound waves recorded from 63 young stuttering children. Inspecting spectrograms of their speech, Stromsta focused attention on the acoustic structure of the dynamics of continuous speech, especially the second formant (F2) transitions, in disfluent speech segments of 63 children who stuttered. He classified the formants in each child's disfluencies either as containing transitions and normal terminations of phonation, or as displaying lack of transitions, irregular termination of phonation, or both. Ten years later, questionnaires were sent to the parents asking about their children's stuttering. Based on 38 responses, Stromsta reported that 89% of the children who eventually became chronic stutterers evidenced abnormal formants at the time of the first recording, 10 years earlier. In contrast, 91% of the children who recovered had evidenced normal second formant transitions. Unfortunately, lack of essential information about the subjects' initial and later classifications, the speech segments used, the acoustic analyses employed, and reliability greatly diminish the credibility of Stromsta's findings. Nevertheless, his approach to the problem has inspired follow-ups.

Nearly 30 years later, Yaruss and Conture (1993) returned to Stromsta's ideas and studied F2 transitions in part-word repetitions of 13 young children who stuttered with a mean age of 49 months. The children were divided into two subgroups, those at high risk and those at low risk for developing chronic stuttering based only on the scores they received on the *Stuttering Prediction Instrument* (G. D. Riley, 1981). Again, spectrograms of disfluent segments were inspected for the attributes of their second formant. The investigators found that "low-risk" children typically exhibited shorter durations of F2 transitions in the early iterations of the attempted utterance as compared with the final production of that utterance (syllable or word). The children at "high risk" evidenced the opposite trend: longer F2 segments in repeated units than in the final production. The authors, however, found no difference in the presence of abnormal F2 transitions between the groups predicted to either recover or become chronic. Thus, Stromsta's conclusions were not corroborated. The Yaruss and Conture (1993) study, however, raises some questions because children were classified by means of an instrument (the SPI) whose power for making accurate predictions is yet undetermined. Furthermore, there were no follow-ups to determine whether their predictions of subjects' classifications were indeed confirmed by direct examination of the children several years later.

The most recent development in the use of speech acoustics information is a study completed by our group (Subramanian, Yairi, & Amir, 2003) that investigated second formant transition rate in fluent speech of preschool children who stutter shortly after stuttering onset. The children were subjected to follow-ups during several years, and their eventual status as persistent or recovered was verified. This study was described in Chapter 8, and it suffices to restate here that the findings are encouraging in regard to the potential prognostic power of this technique. Near onset, children who were eventually persistent demonstrated significantly smaller frequency changes in the F2 transitions in their fluent speech than those of the recovered group.

Our Prediction Factors

The research of early childhood stuttering conducted by the University of Illinois Stuttering Research Program has covered a wide range of aspects of the disorder, including the onset of stuttering, its development, early disfluency and other speech and nonspeech characteristics, phonology, language, genetics, motor skills, cognition, and affective reactions. It has provided a wealth of information summarized and discussed in the previous chapters of this book. The findings have many clinical implications, some of which also have relevance to prognosis. These lead us now to propose guiding criteria that can enhance the work of clinicians in conducting initial evaluations of young children who have just begun stuttering, particularly in relation to assessing the child's risk prospects for developing persistent stuttering and his or her chance for recovery. Following are preliminary outlines and commentary for the University of Illinois Childhood Stuttering Prognostic Guide, which is currently being developed as a part of a comprehensive diagnostic instrument. Three subsets of criteria are distinguished.

Primary Factors

Family History
The child's family history of stuttering has emerged as one of the most powerful risk predictors currently available. The point to remember is that a positive history, in and of itself, is not sufficient. It is the *pattern* of history that is important. Specifically, when the child's family includes relatives who persisted in or still persist in stuttering, chances are greater that he or she will follow this familial pattern and become persistent. Conversely, if the child's family includes relatives who used to stutter but have recovered, there is a greater chance that a child will follow their pattern. Neither of these prognostic alternatives can be made with certainty. Current data indicate that each of these trends occurs in approximately 65% of cases.

Gender

The gender factor is quite strong and by far the easiest to assess. This factor can be used in two ways. First, it is useful in assessing overall risk. Whereas it has been known for many years that boys are at higher risk than girls in terms of stuttering incidence, our data show a tendency for boys to also be at greater risk than girls for becoming persistent in their stuttering. Therefore, all other factors being equal, a girl's overall chance for recovery is better than a boy's. Second, gender information is useful in assessing the length of stuttering history at the time of the examination. Girls tend to recover after a shorter stuttering history than boys. Thus, a 12-month stuttering history without an apparent improvement indicates a greater risk for a girl than for a boy.

Age at Onset

Our findings, as well as those reported by Buck, Lees, and Cook (2002), have indicated a trend for persistence to be associated with later age at onset. Those who persist begin to stutter approximately 3.5 months later than those who recover. The overlap, however, is large. Our current data indicate that the difference is close to being statistically significant and, with a larger sample, might reach significance. Although inclusion of this factor remains uncertain, the age at onset may be considered in light of information about other prognostic indicators. We have kept age at onset under "Primary Factors" because it may be an important factor by virtue of its possible related influences. For example, children who begin stuttering at an older age are more likely to become aware of their stuttering and react to it in a variety of ways, from expressing frustration to crying. We have reported that awareness of disfluencies is sharply heightened between ages 4 and 5 in both children who stutter and normally speaking children. Therefore, in addition to the stuttering children's own reactions, increasing negative reactions from peers should be expected. Furthermore, the older the child, the higher the expectations and various demands are on him or her.

SLD Trends: The Critical Period

We have established that a very large percentage of complete natural recovery in young children occurs within 3 years following onset, with some recovering during the fourth year of stuttering. It is significant, however, that the stuttering of these children, as reflected in the *frequency* of SLD and stuttering severity ratings, almost always begins to subside by the end of the first year. As already reported in Chapter 5, the data indicated divergence between the developmental courses of the persistent and the recovered groups at about 12 months after onset, when the separation of the SLD progress lines becomes statistically significant. This point may indeed serve as an important prognostic factor. What we see is that the children who persist exhibit a rather stable SLD level over time. Children who recover show a definite drop in the level of disfluency, some sharply and some more gradually.

For predicting purposes, then, monitoring recorded speech samples during the first year can provide important clues. This is not to say that if the child stutters after 1 year, he or she necessarily presents high risk for chronic stuttering. Recall that the great majority of children who recover take more than a year to complete the process. The past developmental profile must be consulted. Even if the child still stutters, a *downward* trend in the number of SLD during the first year is taken as a strong positive sign for eventual complete recovery. For example, 8 SLD per 100 words in a speech sample taken 9 months after onset looks rather promising if the speech sample taken soon after onset contained 15 SLD per 100 syllables. On the other hand, 8 SLD at the time of onset and the same number 9 months later should be taken as a sign of higher risk for persistence, although a downward shift still may occur. In short, a flat or inclining SLD curve is a danger sign. The disfluency data should also be checked against clinician and parent ratings of stuttering severity. A close agreement strengthens the basis for the clinical decision.

Duration of Stuttering History

The longer the stuttering history beyond the first year, the higher the risk is for persistence, especially for girls. When other information is unavailable, this factor becomes more influential. For example, we face a difficult case when a child is seen for the first time a year after onset and still exhibits a high frequency of SLD. Although the disfluency may have been declining, the frequent current stuttering, viewed against the absence of quantified data about the child's speech characteristics in the past, places the child in the category of potential risk. Recovery, however, is not ruled out. A child seen for the first time 3 or 4 years after onset already should be considered persistent even if he or she exhibits low-level stuttering. Data on the year-by-year remaining chances for recovery were presented in Chapter 5 (see Table 5.2).

Disfluency Length: Extent and Duration

At the very early stage of stuttering, severity is not a predictor. It is the *continuing* presence of disfluencies with more than one repetition unit, especially those containing three or more units per instance (e.g., "bu-bu-bu-but"), that is a sign of higher risk. Therefore, when monitoring speech samples during the first year, the clinician should consider *extent* of disfluency as well as frequency. Reduction in the number of repetition units typically should occur with the reduction in number of SLD. If disfluencies are still present but become shorter, prognosis is more positive. Children who recover naturally and early do not continue to exhibit multiple repetitions.

The second dimension of length is duration. The total duration of disfluent events does not differentiate the groups near onset or at any later time. In this respect, we disagree with previous claims (e.g., Cooper & Cooper, 1985; G. D. Riley, 1981) that longer blocks and prolongations serve as warnings of persistence. Our recovered group, however, showed a significant *increase,* with time, in the duration of silent intervals between repetition units, indicating a normalization process; that is, the longer intervals reflect iterations that are slower in tempo. Although precise measurements of the intervals between words (e.g., in "and-and-and") require both sophisticated equipment and experience, perceptual comparisons of the tempo of repetitions in previous and current speech samples could be revealing.

Sound Prolongations and Blocks

The early presence of a substantial number of sound prolongations or blocks is a possible risk, although *not* during the first few months of the disorder; in our studies, children who eventually recovered and those who eventually persisted could not be distinguished by this feature close to onset. However, once again, monitoring is important in using this feature for prediction. When the percentage of sound prolongations in the total disfluency begins to shrink over time, even if the child still stutters, he or she is on the recovery path. Conversely, when the percentage of sound prolongations grows, so does the risk for persistence.

Secondary Factors

Stuttering Severity

The disfluency data (SLD) that we have obtained for each child show that the *initial* severity, as reflected in this measure, is *not* a good predictive sign. It is quite understandable why the severity of stuttering has been presumed by many to be an important predictive factor. Naturally, there is a tendency to conceptualize severe overt symptoms as reflecting a more serious underlying pathology, one that is more likely to linger on. The data, however, clearly show that this assumption regarding severity, at least during the first few months of stuttering, is invalid in relation to predicting the future development of the disorder. During that period, even a severe form of overt stuttering is not an indicator of persistence. Children who later recovered exhibited stuttering as severe as, or even more severe than, those who persisted. It is important, however, to consider severity in relation to the length of the stuttering history. If severe stuttering continues for more than a few months or continues unabated, it should be viewed as a risk. It is quite possible, even logical, that 1 or 2 years postonset, after many children have improved along the way to recovery, the stuttering of those who persist emerges as more severe.

Head and Neck Movements

In three of our studies in which secondary characteristics were quantified by means of frame-by-frame analyses, we found no differences in the number of facial and head movements in the first speech samples recorded shortly after onset of children who eventually persisted and of those who eventually recovered. As the process of recovery takes place, there is a decline in the number of secondary characteristics. We also looked at the clinician rating of the severity of these head and neck movements. Again, shortly after onset, such ratings had no predictive power. Within 12 months postonset, however, the ratings of children who later recovered dropped sharply, whereas those of persisting children remained rather stable. Thus, within the first year postonset, children who do not show a substantial decline in the number and severity of secondary characteristics are at higher risk of having chronic stuttering.

Phonological Skills

Early in their stuttering history, children who will eventually persist in stuttering tend to show a lower level of phonological skills than those who recover. In fact, their performance may be lower than normative expectations. These findings suggest that, in at least some cases, stuttering emerges in children who already have poor phonological abilities. There is, however, great individual variability. Nevertheless, when children are evaluated within a few months after onset, phonological skills that are below normal reinforce other risk factors. As we reported in Chapter 6, during the second year of stuttering, much of the difference tends to disappear and the phonological skills lose their predictive power. In general, available information about phonological skills is insufficient to predict stuttering outcome by this factor alone, although it may add to the cumulative impression of the overall prognostic picture.

Expressive Language Skills

In our studies, language skills of those children who eventually persisted and those who eventually recovered could not be readily distinguished from normative expectations or from each other, especially close to the time of onset. Contrary to previous thinking, very young children who stutter tend to demonstrate expressive language skills at or above the average range. These findings may suggest that, in at least some cases, stuttering emerges in conjunction with linguistic abilities that are beyond developmental expectations. These apparent developmental asynchronies may be particularly informative as to the nature of early childhood stuttering, despite the fact that linguistic abilities, per se, do not appear to differentiate the child whose stuttering will persist from the child who will recover. On the other hand, atypical language development patterns were found more frequently (but only in a few cases) in children whose stuttering would persist. To date, our analyses have focused on general measures of language ability. In future studies, more detailed evaluation of language skills should be used to investigate expected patterns of language change over time in young children who stutter, both those who persist and those who recover. In addition, the relationship between young children's language abilities and their skills in related domains (e.g., motor abilities) should be evaluated for potential clues regarding the likelihood of persistence versus recovery. Currently, however, the prognostic power of the child's language development status in the prediction of stuttering pathways is not clear. Although lower than normative linguistic skills cannot be viewed as a risk factor for persistence, delayed language may complicate stuttering.

Acoustic Features

Our data for the second formant (F2) transitions in speech obtained close to stuttering onset indicate that children whose stuttering was found later to persist demonstrated significantly smaller frequency changes in the transition. Perhaps their articulatory movements as reflected in the F2 transitions are more restricted than movement of those who eventually recover. Although continued research for prognostic clues in the acoustic speech signal is warranted, we feel that current data are too limited for practical clinical purposes. Unfortunately, our present data for speaking rate do not provide a sufficient basis for early prediction of the course of stuttering.

Other Factors

Based on clinical experience, we also suggest consideration of the following factors, although no data are available concerning their predictive value.

Concomitant Disorders

The presence of concomitant disorders, such as physical, emotional–behavioral, learning, and speech–language disorders that are associated with stuttering (Arndt & Healey, 2001; G. W. Blood & Seider, 1981), might exacerbate stuttering. Our project was not designed to specifically examine the presence or absence of concomitant disorders. By and large, the children were within normal limits for speech and language skills, with the exception of phonology, and did not have diagnosed psychological or learning disorders. A few children were diagnosed with or suspected of exhibiting mild attention-deficit/hyperactivity disorder, and a very few were reported and observed to have high levels of general anxiety. Some children had asthma, but their course of stuttering was highly variable. Some of the medications they received, in particular theophylline, tended to exacerbate stuttering. This phenomenon also has been noted by other investigators (Rosenfield, McCarthy, McKinney, Viswanath, & Nudelman, 1994). Another interesting condition was reported by one family that had three children with sleep apnea when very young: Two stuttered persistently and one never stuttered. There were additional cases of stuttering in this family, but it is unknown whether other individuals in the extended family were ever diagnosed with sleep apnea. We discussed the more common concomitant disorders of phonology and language previously.

At present, the complex interaction of stuttering and other disorders during the early years of life is far from being understood. Nevertheless, it is logical to assume that any interference with normal development can have multiple effects. Thus, additional complications may increase risk for persistence or may interfere with recovery processes. Although we do not have specific information related to prognosis, extra consideration of concomitant disorders, if present, is warranted.

Awareness and Affective Reactions

We have provided experimental data and clinical observations of awareness of stuttering among a number of very young stuttering children. The percentage of aware children grows with age, especially between ages 4 and 5. Parents of a few children also report awareness and emotional reactions soon after onset. Although there is no evidence that awareness of stuttering, and emotional reaction to it, in very young children at the early stage of the disorder is a predictor of persistence, expressed frustration or other rather strong reactions on the part of either the child or the parents should be considered in the initial evaluation as a factor in recommending intervention. Strong emotional reactions by child or parents might cause further complications, interfering with the potential for recovery, and have secondary effects on the family. For example, one mother said, "My 3-year-old son has developed a stuttering problem within the past few months and recently has gotten much worse. Today he burst into tears when he got stuck on a word and told me, 'Mommy, I just can't say it.' It broke my heart." We should certainly consider the child's and the mother's reactions. As already stated, it is also important to recognize findings that normally fluent children become increasingly aware of other children's disfluency and stuttering at the same ages that the children become aware of their own disfluencies. Therefore, the effect of possible negative comments by fluent children to the stuttering child should be kept in mind.

Examples of Applications

In reviewing all risk criteria, it becomes apparent that their predictive powers vary and that none has sufficient strength to be relied on as a safe prognostic indicator. To arrive at a meaningful risk assessment, the clinician's task is to thoughtfully examine the combination of criteria as they converge in each individual case. Currently, such assessment is an *estimate* of chances. Several examples illustrate different combinations of factors and their interpretations.

(*text continues on p. 358*)

Case A

A 36-month-old boy, first seen 3 months after onset, exhibits rather severe stuttering in terms of frequency of disfluency (e.g., 16 SLD per 100 syllables), moderate tension, and few secondary characteristics. No apparent emotional reactions are noted. There is no known familial history of stuttering. Phonology and language test normal for his age. At this point, there is no reason to view the child as being at high risk. He may be placed under close monitoring for several months. Three months later, there are no signs or parental report of aggravation such as changing symptomatology. Parents report some improvement. Analyses of speech samples reveal 11 SLD per 100 syllables. This is taken as a positive development. The close monitoring is extended to see if further improvement takes place.

Case B

A 50-month-old boy, seen 7 months after onset, exhibits moderate stuttering (10 SLD per 100 syllables), including a few sound prolongations, and moderate tension. Syllable and short-word repetitions consist of one or two repetition units. Phonology is below norms. Onset was moderately gradual in that it took the parents about 2 weeks to determine that the child stuttered. Both parents have no stuttering history but are unable to obtain relevant information for other branches of the family. Reevaluation is recommended in a few months. Four months later, the SLD level remains unchanged, but repetitions now consist mostly of two and three units and sound prolongations are still present. Because of the relatively late onset, continuation of stuttering for nearly 1 year, lack of decline in frequency of SLD, increase in number of repetition units, and continuous presence of sound prolongations, the risk for chronic stuttering becomes higher. Intervention should be considered for this child.

Case C

A 30-month-old girl, first seen 3 months after onset, exhibits moderate to severe stuttering in terms of frequency (e.g., 12 SLD per 100 syllables). Her older cousin has been stuttering for 6 years at a moderate level of severity. In spite of being a female and having a lower level of stuttering than the child in Case A, she should be viewed at potentially high risk because of the familial history of persistent stuttering. Intervention should be considered. Three months later, the parents report slight improvement but still rate the stuttering as moderate. Analyses of speech samples reveal 10 SLD per 100 syllables. In spite of the improvement, the remaining level of stuttering in conjunction with the family history appears to indicate increasing risk for persistence.

Case D

A 55-month-old girl, evaluated 7 months after onset, exhibits a moderate SLD level (9 SLD per 100 syllables), as well as moderately severe secondary characteristics. Her parents report little change since onset. The child was adopted, and the family history of stuttering is unknown. Additionally, phonological skills are below norms. The combination of factors—a female exhibiting late onset (4 years of age), possibly no change in the amount of stuttering since onset, the presence of moderate secondary characteristics, and phonological delay—provides reasons for suspicion. The child should be monitored for 3 to 4 additional months. If the SLD level and secondary characteristics remain stable, intervention should be considered.

Case E

A 25-month-old boy, seen for an initial evaluation 1 month after a sudden onset of stuttering, exhibits a moderate SLD level (12 SLD per 100 syllables), primarily repetitions, and a few secondary characteristics. Phonology is adequate for his age. No apparent emotional reactions are noted. His father stuttered as a child for 2 years before recovering at about age 5. Reevaluation is recommended in 3 months. At that time, the stuttering has increased to 15 SLD, and parents also report that the stuttering has worsened. There is still no apparent reaction on the child's part, and the parents seem to handle the situation adequately. Because we know that stuttering often increases during the first months after onset, prior to the common downward trend, and in view of his young age, good phonology, and familial history of recovered stuttering, we are not alarmed and recommend continued monitoring. Three months later, a considerable decline in stuttering is observed, down to 6 SLD, which is at a mild level of stuttering severity. The child appears to be on his way to recovery. Continued monitoring is recommended.

Conclusions

Diagnosis of early stuttering in preschool-age children by trained speech–language clinicians is a relatively straightforward procedure that involves a low percentage of error. Currently available data on various aspects of the disorder, especially the characteristics of early childhood disfluency, provide sufficient information to make such a scientifically-based determination. Borderline, confusing cases are, and should be, rare. We have provided finer diagnostic procedures and criteria for such cases.

In regard to prognosis, the general knowledge that the majority of children who begin stuttering outgrow the disorder without intervention presents clinicians with questions about important clinical decisions. Should these children receive priority for treatment or receive therapy at all? These questions, in addition to the realities of limited resources, bring to the forefront the necessity to prioritize treatment according to the level of risk for persistent, chronic stuttering; hence, it is important to improve the ability to make predictions concerning the course of the disorder. Information, such as that summarized in this chapter, can be applied in making reasonable risk assessments. The predicting factors listed, however, should be viewed as tools for assessing *chances*. The clinician must always inform parents that, as yet, nobody can accurately predict the development of stuttering in a given child. However, even imperfect prediction instruments are very helpful to clinicians when forced to make triage decisions.

How, then, do these newer contributions of research affect considerations of treatment plans? Selective treatment for high-risk children determined on the basis of clinical prognosis means that some children, those who appear to be at low risk, may not receive therapy. This is not to say that they should be ignored. In addition to comprehensive evaluations, parent counseling might be considered. Although we do not object to providing therapy to those children who are at low risk, we maintain that therapy should be provided when needed and because it helps, not because "it would not hurt." Although partial or complete recovery appears to occur spontaneously, it is possible that treatment can hasten improvement or recovery. Indeed, there appears to be a general tendency to assume, though not always with credible evidence, that treatment does have some effect. Thus, given a case with signs of probable recovery, therapy might be deferred while the child's progress is monitored. Or, depending on the case, the goal for therapy and the approach taken should be conceived with an altered perspective; that is, the goal may be to facilitate and hasten the natural recovery processes.

On the other hand, we cannot say that treatment, even very early treatment, can ensure recovery. Given cases with indications of probable persistence, although some clinicians are set on ultimately achieving cure of stuttering, an alternative perspective might include goals that are more focused on minimizing symptoms, maximizing adjustment, and increasing assertiveness. Certainly, close monitoring of children who begin to stutter is essential. In fact, as pointed out in this chapter, the prognostic process itself necessitates monitoring over time to assess several factors, such as frequency, type, and length of disfluency.

Chapter 11

Parental Involvement and Counseling

Various sources that influenced the emergence of parental involvement as a major method of treating early childhood stuttering are summarized. A review of the literature reveals a wide range of programs within three major approaches: treatment of parents, parental advising, and direct use of parents to facilitate clinicians' treatment of children. The programs within each approach vary in relation to form, theoretical background, objectives, content, procedures, and other parameters. We present the various types of advice given to parents and classify them according to eight categories. We conclude that the many approaches and their theoretical arguments are lacking in sufficient, if at all, supporting data. Although some programs of parental involvement reflect new knowledge about stuttering, their effectiveness has not been demonstrated. Often they have not incorporated recent advancements in models of family dynamics.

Study Questions

1. *What are the three main modes of parental involvement in the treatment of early childhood stuttering? Explain and briefly discuss each one.*

2. *In what ways have parents been used as cotherapists for early stuttering?*

3. *What are the 10 main types of specific advice given to parents of preschool children who begin stuttering?*

4. *What is the research support for advice given to parents of preschool children who stutter? Discuss.*

No other therapeutic approach to stuttering has achieved the consensus of support given to parental involvement in the clinical management of early childhood stuttering. Schuell (1949, p. 251) underlined this point with a statement that "it is impossible to escape the need for working with the parents of the young child who stutters." Nearly 30 years later, Cave (1977) echoed this point of view, saying that "an indirect approach to treatment through parent counseling would seem to be the most satisfactory with the very young child" (p. 411). Although parental involvement is incorporated into the management of various communicative disorders, only in stuttering has it assumed such a central role, often the main, and sometimes the exclusive, mode of treatment. It has maintained significant prominence even though the use of direct speech therapy techniques for early childhood stuttering has increased in recent years.

This chapter attempts to provide a broad perspective of the approaches to parental involvement in the clinical arena of our general focus of interest. Although the term *counseling* has been heavily used in the literature, it represents diverse content and processes, carries several meanings, and includes various forms of intervention. We distinguish three major forms of parental involvement in relation to intervention with early childhood stuttering: (a) parent treatment (parent as client), (b) parent advising (parent as support), and (c) parent training (parent as cotherapist). The pertinent literature is plentiful and has been published in textbooks for practicing clinicians, articles in scientific journals, and booklets and pamphlets prepared for the general public and parents. For our purpose, we analyze only selected parts of this large body of literature.

The Bases of Parental Involvement

Until two decades ago, the extent of parental involvement in treatments of early childhood stuttering resulted from a general reluctance, especially in the United States, to include young children who stutter in therapeutic programs. A number of influences shaped this tendency.

Psychogenic Theories: Resolution of Parental Neuroses

One of the earliest influences stemmed from the psychoanalytic perspective of stuttering as a symptom of the child's unconscious conflicts over unsatisfied needs (Brill, 1923; Coriat, 1943; Fenichel, 1945). Because such conflicts were said to be traceable to the parents' (especially mothers') neurotic personalities and conflict-motivated behaviors, there were strong advocacies of traditional psychotherapies that targeted the parents (e.g., Glauber, 1958). Other proponents of the idea that stuttering is a neurotic reaction emphasized the more tangible aspects of parental behavior, such as overprotective attitudes (Murphy & Fitzsimons, 1960) or rejection and domination (Clark & Snyder, 1955). Problems at these levels did not necessitate in-depth psychotherapy but could be handled through counseling.

Developmental Perspectives: Prevention of Child Awareness of Stuttering

A second influence was Bluemel's (1932) developmental model of stuttering. Bluemel maintained that becoming aware of "primary stuttering" was a necessary element in the child's formation of advanced or "secondary stuttering." It was logical to conclude that preventing the child from becoming aware of his or her already existing stuttering is crucial in preventing or minimizing the development of an advanced disorder. In Van Riper's (1939) view, prevention of awareness was paramount in treating the young stutterer during the primary stage. He and others advocated a strategy of "letting the child alone" while concentrating on treating his or her parents. This concept was later reinforced by Johnson's (1942) claim that calling attention to normal disfluency was the direct cause of stuttering.

Diagnosogenic Theory: Reduction of Parental Pressures

The subsequent emergence of the diagnosogenic theory (Johnson, 1942; Johnson et al., 1959) gave rise to a third influence: the hypothesis that a pressure-creating home environment was in the background of stuttering. Parents were depicted as worrisome, driven by perfectionist attitudes and high standards for both their children and themselves, and as being overly sensitized to their child's speech by virtue of their familial history of stuttering. In such an intense home atmosphere, according to Johnson, parents' intolerance of the child's normal disfluencies was the immediate cause of stuttering. Parents were identified as the prime target for intervention, with the parallel objectives of modifying their pressure-inclined attitudes and keeping the child from becoming aware of disfluencies.

Home Environment Research: Reduction of Parental Pressures

The extensive findings regarding the families of children who stutter, based on research inspired by the diagnosogenic theory, constituted yet another source of influence. With a few exceptions (e.g., Quarington, 1974), the findings were generally interpreted as indicating that children who stutter, as a group, were subject to more adverse parental pressures and negative attitudes than normally fluent controls. Domination, over-protection, high expectations, and perfectionism in child rearing, as well as the parents' feelings of rejection toward the child and undesirable evaluations of his or her personality, were identified as characteristic parental behavior patterns (see review by Yairi, 1997a). Such findings reinforced the already prevailing inclination to focus intervention on parent counseling.

"Spontaneous" Recovery: Remediation of Speech by the Parents

A completely different influence has emerged from interpretations of data on natural or spontaneous recovery. As elaborated in Chapter 5, some investigators rejected the notion that the frequent recovery observed in young children who stutter is spontaneous (R. J. Ingham, 1983; Martin & Lindamood, 1986; Wingate, 1976). In their view, the recovery, far from being spontaneous, was at least partially effected by parental intervention in correcting their children's stuttering. The implications to parental involvement were quite different from those of the previous sources, as they encouraged systematic use of parents in actively correcting their child's stuttering.

Modes of Parental Involvement

Historically, parental involvement in the treatment of childhood stuttering took several forms and varied along several dimensions. Objectives differed from that of changing parents' personality to that of training them in treating their children. The counseling style ranged from authoritarian to client-centered, and its level of intensity from supportive to reconstructive. There were variations in the format of treatment (individual or group), frequency of contacts, type of therapists, and so on. Furthermore, programs often combined elements from several approaches. It is difficult, therefore, to apply single classification to all intervention methods found in the literature. Following, we present several programs representing the three different modes of parental involvement in treatment of childhood stuttering: parent as client, parent as support, and parent as cotherapist. Our purpose is to provide readers with a perspective of the range of thinking and practice in this aspect of clinical intervention. We caution in advance that many of the intervention programs have not been substantiated with data.

Parent Treatment (Parent as Client)

Treatments outlined by clinicians holding to the psychogenesis point of view have strived to achieve a greater degree of parents' emotional adjustment and insight into the psychodynamics of their allegedly disturbed relations with their child. In this group, traditional psychoanalysts have been extreme in zeroing in on the parents, sometimes advocating that parents alone should be treated. Among those who prescribed psychoanalysis was Glauber (1958). He advocated treating several members of the nuclear family using a different therapist for each one; however the mother of the young stutterer, viewed as the prime source of conflict and anxiety, was the focus of therapy. Resolving the mother's strong psychoneurotic anxiety of separation from her own mother as well as from her stuttering child was deemed crucial. Fathers' involvement in the treatment was usually limited to counseling regarding specific harmful behaviors toward the child. Glauber (1958) reported that concern in the family about stuttering was greatly diminished after 2 to 6 months of intensive treatment, and that psychoanalysis for the mother was sufficient to eliminate stuttering in young children.

A less extreme approach was taken by Glasner (1947, 1962). Despite believing that many young children who stutter and their parents exhibited neurotic symptoms, he was not of the opinion that deep unconscious conflicts should necessarily be implicated. Home atmosphere created by overprotective, perfectionistic parents could be conceived as sufficiently traumatic to impair the child's emotional growth. In some cases of early childhood stuttering, his treatment included extensive psychiatric guidance for several family members. In the majority of cases, however, parents received a short counseling session with the same therapist who treated the child. Both parents underwent an extensive initial interview, and at least one of them had to be seen at each subsequent child's therapy session. To free a stuttering child of neurotic patterns, parents had to recognize their own problems and the direct relationship of their interpersonal attitudes to the child's stuttering. Glasner also believed that parents often were unable to contribute constructively to progress not because of resistance, but due to ignorance of emotional disturbances and how they should be handled. Therefore, the treatment was also geared to counseling–educating parents regarding principles of emotional hygiene and the possible causes of stuttering.

Murphy and Fitzsimons (1960) viewed stuttering as a tension-reducing symptom but thought that parents of children who stutter rarely presented problems of deep psychological origins. In their view, parents contribute to the development of stuttering by exercising perfectionistic, critical, and domineering attitudes. The authors advocated a concomitant child therapy and parent counseling program with two separate clinicians (a single clinician could have been perceived by a child as the parents' ally). They strongly objected to a directive, advice-giving type of counseling in which the clinician acts as regulatory authority. Thus, their counseling was more psychotherapeutic and client-centered in character, providing parents with ample opportunities to vent feelings. Because the overall objective was to strengthen the child's self-concept to diminish his or her need for stuttering symptoms, it was important to help parents develop a sense of competence and create an atmosphere of acceptance and faith. It was assumed that parents, by venting feelings, learned to neutralize their own anxieties and effect necessary changes in their tension-creating reactions.

An interesting variation in this general direction of parental involvement can be seen in the work of Clark and Snyder (1955). Whereas many who addressed the issue of parent therapy or counseling in cases of childhood stuttering tended, either explicitly or implicitly, to emphasize the mother's role in the child's adjustment difficulties and geared their counseling toward her, Clark and Snyder reminded us that "fathers are parents too" (p. 226). Claiming frequent revelations of hostility toward and strong rejection of stuttering children by their fathers, the authors contended that such attitudes were reflected in the children's display of basic disturbances in child–father relationships, such as inordinate fear of authority figures and lack of well-defined masculine identification. Consequently, Clark and Snyder advocated the inclusion of fathers in group therapy, which was deemed the best medium for parent counseling. Both father and mother were encouraged to participate in small groups of up to 12 parents. The sessions had a psychotherapeutic character in which free expressions of feelings and concerns were encouraged, including, of course, those about the stuttering child and the parents' relationships with him or her. The clinician's participation or interpretation of comments was minimal. Clark and Snyder rationalized that, in discussing each other's problems, parents gain insight into their own feelings and interactions with their child. Seeing the faults in others reduces the parents' guilt about their own, making it easier to admit problems and cope with them. The authors stated that marked changes had occurred in many parents' attitudes toward their child and in the general emotional tone at home. No data were provided to support their conclusion. Nevertheless, Clark and Snyder's ideas appear to have influenced more recent therapies, such as Conture's (2001) parent group program (see Chapter 13).

In summary, various parent treatments characterized by psychogenetic orientations to stuttering have been offered. Whereas the concept of parent counseling is widely accepted by speech–language clinicians who treat stuttering in young children, the notion of parents as the *primary recipients* of therapy, especially psychotherapy, is not. Some of the programs reviewed, and their influence on more current ones, appear to be unfamiliar to many clinicians. It is imperative to state at this point that adequate support for the psychogenetic theoretical bases is lacking. Current data are insufficient to assume a priori the presence of clinically significant personality deviations in parents of young stutterers. Both Adams (1993) and Yairi (1997b) concluded that children who stutter do not grow up in a home environment that is blatantly pathologic. There also is no credible evidence of the effectiveness of the treatments described. Nevertheless, in the clinical setting, we confront the individual case, not group data. Some parents of children who stutter may have clinically significant emotional problems that warrant treatment, as do some parents of normally fluent children. Although we do not assume that such problems are the cause of the child's stuttering, the stuttering and its treatment may be further complicated by them. Thus, in some cases, clinical impressions may suggest additional expert input concerning the need for parent therapy.

Parent Advising (Parent as Support)

Some Classical Programs

Another mode of parental intervention broadly referred to as counseling includes programs whose main objective is the modification of specific parent–child relationships, particularly various forms of pressure, and other environmental factors presumed to influence the occurrence of stuttering. Combining general principles of good parenthood with knowledge of stuttering, these programs were typically developed by speech pathologists oriented to learning theories. Their parent counseling is characterized by more direct guidance and advice, and thus by greater emphasis on intellectual understanding of stuttering than in the approaches described in the previous section.

As mentioned earlier, Wendell Johnson's views on the origins of stuttering were instrumental in placing parent counseling (advising) at the center of therapeutic programs for incipient or suspected stuttering in young children. His own style (Johnson, 1948, 1961) was directive and authoritarian, and consisted of three distinct parts. Advising began with an extensive case history interview, often using a lengthy standard questionnaire of more than 800 items. Johnson held that leading parents through 3- to 5-hour periods of detailed systematic questioning forced them to recapture a necessary perspective of stuttering and become highly aware of their contribution to its creation and perpetuation. He actually believed that in some cases this process, in and of itself, was sufficient to bring about parental behavioral change that resulted in substantial improvement, or even remission, of the child's stuttering problem.

The next, perhaps most important, part of Johnson's advising consisted of parent education. It involved imparting information about speech development, the normalcy of disfluencies, and the causes of stuttering according to Johnson's own theory (overreaction of overanxious parents to normal disfluency). The objectives of this education were to "improve" the evaluation made by parents of their child's speech as stuttering and to alter their negative reaction to it. Although Johnson recognized the strength of personality dynamics that govern parents' preconceptions and emotional reactions, his writings reflected a belief that the clinician's power to convince on one hand, and the parents' potential for intellectual understanding of "the facts in the case" on the other hand, could bring about a desirable change. His authoritarian style in the process required total changes in beliefs as well as in action. He stated, for example,

> This does not mean that the parents should not let the child know they
> are concerned about his speech. They *must not* be concerned about him.
> Nor does it mean that the parents should suppress their desire to correct
> the youngster's speech, to have him stop and start over again, go slowly,
> etc. They *must have no* such desires. Neither does it mean that the parents

should be told merely to pay no attention to stuttering. *There is no stuttering.* (Johnson, 1948, p. 249 [italics added])

The third stage of Johnson's advising focused on altering those environmental conditions presumed to be causing the child's feelings of insecurity and resultant hesitancy in speech. Parents were guided to identify adverse conditions specific to their own child. The clinician then provided practical suggestions for day-to-day practices. Clearly, this part of the counseling also was very directive, often down to specific details of planned parent–child activities.

Johnson's ideas on advising parents of beginning young stutterers left their mark on the writings of several of his contemporaries, as well as on current common practices. Schuell (1949), for example, also believed that the child's speech should not be of primary importance. Instead, what must be changed is the child's belief that something is wrong with his or her speech. The main objective of Schuell's counseling was to alter parents' perceptions and attitudes so as to promote in the child a strong feeling of acceptance, a feeling necessary for him or her to communicate without apprehension.

Schuell's (1949) outline for parent advising included a structured series of at least four sessions, containing a stronger element of client-centered approach but still retaining Johnson's method of providing specific "do" and "do not" advice about stuttering and his guided corrective home assignments. It began with a free interview with only one parent, with the clinician remaining relatively passive to allow free verbalization of parental concerns. The second session, held with both parents, was used for conveying information about stuttering, discussing questions, and assigning specific home observations about the child's stuttering and parents' interactions with the child. Information gathered by parents from home observations was analyzed in the third session, and specific suggestions to modify their behavior with the child were given. The fourth, and any subsequent sessions, were planned to analyze progress and make further suggestions. Similarly, at about the same time, S. Brown (1949), a physician and a speech pathologist, suggested that pediatricians also counsel parents of young stutterers. He advocated an initial series of sessions 2 to 3 weeks apart and follow-up conferences at 3- to 6-month intervals.

Among others who followed Johnson's counseling framework, but with some notable deviations, were Bloodstein (1958) and Sander (1959). Bloodstein's counseling centered on reduction of speech-related pressures and general pressures at home. In contrast to Johnson, however, he pointed out that any effort to change parental behavior must begin with removal of their guilt about the child's stuttering. Regular, sometimes intensive, counseling sessions were conducted. Periodic reexamination of the child was used to assure parents that they were not left alone and that the clinician shared responsibility for the child's improvement. Similarly, Sander (1959) warned against the risk of pointing to parents' past mistakes. Unlike Johnson, he believed that advising parents on an intellectual level when they were not emotionally ready to accept such advice was futile. Like Johnson, however, he emphasized the importance of case history interviews as vehicles for parents to reevaluate their thinking in more concrete, vivid terms as they recalled their children's past.

Although Schuell (1949), Bloodstein (1958), and Sander (1959) cautioned against superficial advice and favored comprehensive counseling, it was Zwitman (1978) who published such a comprehensive, detailed, step-by-step program that may especially appeal to beginning clinicians. His theoretical assumptions were also different and contained elements of ideas that reflect current thinking. Assuming that stuttering results from delayed maturation of speech and language skills combined with environmental pressures, and knowing that early stuttering tends to dissipate with age, Zwitman thought that counseling should provide a child with the most favorable environment for fluency so that maturation and stabilization of the communication system can take place. That means introducing consistency into the parent–child relationship in the daily routine by creating a reasonably tolerant environment, yet one that also recognizes rules and consequences. Part I of the advising consists of three sections: (a) parent reaction to disfluency, (b) handling of speaking demands, and (c) improving the child's self-concept and security. Part II draws heavily on behavior modification principles and comprises four sections concerned with everyday routines: (a) parent reaction to child's unintentional misbehavior, (b) reaction to intentional misbehavior, (c) establishing consistent responses, and (d) rewarding the child for desirable behavior. Zwitman's primarily didactic program also includes procedures for parent monitoring using detailed questionnaires, rating scales, and checklists. It allows flexibility in choosing specific sections according to each child's needs, a detailed discussion for implementation of each step, and examples of answers to common questions raised by parents. In general, neither Zwitman nor others provided scientific data regarding the effectiveness of their counseling.

More Recent Programs

Additional writing about and programs for advising parents of preschool-age children who stutter, sometimes as components of more comprehensive treatment programs, have continued to appear with some variations in orientation, general structure, and step-by-step details (e.g., Gregory & Gregory, 1999; Rustin, Botterill, & Kelman, 1996; Starkweather, Gottwald, & Halfond, 1990; Zebrowski & Schum, 1993). A rather detailed program was published by Fosnot and Woodford (1992). In *The Fluency Development System for Young Children,* the authors include a significant component of parent advising consisting of two parts. The first, *behavioristic counseling,* begins with an individual session, continuing later in a group format. It is instructional in character, aimed at assisting parents in modifying their behaviors. For example, parents are informed about speech and language development, normal and abnormal disfluency, theories of stuttering, and ways to handle discipline with a disfluent child. Parents are also given home assignments, such as observing the child's fluency at home and keeping charts, engaging in smooth versus bumpy speech, and learning to speak slowly. The second part, *humanistic counseling,* is nondirective and is oriented toward encouraging parents to vent and share their emotions and develop more confident and positive attitudes. The clinician may use open-ended questions or statements, such as "Now when I see my child disfluent, I tend to feel …," to stimulate group discussions.

Summary and Critique of Parent Advising Programs

The few programs we reviewed in this text appear to reflect not only past thinking but also significant portions of current practices in advising parents. As with parent treatment, questions must also be raised regarding the counseling–advising bred by learning theories of stuttering, especially Johnson's ideas (Johnson, 1942; Johnson et al., 1959) concerning the immediate cause of stuttering (i.e., parents' reaction to normal disfluency) and the function of awareness of disfluency or early stuttering in precipitating or aggravating the problem. (The role of awareness was also emphasized by Bluemel, 1932, and Van Riper, 1939.) As elaborated in Chapter 3, however, this theory has been basically discredited. Thus, advising should not contain information that implicates parents' behavior as causing the child's stuttering.

The circumstances are different, however, in regard to home environment factors that might contribute and complicate an *already existing* stuttering problem. The difference between cause and aggravating influences should be clearly explained to parents. As we mentioned earlier, although children who stutter, as a group, do not grow up in a home environment that is blatantly pathologic, there is no question that environmental factors influence stuttering. Bloodstein's (1981) analysis of the literature led him to state that much of the variation in the frequency of stuttering can be accounted for by communicative pressures. In a comprehensive review of the literature on the home environment of children who stutter, Yairi (1997b) concluded that there are consistent reports that these children are raised more frequently in less harmonious families, by parents who tend to be overprotective and anxious more frequently and to a greater degree than parents of normally fluent children. Those parents may also have negative evaluations of their child's personality, and sometimes react overtly in negative ways to the child's stuttering. Yairi stated, "Keeping in mind reservations about the quality of current data, my overall conclusion is that children who stutter have higher chances than do normally-speaking children of encountering unfavorable home conditions" (p. 42). Therefore, it would appear logical to provide parents with advice about improving the home environment and specifically their interaction with their children. Nevertheless, we caution readers that, in spite of wide support in the clinical literature for advising parents accordingly, our knowledge, based on carefully controlled scientific studies, is limited regarding the true effectiveness of advising parents, either on their own behaviors or the child's stuttering.

Among the few who addressed the parent counseling issue, Johnson (1961) credited 85% of improvement in the stuttering of 164 young children to the single extensive interview and brief counseling given to their parents at the initiation of his studies concerning the onset of stuttering. Furthermore, the rate of complete recovery for children whose parents received counseling was 45%, compared with 23% for children whose parents were interviewed but did not receive counseling. Similarly, Jameson (1955) concluded that "there is a greater chance of speech recovery if the mother attends for advice when the child is still under the age of 5 years" (p. 67). She reported that among 41 recovered stutterers, 12 received parent counseling only. In a group of 28 stutterers who did not recover, 2 received parent counseling only. Johnson's and Jameson's conclusions, however, were based on impressions of parents and interviewers, not on controlled procedures, such as careful descriptions of the children in groups, or objective data that document improvement.

In 1978, Zwitman reported on the effectiveness of parent counseling for 15 three- and four-year-old children who stuttered. Pre- and posttreatment speech samples were compared in terms of number of disfluencies for individual programs lasting 8 to 12 weeks. Six children stopped stuttering, 6 had notable reduction in stuttering, and 3 showed no change. A 6-month follow-up revealed that 1 of the 6 recovered stutterers was again abnormally disfluent. Of the children who had different degrees of speech improvement at the termination of the program, 1 showed complete recovery at follow-up, whereas the other 8 showed improvement. No control subjects were used. Several years later, Boada and Meyers (1990) reported on the effects of counseling for parents of preschool-age children at pretreatment, posttreatment, and follow-up. Parents were more positive than negative in all interactions, suggesting that the advice for them to be more positive had some effect. However, there were no significant changes in reducing negative comments or interruptions. Fortier-Blanc, Labonte, Beauchemin, and Jutras (1997) reported data that questioned the effectiveness of indirect intervention with preschool children who stutter. In our opinion, considering the high rate (up to 80%) of natural recovery from stuttering in early childhood (Andrews, 1984; Yairi & Ambrose, 1999b), any conclusion of such research must be based on tightly controlled studies comparing the effect of a particular counseling program to that of other forms of treatment and to no-treatment conditions.

Fosnot and Woodford (1992) took another direction in their questionnaire survey of 20 parents who regularly attended counseling that was designed to study parents' evaluation of the counseling. They reported high percentages of parents' satisfaction with various aspects of the instructional counseling. The humanistic counseling procedures, especially sharing of feelings, received the least favorable responses. These results, however, do not provide data about the effectiveness of counseling on actual parent behavior or on children's stuttering.

Specific Advice Given to Parents

A considerable portion of the literature on parental involvement has been designed to communicate directly to the general public at the lay level, using letter formats, pamphlets, and books. Typically this literature presents information about stuttering and lists suggestions for parents to follow. These sources vary in scope and orientation from being brief, general, more objective, and informative (National Institute of Health, 1981), to being wordy and specific (Murphy, 1962), to being rather dogmatic (Johnson, 1949). Specific forms of advice for parents can also be found in sources intended for speech pathologists, physicians, or other professionals (Bender, 1943; Sander, 1959). We thought it would be helpful for practicing clinicians and students to consider this extensive material, organized into several categories, most of which can be found in one or several of the following sources, as well as others: Ainsworth and Fraser-Gruss (1977, 2002), Bender (1943), Bloodstein (1958), Bluemel (1959), S. Brown (1949), Conture (1999), Cooper (1979), Curlee (1999a), Eisenson and Ogilvie (1957), Glasner (1962), Gregory (1999b), Gregory and Gregory (1999), Guitar (1999), Irwin (1980), Johnson (1949, 1959, 1961), R. Lewis (1949), Luper and Mulder (1964), Murphy (1962), National Institute of Health (1981), Paterson (1958), Perkins (1999), Sander (1959), Schuell (1949), M. Schwartz (1979), Starkweather (1982), Van Riper (1948), Wingate (1976), Wood (1948), Wyatt and Herzan (1962), Yairi (1982b), and Zwitman (1978). Except in a few cases, specific sources for each item will not be repeatedly cited.

Information About Stuttering and People Who Stutter. Sharing information with patients regarding any disorder has become increasingly common for various purposes, such as deciding upon treatment choice. In childhood stuttering, an important assumption has been that knowledge about the disorder reduces parents' apprehension. What information did various authors deem as important to share with parents? We were able to discern two major areas.

1. *Possible causes of stuttering.* The information that various authors share reflects large differences in theoretical orientation. Several older sources include statements about a single environmental or psychological cause. Others present a more balanced view of organic, psychogenic, and learning etiologies. A National Institute of Health publication from 1981 places a greater emphasis on physiological findings. One of the most recent sources (Ainsworth & Fraser, 2002) lists genetics as the etiology in 50% of cases, as well as emotional stress and muscle discoordination. Conture (1999) emphasizes multiple etiologies, and also suggests delays or differences in brain functions concerned with speech planning. Many sources expand also on what does not cause stuttering (e.g., imitation, starting school).

2. *Facts about the population of stutterers.* The most common information that authors deemed important concerns incidence, age at onset, gender ratio and its meaning, familial incidence, natural recovery, and the general normalcy of those who stutter (except for their stuttering). There has also been a change in interpreting familial incidence of stuttering, away from past psycho-sociological explanations to recognition of genetic factors.

Normal and Stuttered Speech. Information that compares normal and stuttered speech is typically more detailed and less guarded or qualified than information about the etiology of stuttering. Parents are advised about the following topics.

1. *Norms of speech and language development.* This information relates to milestones and processes in the acquisition of speech sounds, words, and sentences. The emphasis is often that in many cases the child who begins stuttering is still in the process of learning new speech and language skills.

2. *Disfluency norms.* Many sources make the point that speech disfluencies are normal and common, part of normal development. The normalcy of disfluency tends to be overemphasized and exaggerated to the point of providing erroneous information. For example, Ainsworth and Fraser (2002) suggest that it is not uncommon for 3-year-olds to say, "Can I have my ba-ba-ba-baby?" when, in fact, current data indicate that it is rather rare for a normally fluent child to emit three extra repetition units.

3. *Symptoms and "warning signs" of incipient stuttering.* Parents are informed what they should be watching for in their child's disfluency that signifies stuttering rather than normal disfluency. Multiple repetitions of syllables and words, use of the schwa vowel in syllable repetitions, prolongations of sounds and tension, and effort in getting through the disfluencies seem to top the list. There seems to be some confusion between warning signs for the presence of stuttering and risk factors for chronic stuttering (e.g., Ainsworth & Fraser, 2002).

4. *Patterns, fluctuations, and development of early stuttering.* Authors provide information about changing symptomatology, such as easy repetitions developing into tense prolongations and blocks, situational influences on the frequency of stuttering, and the

up-and-down cycles of the disorder. Ainsworth and Fraser (2002) incorporate recent information concerning factors that seem to increase chances of natural recovery. Guitar (1999) writes about issues that may concern parents of children who persist in stuttering (e.g., the effects of stuttering on future dating and marriage are minimized). Parents are advised to be accepting, provide a lot of support, and continue with behaviors recommended during past treatment or counseling.

General Health. Health-related advice is relatively uncommon. Such limited interest probably reflects the generally accepted notion that preschool children who stutter, as a group, do not exhibit unusual health history. Some experts recommend a medical examination only to alleviate parents' concerns that something is physically wrong with the child. Bender (1943) and Eisenson and Ogilvie (1977), on the other hand, believed that poor health may have precipitating influences on the young child's speech and encouraged active parental attention. The advice of a few authors who took more interest in health matters can be summarized in the following statements:

1. *Resolve common childhood health problems* such as malnutrition, indigestion, sleeplessness, and various diseases.
2. *Regulate rest and bedtime.* Suggestions include consistent or early bedtime and even confinement to bed for a few days, especially immediately after onset (Bender, 1943; Bluemel, 1959; Johnson, 1961; L. Nelson, 1999).
3. *Regulate diet* (i.e., eliminate refined sugar and caffeine, supplement with vitamins and minerals) (Bender, 1943; R. Lewis, 1949, M. Schwartz, 1979).
4. *Promote regular physical exercise* (Bender, 1943).

Relaxation and Reduced Stimulation. Several sources emphasize the importance of creating a relaxed, tranquil atmosphere around the child, a position based on the common clinical observation that stuttering in early life occurs chiefly under conditions of excitement, often when the child feels hurried or under stress. The advice that parents receive can be summarized as follows:

1. *Reduce the pace of everyday life.* Engage the child in fewer activities, allow more time for each one, move slowly, and avoid rushing the child.
2. *Reduce environmental overstimulation.* Auditory, visual, or other stimuli result in irritation. Periods of quiet (even without conversation) should occur at home to promote inward composure. The child's surroundings should be kept organized.
3. *Avoid excess physical stimulation.* Restrict vigorous play activities that build excitement and exhaustion. Control shouting and teasing.
4. *Minimize psychological excitement.* Keep preparations low key in relation to upcoming holidays, vacation trips, birthdays, and so forth.

Environmental Pressures. Perhaps the most common belief expressed in the literature is that various environmental pressures are responsible for maintaining stuttering (some authors hold that they may cause stuttering) and that parents should change their behavior to reduce these pressures. Bloodstein (1958) regarded parental pressure and anxiety imposed on the child as the most important factor capable of turning a young child's disfluencies into chronic stuttering. Although the diagnosogenic theory of stuttering was seriously questioned rather early (Wingate, 1962) and eventually lost credibility altogether (Ambrose & Yairi, 2002), the belief in the importance of controlling environmental pressures through parent counseling has been upheld. It has probably been sustained as a result of increasing research data on the characteristics of the home environment of children who stutter, as mentioned earlier.

In addition to recommending lessening pressure in general, the literature has addressed advice related to three major area-specific pressures:

1. *Speech-related pressures*
   a. Keep a log of the child's stuttering to identify pressures that influence its occurrence.
   b. Do not express anxiety about, disapproval of, or negative reaction to the child's stuttering.
   c. Do not interrupt the child. Reduce time pressure on the child's speech.
   d. Do not press the child to speak in any situation, especially when he or she becomes the focus of attention.
   e. Do not advise the child how to speak by saying, for example, "be fluent," "slow down," "think," and so on.

2. *Biological function pressures*
   a. Minimize concerns about how much the child eats and about his or her eating manners.
   b. Keep bedtime a simple event; avoid rigidity.
   c. Do not unduly push toilet training.
3. *Behavioral–social–family pressures*
   a. Be less restrictive of the child's behavior; scold less.
   b. Reduce criticism and correcting; be less demanding and accept the child's level of performance.
   c. Reduce competition for attention and sibling rivalry.

Emotional Health. Although only a few authors, particularly Glasner (1949, 1962), thought that young children who begin stuttering, as a group, suffer emotional problems, the literature contains frequent suggestions that parents should attend to the task of improving the child's emotional stability. Specific suggestions follow:

1. *Reexamine discipline methods* to prevent formation of deep fears in the child. Maintain consistency in approach.
2. *Improve interactions with the child.* Be a good listener, spend time with the child, and help him or her express feelings.
3. *Provide feelings of security* by showing the child tangible affection and reducing the intensity of family quarrels.
4. *Develop self-confidence* by giving the child responsibilities and proper praise; do not pamper the child.

Handling Moments of Stuttering. A definite change of attitude toward handling moments of stuttering—from passive denial of stuttering to an open recognition of its occurrence and even to its active correction—has been taking place over the years. Still, opinions are diverse, sometimes conflicting, on this issue. The most common advice follows:

1. *Wait for the child to finish the stuttered word.* Be a patient listener, do not help the child say a word, and accept or ignore the stuttering.
2. *Reassure the child* after instances of pronounced stuttering; show that the difficulty is recognized and understandable.
3. *Remind the child to slow down* and repeat the word easily (Ainsworth & Fraser-Gruss, 1977; Irwin, 1980; Yairi, 1982b).
4. *Model for the child by repeating the stuttered word* in an easy manner but without further comment.

5. *Minimize the child's talking;* redirect the child to activities that do not require talking.

Speech Models. The idea that parents' speaking patterns may influence the child's stuttering has been mentioned in many sources, the rationale being that children learn by imitating the adult models they hear. By listening to and repeating good models, the child is more likely to develop correct speech. Whereas some authors feel this is particularly important for the child who is at the juncture between normal disfluency and early stuttering, others have applied the principle to all young children who stutter. Advice on this point varies from vague statements to detailed specification of speaking rates for the parents. The following are examples of specific advice:

1. *Habitually demonstrate good voice and speech,* including smooth speech, nice quality, melodic voice, and soft voice.
2. *Provide realistic language models.* Use simpler words and short phrases proper for the child's age.
3. *Slow down conversational pace* and turn-taking style; pause before answering.
4. *Speak at a normally slow rate;* avoid hurried speech.
5. *Speak at a slower rate than normal;* use stretched speech.
6. *Practice speech directly with the child.*

Both Bluemel (1959) and M. Schwartz (1976) advocated home programs to facilitate the child's adoption of slow speech. Bluemel suggested planned activities of reading aloud, telling stories, singing, and so on, with the child repeating or joining in. Schwartz advocated daily practice with stretched speech.

Professional Help. Urging parents to enlist professional consultation is one of the most common recommendations found in pamphlets. Specific suggestions include these:

1. Seek professional help, especially of a speech–language clinician experienced with stuttering.
2. Pursue intervention soon after stuttering onset.
3. Obtain information about the nature of clinical intervention and expected parental involvement.

Summary of Specific Advice

The preceding review of the many kinds of specific advice for parents of preschool-age children who stutter reflects the overall "wisdom of the field." Interestingly, except for conflicting views on how to handle instances of perceived stuttering, and the relatively little enthusiasm for diet-related items, this portion of the literature reflects reasonable agreement among many expert clinicians as to what parents should be told. Differences are more in terms of emphasis than substance. The variations in advice that may be confusing can be simplified and made more useful to clinicians to consider when compressed into only 10 items. Thus, parents should be advised to do the following:

1. Seek professional help and obtain basic information about stuttering to correct unfounded assumptions and alleviate misplaced anxiety and guilt.
2. Become informed about the prognosis of stuttering and factors that may facilitate or impede progress.
3. Become informed about normal speech and language development and the differences between normal and abnormal disfluencies.
4. Reduce general tension at home. This can be done through identifying and decreasing routine frictions in everyday parent–child relations.
5. Reduce pressures directed toward the child who stutters. This can be done by analyzing their own expectations, demands, and restrictions.
6. Minimize situations likely to elicit pronounced stuttering in an effort to prevent the child's frustration and growing fears of stuttering.
7. Avoid negative comments or other types of verbal or nonverbal reactions that convey disapproval of the child's stuttering.
8. Learn how to constructively handle moments of stuttering: Wait patiently without reacting, or kindly acknowledge the problem, assure the child, and suggest or demonstrate easy speech.
9. Create a home atmosphere conducive to slow speech and fluency. Strive to reduce physical stimulation, excitement, and the pace of activities, and to maintain quietness.
10. Facilitate fluency by providing the child with a model of uncomplicated language and slow speaking rate.

Critique of Advice to Parents

In spite of the common appearance in the literature of many of the recommendations listed in our review, and the popularity they have maintained among speech–language clinicians, their practical merit awaits sound scientific basis. There are virtually no data on the effect on children's stuttering of, for instance, being a good listener, toilet training, and early bedtime. Although relatively limited scientific evidence has been reported in support of the clinical effectiveness of much of the advice, interest in these aspects of intervention has been growing, particularly in the potential relevance of several items concerned with the speech and language patterns modeled by parents. For example, Miles and Bernstein Ratner (2001) reported that the language input of mothers of preschool-age children who stutter was not different from that of control parents. Furthermore, there were no differences between the language of parents of children who recovered from stuttering within 1 year and those who persisted. The authors concluded that the premise underlying admonition for parents to reduce the length and complexity of their utterances (e.g., Bloodstein, 1995; Conture & Melnick, 1999) should be reconsidered. Miles and Bernstein Ratner also cautioned about the potential long-term harmful effect of such advice to the child's language development. Weiss (2002) reported a preliminary investigation on the language recast behavior of parents of school-age children who stutter and control parents (i.e., the parents' accurate reformulation of the child's utterances). No significant differences or specific relationships to the occurrence of stuttering were found.

An important impetus for research in this domain was made in a series of articles by Meyers and Freeman (e.g., Meyers, 1989, 1990; Meyers & Freeman, 1985). Among other factors on which these two authors, as well as others, focused was the speaking rate of parents. As the case has often been, conflicting findings have been reported. Meyers and Freeman (1985) measured the speaking rate of mothers of 12 four- and five-year-old boys who stutter and mothers of a matched control group. Mothers of stuttering children exhibited rates that were significantly faster by a half syllable per second, on average, than the rates of control mothers. Others, however, reported no differences (e.g., Kelly, 1994; Schultze, 1991).

Overall, current information does not provide sufficient support for any hypothesis that parents of children who stutter talk in ways that present more complex or faster speech models that could be viewed as stressful or having other negative influences (Bernstein Ratner, 1993; Nippold &

Rudzinski, 1995; Yairi, 1997a). This lack of evidence, however, does not mean that reducing parents' language complexity or speaking rate to below normal would not also reduce the children's level of stuttering. Such simplification in parent modeling may work in ways that are still not apparent to us. Current ideas about the central speech and language processes underlying stuttering would seem to enhance advice for slower speech and simplified language. Zebrowski, Weiss, Savelkoul, and Hammer (1996) noted that, in two cases in their dyad sample, the mothers' language usage appeared to be related to the child's level of fluency. Stephanson-Opsal and Bernstein Ratner (1988) showed that the mother's slower rate had the effect of reducing the child's stuttering, although the child's own rate actually increased. Researchers also have studied the gap between the speaking rates of adults and of children. Kelly (1999) found that reduction in the adult–child speaking rate gap facilitated fluency in some children who stuttered, and, as discussed further in Chapter 13, evidence for the influence of the parent's slow speaking rate on the child's rate has been reported by Guitar and Marchinkoski (2001). Our main conclusion is that much more research is needed, with larger numbers of children and in which each type of advice given to parents is investigated in isolation using sophisticated design and controls.

A Sample Outline and Narrative of Parent Advising

A distinction should be made between the immediate advising in conjunction with the initial evaluation and in-depth counseling provided as part of comprehensive intervention. We focus here on the first. Although this "counseling" often ends up largely as the clinician's monologue, after the completion of a lengthy evaluation lasting several hours over two or three sessions, sharing information with parents about findings, impressions, and reasons for recommendations, as well as allowing them special time for questions, is a must. The clinician should consider that this may be the last contact with the family (not a rare situation if the family resides in a distant community) and, therefore, select the essential information and advice he or she would like to provide the parents. Although some parents may be comfortable with their child in the room during presentation of general information about stuttering, we feel that discussion about the child requires the parents to come alone. A special visit without the child affords a more relaxed and open session in which parents can freely discuss concerns and problems regarding their child. Because many new clinicians are a bit overwhelmed with the task of summarizing and presenting basic feedback and information for parents, we offer an outline and a sample narrative for the initial parent advising. (In this hypothetical case, the child is a boy.) Clinicians, however, should be keenly aware of reservations regarding the actual scientific support for the merit of specific parental advice.

I. Results of Evaluation. Typically, at the conclusion of the evaluation, the clinician is in a position to confirm the parents' diagnosis of stuttering and provide them with a general assessment of the current status of the disorder. Furthermore, findings from other domains covered in the evaluation are considered, with special reference to their impact on, or interaction with, the child's stuttering.

    A. *Findings Concerning Stuttering.* The clinician may start by saying, "Yes, our evaluation confirms your judgment that your child indeed exhibits stuttering. In our opinion it is mild but still unquestionably different from normal disfluency. Although his speech is at times fluent, eventually he slides into periods of talking during which he stutters. As you have reported, he exhibits quite a few repetitions of syllables and short words; in some instances he repeats syllables and short words three or four times. These are associated with some physical tension at a moderate level. Normally fluent children repeat considerably less frequently, and they typically repeat a syllable or word only once. Once in a while, we also heard very brief prolongations of vowels in your child's speech, like on the word 'and,' and we also noticed a few instances of eye squinting during stuttering. Generally, however, the speech and other characteristics we have noticed are common in early stuttering." With a different child, however, the conclusion can be summarized as follows: "What we have observed would seem to indicate that his stuttering is quite severe and complex. In fact, it is now beyond the typical early stage of the disorder."

    B. *Other Findings.* At this point, the clinician reviews for the parents results of language, phonology, motor, hearing, and any other tests and observations. An example follows: "Your child's speech and language skills are typical for his age. This means that he understands and can express language at the level we would expect for his age. He has errors in the way he makes a few speech sounds but not at a level of concern at this point. We will send you a brief report with results of formal tests and other pertinent analyses of speech and language." In another case, however, the clinician might say, "In addition to the stuttering, your child also has some difficulties with making speech sounds. He is a bit behind where he should be for his age, although it is not hard to understand his speech. He may need a little help with this later if he doesn't improve on his own. We also noticed that your child had some difficulty staying on task. Are you aware or concerned about this? Have you sought professional opinions?" A positive comment about some of the child's strengths is opportune during this discussion, such as, "Overall your child is a good communicator and has many interesting things to say."

II. Information and Prognosis. Having presented the findings for the child, the clinician may wish to continue by providing general information about the incidence, onset, and possible developmental paths of the disorder. Statements about the commonality of stuttering in young children and its generally positive prognosis also serve to alleviate some of the parents' worries.

A. *Incidence.* "You should know that stuttering is quite common in young children; about 5% of them stutter for some period during childhood, primarily between ages 2 and 6. The majority of those children begin to stutter between ages 2 and 4. So, your child is a bit below the middle of this range. More boys than girls stutter, and this difference has some implications concerning what may happen with the stuttering in the near future."

B. *Recovery and Chronicity.* "The good news is that our current scientific information is quite encouraging, showing that a large majority of children (about 75%) who begin stuttering also stop stuttering without treatment. This appears to be a natural development. From a practical point of view, the percentage is higher (perhaps 85%) because many children who persist show very mild, or near recovered, stuttering. Therefore, your child's chance of getting better, or even of stopping his stuttering, is considerably better than his chance of developing persistent stuttering. Children who recover do this at different times. Some recover rather quickly, within a few months to a year after onset, but most recover between 1 and 3 years after onset. A few even recover after 4 years or longer. Still, 15% to 25% of children who stutter develop a chronic stuttering problem that lasts for several or many years."

C. *Prediction.* Continuing with this line, the clinician may then proceed: "Currently, we cannot make an accurate prediction about the future course of the stuttering of each child seen in our clinic. This is true also for your son. But we can estimate the relative chance of recovery. For example, the longer the time after onset, the smaller are the chances for recovery. Girls have better chances. The age at onset may be a factor. Those who begin at young ages may have a better chance. The past family history is a factor. If members of your family used to stutter and recovered, your child's chance to recover is also quite good. On the other hand, if other relatives stuttered for a long time, your child also has a good chance of following this pattern. You told me earlier that you have no relatives who have ever stuttered. You have expressed your concern because your child stutters quite severely. The stuttering severity at onset or a short time after, however, is not a good sign of persistence. We have seen many children with severe stuttering who have recovered. Severity is a much more important factor at a later stage, say 1 or 2 years after onset.

"So, let's see what we can suggest about the future course of your child's stuttering. Your son is now 36 months old, and we have evaluated him only 3 months after onset. He exhibits rather severe stuttering in terms of frequency of disfluency (16 Stuttering-Like Disfluencies per 100 syllables), moderate tension, and a few secondary characteristics. We did not detect any emotional reactions to the stuttering. You reported no known familial history of stuttering. He tested normal on the phonology and language tests. At this point, there is no reason to view him as being at high risk. He should, however, be closely monitored for several months. We would like to see him again in 3 months. If there are signs of improvement, good. We will continue monitoring. If things do not change, we'll then consider the option of intervention."

III. Intervention. At this point, it makes sense to continue talking with parents about intervention options and the current views about them, even if a waiting period is recommended. Parents should be informed consumers, better able to make decisions or seek additional advice. Certainly, this topic is essential in cases when parents raise the issue of therapy, or when the clinician recommends immediate intervention.

A. *Intervention.* "You ask about therapy options. This is a rather complicated issue, and as in many other health conditions, experts vary greatly in their opinions about the best course of treatment. For example, when one of us had an extremely painful condition of a herniated disk, two doctors recommended surgery but a third one insisted on waiting a while for natural healing, which has an approximate 70% chance of success. All three consulted the same test results and other medical data. As for early childhood stuttering, until 20 years ago or so, the standard 'rule' was that the child should not receive direct therapy for fear that early intervention might cause more damage by drawing attention to the stuttering. Treatment focused on the parents, who received counseling. The situation, however, has changed. At the present, many clinicians advocate early intervention. On the other hand, some do not believe that each child should begin therapy right away if it is only a matter of months after onset, because the risk factors vary greatly. They think it makes sense to wait a while, to give natural recovery a chance. The child's progress is monitored, and decisions about intervention are made accordingly. Of course, your feelings and wishes in this respect are an important consideration in deciding what to do and when. Parents, too, are different in their opinions. Some wish to wait whereas others are anxious to begin therapy as soon as possible."

B. *Types of Therapy.* "Although many treatment programs have been developed by speech–language clinicians and other professionals, there seem to be six major approaches involving the child in treatment[a]: (a) encouraging the child to use slow speech through modeling and practice (Pindzola), (b) gradually increasing the length of fluent speech the child can make by means of systematic positive reinforcement (Costello Ingham), (c) discouraging and correcting instances of stuttering while also reinforcing instances of fluent speech (Onslow and associates), (d) practicing on improvement of oral movement skills (G. D. Riley & Riley), (e) improving the child's interpersonal communication skills (Conture), and (f) involving the child in play therapy (Wakaba). Most programs provide some individual or group parent counseling, and some use parents in helping with implementing the child's treatment. Other programs focus on improving parent–child interactions (Rustin)."

C. *Effectiveness of Treatment.* "Are these therapies any good? We tend to think that they help in various ways, either in reducing the child's stuttering or in creating better parent–child relationships. Nevertheless, only a small amount of good data is available on the successes of treatment for early childhood stuttering. Several clinicians who conducted studies in this area reported what appear to be good results. There are, however, several reservations about the findings of these studies. For example, much of the reported success may be a function of the high level of

---

[a] More information about these programs can be found in Chapter 13.

natural recovery that I explained to you earlier. No sufficient controls have been employed in several critical aspects of these studies. Nevertheless, there is a choice, should you decide to seek additional help. We would be happy to further advise you about availability of clinical services."

IV. Causes of Stuttering. The clinician should, at this point, make yet another shift in the discussion and answer questions that parents asked earlier or additional questions that arose while the clinician was talking. Almost always parents want to hear about what causes stuttering. We aim at providing a broad view without confusing the parents, and also use the opportunity to alleviate preconceived erroneous beliefs that often cause undue concerns. Thus, the clinician may continue as follows: "There have been many diverse ideas about the cause of stuttering, but we are still not too clear about what makes a child stutter. It is possible to distinguish four major groups of theories or explanations.

"First are *psychogenic explanations.* These suggest that the stuttering that we hear and see is only a symptom of something else that is the real problem. In the past, some people theorized that deep emotional difficulties, often called 'conflicts,' were created in early childhood. They think that the problems are unconscious and, therefore, often impossible for the child to deal with. When the conflicts are not recognized and resolved, they lead to the speech difficulties. A good comparison here is fever. Fever is not a disease, but a symptom of an infection somewhere in the body. When the infection subsides, the fever disappears too. I want you to know, however, that although people have thought that stuttering is 'psychogenic,' these explanations are not accepted by most experts today. The best research has failed to show that people who stutter, as a group, are more neurotic or have more other psychological disorders than those who do not stutter. We do not think that your child began stuttering because of any serious emotional difficulties. It is true, however, that when stuttering continues, the child may eventually develop all sorts of emotional reactions. These are the results, not the cause, of stuttering.

"The second group is that of *learning explanations.* These are quite different from ideas about psychogenic causes. By 'learning' we mean a behavior that the child develops in a complex manner; some people refer to it as a habit. There have been many explanations as to how children acquire stuttering behavior as a habit. A popular theory that you may have heard is that stuttering begins as normal speech repetitions, for example, 'and-and' or 'Mo-mommy'—the kind of repetitions that all children do as they learn how to talk. The theory says that if parents worry about the repetitions and frequently react to them in negative ways, the child may get quite tense while talking, and the easy normal repetitions become tense—what we call stuttering. In this scenario, without treatment, stuttering gets progressively worse over time. Again, the great majority of experts nowadays do not accept this explanation which, unfortunately, puts the blame on parents. The scientific data do not support it. We believe, however, that once the child begins stuttering, for whatever reason, the way people respond to it is likely to have considerable influence.

"The third group consists of *organic explanations*. These, too, are very different. They convey the idea that, in people who stutter, something is wrong with the biochemistry, brain anatomy, or movement coordination of speech muscles. Various organic reasons have been suggested as causes of stuttering. Long ago, it was thought that perhaps a large tongue or that being left-handed and forced to write with the right hand were causes of stuttering. In spite of much research, for a long time it has been impossible to identify a particular, consistent abnormality. More recently, several investigators reported findings of various differences in brain functioning between adults who stutter and normally fluent people. Although it appears that adults who stutter are somewhat different from those who do not stutter, there is not enough information and little is definitive. Furthermore, differences in brain function in adults may be the results of years of stuttering, not the cause of stuttering. So far, no data have been reported for young children who stutter.

"Finally, there have been *complex explanations*, combining some of the above as well as other notions. These explanations reflect current thinking. Although we do not know what causes stuttering, we are quite sure that in most cases stuttering is genetically transmitted in families. But we do not yet know what it is that is being genetically transmitted. Perhaps there is an organic factor, structure, or function that is inherited, for example, a genetically based flaw in the speech planning process. It may surface and become apparent during the period of rapid expansion of the language system in young children. Perhaps such a flaw requires certain environmental conditions to be triggered in order to produce stuttering. Indeed, there are strong indications that environment may play a substantial role, and that there is a complex interplay between genetic and environmental contributions. In short, regardless of what you may have read or heard, there currently is no satisfactory answer to the question of what causes stuttering or why many children stop stuttering on their own accord and some do not."

V. Parents' Involvement. Having briefly brought parents into the midst of the big questions that have fascinated investigators of stuttering for many years, the clinician should then return to the practical level and focus on what can be done now to alleviate the child's stuttering regardless of whether the child is recommended to receive professional treatment. The clinician should attempt to suggest what parents can actively do. Because most parents are confused, and many experience guilt, this aspect of the counseling is very important.

Prior to providing specific advice, the clinician should share some caveats about what he or she is about to suggest: "We want to share with you some advice that many clinicians have recommended to parents of preschool children who have begun stuttering. Again, it is important to emphasize that, although these may make sense, too often there is no adequate scientific evidence, if any, showing that if parents follow any, some, or all of the advice, their child will improve or stop stuttering. Nor is there evidence that, if the child stops stuttering, the change was indeed enhanced by parents' acting on the advice. Nevertheless, this is the collective 'wisdom of the field,' and if it makes sense, you may wish to implement the suggestions and judge for yourself. We will focus on two aspects: general home management and handling instances of stuttering."

A. *General Home Environment.* "Concerning home environment in general, if your child is one of the majority who has a predisposition for natural recovery from stuttering, then you may wish to ensure that conditions surrounding the child will not hinder the recovery process. If your child is heading into the chronic stuttering pathway, attention to the following may reduce his level of stuttering, as well as other problems that often come to be associated with stuttering. So, here is perhaps the most common advice given to parents by many clinicians.

"*Decrease undue pressures.* We know that stuttering is sensitive to various types of pressure. We often see this in older children and adults. Many clinicians feel that such pressure contributes to the aggravation and persistence of stuttering. If true, the logical conclusion is to identify and reduce sources of pressure. Of course, what is pressure to one child is not necessarily pressure to another. Quite likely, however, you have already recognized a few of your behaviors or home situations: various demands, expectations, rules, restrictions, and so on, that you may wish to change. Can you tell me one example? One good way is for you, as parents, to get together a few times and identify home situations that perhaps put undue pressure on your child. Review a typical day. Are there consistent situations that create conflict with the child and cause you or him to get upset: waking up, getting dressed, eating breakfast, playing, dinner time, bedtime, and so on? Can you do something to change your habitual reaction? Can you allow yourself wider margins of flexibility before reacting to the child's behavior? Is there an alternative response on your part to resolve the situation? Do not set high goals in pursuing this issue. A few limited changes, with realistic chances of success, are good enough to begin with.

"*Work on slowing down the pace of life.* One of the most frequent observations related by parents about their child who stutters is that he or she stutters when or stutters more when stimulated (physically or psychologically), excited, irritated, and in a hurry. Thus, it makes sense to reduce physical and emotional stimulation, pursue slow-paced activity, slow down play activity, and do things in a more relaxed fashion. For example, take the child for a walk rather than playing roughly with him to the point that he huffs and puffs and starts stuttering. Aim for small changes. For example, if getting the child ready in the morning is a pressure point in your day, plan ahead to reduce conflict. You might tell the child to find socks and shoes and place them by the door before the timer rings (set for 5 minutes). Tell the child that lunch menus will be talked about after he gets into the car. Get up 10 minutes earlier than usual. Realize that the goal is not to eradicate time pressure or stress from your household, but to define and change certain pressure points. Children need to be excited and active, but not all the time. Reducing excitability even by 5% or 10% may keep the child below the threshold of behavior that may trigger stuttering.

"*Slow speech.* It has been shown that a slow speaking rate reduces stuttering. Slow speech is one method that is used in stuttering therapy, for both adults and children. It is difficult to expect a child to slow down when everybody else around him speaks fast. Therefore, clinicians believe that if parents talk slower to their child, their model may influence the child to follow suit. In fact, a recent study has provided initial data that support the idea. Talking slowly, however, is quite difficult for many parents and takes time to get used to. For example, you might talk slowly for a short time when you tell a story, about as slow as I will be talking for the next minute or two. Or, you might speak slowly for a short time when you help your child build with blocks or make things. You may then extend this slowing down to other situations, such as when you are driving in the car. In general, doing things slowly facilitates slower speech, and vice versa; talking slowly is not conducive to fast movements and excitability.

"*Improve self-confidence.* It is important for every child to feel good about himself. Unfortunately, a child who stutters is more likely to fail in maintaining self-confidence than many other children, especially if he persists in stuttering. Sooner or later he will experience some negative reactions from others, or experience frustration about his own speaking difficulties. In this case, it is especially important to help him develop confidence and a positive self-image. You can accomplish this in many small ways. Enlist your child in daily chores—picking up sticks in the yard while you rake, carrying some of his clean laundry to his room, putting toys away, or any small task that he can help with. Be sure to praise him for his cooperation and the good job he has done. Also, help your child develop or pursue a pleasurable hobby or activity in which he is good but that does not depend on speech. This promotes self-esteem and ensures that the child realizes he can be good at some things. Athletic and artistic outlets are good examples."

B. *Handling Moments of Stuttering.* "You asked what you should do when your child stutters. Although many clinicians suggest a generally passive parent behavior, others suggest a more active one. We think that some mixture is warranted. Here are a few types of things you can do.

"*Wait patiently.* In many instances of mild stuttering, perhaps the best thing you can do is wait patiently without reacting directly to the stuttering. This is the passive approach.

"*Use echoing.* When stuttering is moderate to severe, sometimes you may become more active by echoing or repeating the word on which the child stuttered. Repeat the word in an easy, somewhat prolonged, but fluent manner. No need for you to comment, just do it. This way, you show the child how stuttering can be corrected, and you do it without bothering him too much with suggestions. For example, the child says, 'I w-w-w-want another cookie.' You reply, slowly and easily, 'Oh, so you wa→nt another cookie.'

"*Use direct instruction.* At other times, you might suggest to the child, 'Let's say this word again easily together,' proceeding as described above, with an easy reproduction of the word. Or, you can say, 'Try saying this again easily,' and let him repeat the word alone.

"*Show empathy.* When stuttering is severe and the child seems to be frustrated or to react negatively in other ways, it is okay to recognize the problem and utter an encouraging word. For example, you might say, 'Sometimes speech is difficult, but we can learn to make it easier. Let's say it easily together.' From very early, make it easier for the child and you to talk about stuttering. Many parents and children never talk about it, even as the child continues to stutter. Think of how you would handle a minor cut or scrape. The child is upset, and you acknowledge that, saying, 'That's too bad; I'm sorry it hurts.' You proceed to wash it off, and provide a kiss or bandage. Then you move on to the next activity. You let the child know that you recognize his discomfort, and also that it's not something terrible that should be dwelled upon."

VI. Conclusion. The clinician should end the session with a summary of what he or she said previously, highlighting the main points, and outlining a clear plan of action for the near future. The clinician should advise parents to closely monitor the child's stuttering, taking notes of specific disfluency and secondary characteristics, emotional reactions, and changes in severity that they observe. We suggest that parents keep a diary or notebook in a kitchen drawer for handy access. If immediate therapy is not recommended, a follow-up visit within 2 to 3 months should be scheduled. Parents' attention may be drawn to additional sources of information and support, such as the Stuttering Foundation of America (www.stuttersfa.org or www.stutterhelp.org) and the National Stuttering Association (www.nsastutter.org or www.westutter.org). They should be encouraged to contact the clinician again should a substantial increase in stuttering occur. Finally, the clinician should assure the parents that they have already taken the most important step in optimizing their child's potential to be a good communicator with strong self-esteem: They have had an early evaluation.

Parent Training (Parent as Cotherapist)

A third category of counseling programs can be distinguished by its main objective of providing parents with *concrete training* in modifying their behaviors or with training to transfer therapeutic procedures to the home environment. Characteristically, parents are also encouraged to participate in the child's therapy sessions. Several early programs that have left a strong mark on more current programs (described in Chapter 13) are briefly reviewed in this section.

A unique form of what we have referred to as parent training as a cotherapist is filial therapy, which engages parents in their child's treatment by learning to conduct nondirective play therapy at home (Guerney, 1964). Application to stuttering was first reported in 1974 by Andronico and Blake. The objective is to have parents show the child understanding and acceptance of his or her feelings. Emphasis is placed on empathy. Following the clinician's demonstrations, the parent assumes the play therapist role while being observed and supervised. Carryover to home therapy sessions begins after a 6- to 10-week training period. Parents learn to demonstrate their understanding by "reflecting" on the child's verbal or play expressions without imposing their own feelings upon the interaction. The training program is also extended to meet parents' emotional needs through group discussions.

A different direction of parent training was taken by Wyatt and Herzan (1962). Their assumption was that stuttering in young children represents a primary disorder of language. Specifically, it was considered to be the result of "disruption of the complementary pattern of verbal interaction between mother and child" (p. 650). Parent–child interaction might have been either unsatisfactory in nature or not frequent enough. Consequently, Wyatt and Herzan's program aims at establishing normal, successful patterns of interaction. Preschool children and their mothers are seen together by the therapist, and both undergo learning experiences. Mothers are taught to attune themselves to the child's level of verbal and nonverbal communication, become alert to the child's messages, and respond correctly. An additional emphasis is on mutual imitation of linguistic expression and on incorporation of the child's frequent expressions into parent's speech. This training is viewed as facilitating not only language skills, but also close interaction. The therapy is basically a form of "mother guidance" in behaving and talking. The therapist teaches the mother first through explanation and analysis, then through actual demonstration. Next, the mother takes over much of the therapy time. She is not to be replaced by the therapist; she must fulfill her roles as the primary speech model and must have the satisfaction of being competent in helping the child improve his or her speech.

Egolf, Shames, Johnson, and Kasprisin-Burrelli (1972) also described a training program designed to improve parent–child interactions, which they presumed to be the factors that maintain stuttering. We include it here although they described use with school-age children. Samples of parent–child interaction are scrutinized to identify and analyze major parent behaviors, such as verbal aggression, silence, interruption, and so on. Therapy consists of two stages. First, the child speaks in the presence of the clinician, who deliberately acts in a manner that contrasts with that of the parent, a manner that the authors determined to improve the child's fluency. Second, the child speaks in the presence of the clinician and parent. The parent joins in and participates in the conversation. The major assumption is that if the child speaks fluently in the presence of the parent, fluency is generalized. The child should observe, follow the clinician's model, and make corresponding changes in his or her own behavior, which, in the past, perpetuated stuttering.

Several developments in the 1970s and 1980s began influencing the content and form of parental involvement in the treatment of young children beginning to stutter. These included research findings that implied inferiority of the motor speech system as a significant factor in stuttering (e.g., G. D. Riley & Riley, 1985; Zimmermann, 1980b), a growing interest in rate control techniques in stuttering therapy with adults (Perkins, 1973), and the assertion of a few scientists that natural recovery from stuttering in preschool ages is actually the result of parental encouragement of slow speech in children (R. J. Ingham, 1983; Wingate, 1976). Consequently, there has been an inclination toward training parents to talk slowly as a means of inducing slow speech in the child, or encouraging parents to suggest slow speech to the child in the most direct ways. Thus, although Gregory and Hill (1980) involved parents in group and individual advising that focused on traditional objectives, they also provided parents with concrete demonstration of interactive behaviors and helped them acquire and use better speech models at home. They employed role playing, observation of therapy and films, and analyses of videos of parent–child interaction. Prins (1983) emphasized the role of counseling in using parents as basically trained observers assigned specific tasks to provide essential data for making clinical decisions. In their home observations, parents were asked to focus on four dimensions: (a) child speaking—amount, situations, fluency variations, and language complexity; (b) parent speaking—rate, complexity of language, number of questions, and number of explanations; (c) parent listening—amount of exclusive listening, behavior during listening, and frequency of interruptions; and (d) daily routine—meals, bedtime, and their interaction with the other factors.

Costello (1999) trained parents to acquire specific behaviors through participation in the child's therapy session. First, parents observe therapy sessions that focus on direct speech modification (e.g., the Extended Length of Utterance program described in Chapter 13). Once a workable procedure is developed for the child, parents are invited to become active participants and actually practice those skills, which they are required to exercise at home.

L. Johnson (1980) described a parent training program consisting of two basic procedures: selective attention and speech pattern modification. The first focused on training parents of children with incipient stuttering to eliminate attentive responses to stuttering and increase them consequent to fluent speech. The second procedure aimed at training the parents to talk at a slowed speech rate of 160 to 180 syllables per minute, maintaining continuous flow and short phrases. This rate is employed at home initially in selected situations and later as often as possible. Parents are closely monitored through logs, weekly tape-recorded conversations at home, and biweekly conferences with the clinician. Other clinicians either have advised parents to slow down their speaking rates considerably (M. Schwartz, 1976) or have included in the counseling programs active training of parents in controlling speaking patterns, rate, and voice intensity (Shine, 1980; Yairi, 1982b). As we discuss in Chapter 13, several current therapy programs, perhaps influenced by some of these earlier ideas, also make extensive use of parents as adjunct clinicians.

In summary, training parents as cotherapists was the last to emerge of the parental involvement approaches to the treatment of early childhood stuttering. Unlike the other two forms (parent as client or parent as support), the programs in this group vary widely in theoretical background. They also vary quite widely in the clinical procedures employed, using parents as play therapists, facilitators of language skills, conditioners of fluency and stuttering, and inducers of slow speech. It stands to reason that treatment can be more effective if expanded both in the amount of time devoted to it and the environments in which desired changes are achieved. Again, clinicians should be aware that credible data on the effectiveness of these particular programs, based on controlled studies, are lacking. L. Johnson (1980) reported "encouraging" results of her home intervention–parent counseling program. She presented some quantified data for a small group of 7 children, but not for a control group. As we discuss in Chapter 13, the use of parents in treatment programs has been on the rise in recent years, with a few clinicians reporting either positive or mixed results.

Conclusions and Clinical Implications

This chapter attempted to provide a broad, and in some respects historical, perspective of the approaches to parental involvement in the clinical management of early childhood stuttering. The sheer number of publications addressing the issue over several decades indicates a widespread, long-sustained belief in the importance of this mode of clinical intervention. Our analysis reveals that the common usage of the term *parent counseling* in relation to early childhood stuttering does not encompass the wide scope of parental involvement in the clinical management of the disorder. We have identified three different forms of parental involvement: parents as direct recipients of formal therapy; parents as recipients of advice on how to modify the home environment in ways that may help the child cope with, and alleviate, his or her stuttering; and parents as active coclinicians in carrying out their child's professional therapy. In regard to specific advice to parents, the literature provides many suggestions, from how parents should respond to stuttering events, to the general management of the parent–child interaction, to taking care of the child's diet and long-term emotional growth.

For the most part, but not always, the approaches to parental involvement and advice offered to parents have not been haphazard, but logically reflect the various authors' theoretical positions about the cause of the disorder and factors that influence it. We concluded that psychogenic-oriented approaches, as well as those that put the onus of the direct cause of stuttering on parents' attitudes, are the least defensible. Also, we made the case that the presence of environmental influences in stuttering are indubitable. In fact, genetic findings, discussed in Chapter 9, indicate that there are additional environmental contributions. Still, we take a skeptical view in regard to what this means for parent advising and counseling. While pointing out the evidence for problems in the home environment of children who stutter, Yairi (1997b) also cautioned that "no credible evidence … has been reported to support the contention that such reactions have either positive or negative influences on recovery from stuttering" (p. 42). In other words, one weakness of tying environmental factors to specific parent treatment or advising lies in insufficient demonstration of the direct cause–effect relationship of those environmental factors and young children's stuttering. For example, although research findings have indicated that parents of children who stutter tend to be overprotective, the direct effect on stuttering of an increase or decrease in overprotectiveness has not yet been demonstrated. Costello (1983), directing her discussion specifically to environmental variables frequently invoked in parent counseling, also concluded that none of these variables had been shown to be functionally related to stuttering. She stated that "no rigorous experimental evidence exists to demonstrate that the presence or absence of any particular family–environmental variable, or a composite of variables, is a functional antecedent to stuttering" (p. 72). Although such conclusions are a bit too harsh, her point should be well taken both as a judgment still suitable to current knowledge and as a thoughtful statement of the needs for future research.

Regardless of the said environment–stuttering relationship, we also concluded that the merit of many of the clinical procedures reviewed in this chapter is far from being evident because the available data to support a tangible clinical effectiveness of these parental-involvement procedures are sparse. The little that has been reported lacked in basic experimental controls. Andrews, Guitar, and Howie (1980) did not include parental counseling and involvement in their analysis of the effectiveness of stuttering therapy. One probable reason for their omission was the dismal pertinent research data at the time. We are not suggesting that parents' involvement as described in this chapter is not necessary or ineffective. Clinicians offer their best at a given time based on their understanding of the nature of the disorder, the available research data, clinical experience, and clinical intuition. There should, however, be a constant drive to increase the weight of the data factor in the total formula. One should be skeptical about untested assumptions and clinical procedures that are being advocated simply because they bear the signatures of "authorities" in the field.

The foregoing discussion should not be construed to mean that there has been no progress in programs of parental involvement. Quite to the contrary, the review of the literature reveals an appreciable measure of vitality. Changes and adaptations relevant to new information and theoretical concepts of stuttering have been taking place. For example, as a result of data indicating that stutterers may be suffering certain motor speech inferiorities or that such inferiorities reflect problems in central speech planning, there has been a noticeable increase in the advocacy of using parents for manipulating the child's speech, especially in slowing it down to generate fluency. Thirty years ago such advice was, by and large, a taboo. Growing information about the possibility of genetic factors in stuttering and data about natural recovery has also been filtering down to the level of advising. J. Riley (1999) has attempted to present parent counseling within a component model of stuttering (see G. D. Riley & Riley, 2000). We cannot help, however, but form a general impression that the counseling–advising better reflects current knowledge of stuttering than current knowledge of the interplay of family forces, as well as the interplay between family forces and stuttering. Indeed, much of the past research on families of stutterers that supported the speech-noninterference and pressure-reduction themes—two of the most common objectives of traditional advising programs—was conducted with theoretical motives to show the effects of parents' personalities and their child-rearing habits on the stuttering child. With a few exceptions (e.g., J. Andrews & Andrews, 1986; Mallard, 1991; Rustin & Pursure, 1991), the reverse—that is, the continuous *influence of stuttering,* once formed—on the child's family has largely been overlooked by investigators. Perhaps for this reason, the counseling has typically centered on what parents can do to help their child, not on the crisis created for the family by the presence of a child who stutters.

Since the 1960s, several concepts and models of family relationships that enhance research of family dynamics have been developed. Schaefer's (1965) three-dimensional model and Moos's (1976) three-factorial model of family styles are good examples. They allow comprehensive approaches to the understanding, on several dimensions simultaneously, of life situations as perceived by the family members. Schaefer's model included the dimensions of acceptance–rejection, psychological control, and lax control–firm control. Moos's (1976) model included three underlying domains of variables, each assessed by several scales: relation domain—the way in which family members relate to each other; personal growth domain—the personal growth goals toward which the family is oriented; and system maintenance domain—the degree of structure and openness to change that characterizes the family setting. Margalit, Leyser, Ankonina, and Avraham (1991) viewed families of exceptional children as living under prolonged stress that would introduce change in the family system, forcing its members to develop new roles and adapt their coping skills to the situation. Therefore, the interrelationship between parent perception of the child's difficulty, the family climate, and the child's perceptions about him- or herself and his or her parents should be major considerations in the rehabilitation process. In-depth examinations of mothers' self-confidence predicted their attachment interactions with their children, as well as outcomes in terms of the children's experience of loneliness and social difficulties (Al-Yagon & Margalit, 2002). The loneliness experience of children with learning disabilities was documented by Al-Yagon and Margalit through different age groups as related to personal and interpersonal factors. Such interpersonal difficulties should be further explored within the expanding models of resilience. Recent resilience research (Margalit, 2003) pinpointed the need for exploring the conditions that will predict the capacities of children with special needs to identify inner energy for considering their difficulties as challenges and to focus effort at negotiating positive adaptation processes and future outcomes in the context of significant personal adversity, such as learning disabilities or stuttering.

Unfortunately, there has been little research on the dynamics of families of stutterers using such models. (Yairi & Williams's, 1971, study on children's perception of their parents' attitudes was concerned with older, confirmed stutterers in Grades 6 and 7.) This is perhaps why much of the counseling and advising described in the literature appears to be rather limited, frequently consisting of information about stuttering and speech development, as well as advice in the form of lists of do's and don'ts. In several sources, advice covers so many facets of parent–child relationships that, in our opinion, it might actually hinder constructive action by presenting parents with an overwhelming task. Comprehensive, in-depth counseling programs that integrate the unique situation of families of stuttering children with modern models of family functioning need to be further developed. In our opinion, a period of 45 years characterized by a scaled-down interest in the psychological aspects of stuttering has created a significant gap in both basic and applied knowledge. Parental involvement is one of these aspects. Wide-ranged research activities concerned with the families of people who stutter, the effectiveness of programs, or the usefulness of specific information items should be encouraged.

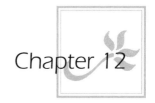

Chapter 12

Treatment of Childhood Stuttering

General Considerations

A large number of diverse therapies for stuttering have been offered, which, together with other complicating factors, create confusion regarding treatment selection. The rich therapeutic field, however, can be meaningfully subdivided into a manageable number of major approaches that reduce confusion and enhance understanding of options. We advocate the view that treatment of stuttering should be theory-driven, reflecting the clinician's beliefs about the nature of the disorder, with clear understanding of why specific procedures are applied and a clear rationale for sensible alternatives. At present, many therapy programs are characterized by large gaps between theory and practice. Treatment of early childhood stuttering raises several important issues, including these: Can stuttering be prevented? Should it be treated? Who should be treated? The past 25 years have seen important changes in the general approach to therapy taken by speech–language clinicians. Controversies about who should receive therapy and when it should be received have remained unresolved.

Study Questions

1. What are the reasons for the proliferation of therapies for stuttering, and what additional problems complicate selection of treatment regimen?

2. What are the major stuttering therapy approaches suggested as classified in this chapter? Explain each one and emphasize the differences.

3. What are the controversial issues regarding stuttering therapy for preschool-age children? Discuss.

A Perspective on Stuttering Treatment

The Richness of Treatment

A large number of widely varied therapies have been employed in the treatment of stuttering over the centuries. As a school-age child and as a young adult during the 1940s and the 1950s, one of the authors (Yairi) who exhibited severe stuttering had the following therapies, among others, prescribed by clinicians: (a) dipping legs in a pail of cold water for 15 minutes every night; (b) looking out the window at a tree, breathing in all the "good spirits" and breathing out all the "bad spirits"—that is, breathing in beauty and relaxation and breathing out ugliness and tension; (c) reading out loud while penciling a circle around each word in old magazines; (d) enduring injections of an unknown medication in the buttocks to induce relaxation; (e) speaking to the rhythm of desk metronomes; (f) having the face and neck muscles electrically stimulated; (g) speaking while moving the right thumb from side to side in a metronomic motion (hiding the hand in the pants pocket); (h) phonating different vowels in a siren-like fashion; (i) being hypnotized; (j) practicing self-induced deep relaxation; (k) speaking while folding in the right-hand fingers, one at a time, for each word; (l) receiving traditional psychoanalysis; (m) being injected with sodium pentothal to help reach the unconscious; (n) practicing diaphragmatic breathing; (o) identifying stuttering; and (p) making easy repetitions of stuttered words.

This list of 16 treatments is by no means a complete account of therapies experienced by Yairi. Similar personal experiences were not uncommon earlier in 20th century when the profession of speech pathology either did not exist or had just taken early root. Johnson (1946) and Van Riper (1973) described similar personal histories. The fact that an enormous diversity of clinical procedures has been attempted by people who were sincerely intent on curing the same disorder, as they understood it, is indeed puzzling. Such proliferation could probably be attributed to the multifaceted nature of stuttering, the large number of explanations or guesses about its causes, and the contributions of professionals from various fields, especially medicine and psychology, before speech pathology took over the treatment of this disorder. Regardless of the reasons, the rich repertoire is confusing, not only to many students struggling to make sense of an apparent chaos of past and present therapies, but also to experienced clinicians. It is possible, however, to clarify the picture and establish some order in the chaos. As discussed in this chapter, there are certain commonalities among various techniques that permit a meaningful and substantial reduction in the apparently endless list of therapies for stuttering by organizing them into several general approaches to the treatment of the disorder.

Problems in Selecting Treatments

A review of past and contemporary treatment programs for stuttering, including those used to treat Yairi, as well as therapies for early childhood stuttering, some of which are discussed in this chapter and in Chapter 13, illustrates the wide range of general approaches and specific techniques available to clinicians. Selecting a particular treatment, however, presents difficulties for two primary reasons. First, there are no current, comprehensive, widely accepted theories of stuttering that provide clinicians with basic understanding of why they do what they do in therapy in light of the nature of the disorder. Second, as of today, the clinical efficacy research in stuttering, especially pertaining to young children, has not been conducted in a manner that permits a scientifically based endorsement of specific methods.

An additional issue is the need for clinicians to clarify for themselves what aspects of the disorder should be included in the therapeutic regimen. Should clinicians be concerned primarily with possible etiologies, with the main characteristics of stuttering (i.e., disfluencies), or with the wide range of aspects and consequences of the disorder? In 2001, the International Classification of Functioning, Disability, and Health, known as ICF, was adopted under the umbrella of the World Health Organization (WHO), replacing its old classification code, the International Classification of Impairment, Disability, and Handicap (ICIDH). The ICF is structured around two broad components of health: Part 1, Functioning and Disability, including (a) body function and structure and (b) activity/ participation (involvement in life situations), and Part 2, Contextual Factors, including (a) environment and (b) personal factors. Function and disability are viewed as a complex interaction between the health condition of the individual and certain contextual factors (including the environment and personal factors), and impairments are defined as problems in body function or structures, such as a significant deviation or loss.

Yaruss and Quesal (2004) have made an important contribution by suggesting a model that adopts the ICF to stuttering. According to the model, a person who stutters is viewed as exhibiting an impairment of body function that is limited to fluency, but not impairment of structure (except in cases of neurogenic stuttering). In terms of activities, however, a broad range of components might be affected, mostly related to communication, including various types of verbal interaction. Yaruss and Quesal point out that the code also includes other aspects of activity and participation that can be affected by stuttering, such as domestic life, and major life areas such as education, employment, community and civil life, and relationship-forming. In our view, by reflecting on and emphasizing the various domains and components of disorders, these concepts and the accompanying terminology could improve communication among professionals and assessment of the results of treatment. They could also influence the actual choice of treatment or combinations of treatment, including those employed for early childhood stuttering.

Major Approaches to Therapy: A Classification Synthesis

Thus, we are back to the question of selecting a treatment. Realistically speaking, there are two primary ways of approaching this task. The clinician can (a) choose one of the numerous published and unpublished programs that is most suitable for the client's needs and the clinician's comfort, or (b) select various components of these programs that are desired for treatment and assemble them into a meaningful new program. Any review of past and present literature shows that the numerous techniques and complex programs are very confusing. Upon review, however, the diversity is not as wide. Often several techniques are similar in what they purport to accomplish. In our opinion, this expansive, rich therapeutic field can be meaningfully subdivided into a small number of subsets that can be viewed as major approaches, each containing several techniques that share certain commonalities. To classify stuttering treatment in general, applied to all, we propose a system of nine major approaches based on the common theme of the specific clinical techniques that have been employed. They are listed in Table 12.1, along with a few examples of each procedure.

Two approaches (1 and 9) focus on physiological aspects, three approaches (4, 6, and 8) are speech oriented, three (2, 3, and 5) focus on attitudes and emotions, and one (7) on motor skills. It is interesting to note

Table 12.1

Nine Major Approaches to Stuttering Treatment and Examples of Procedures

Type of Approach	Examples
1. Reducing tension/inducing relaxation	EMG feedback, deep relaxation, sedation, antianxiety drugs
2. Modifying evaluative sets	Using descriptive language for stuttering, observing normalcy of disfluent speech, behaving like a normally fluent speaker
3. Modifying emotional reactions	Lessening fear of stuttering, elevating self-confidence, increasing assertive behaviors
4. Modifying stuttering	Altering habitual patterns into more normal forms (cancellations, pull-outs, bouncing)
5. Modifying environment	Parent counseling, removing child from home
6. Reinforcing fluency and extinguishing stuttering	Punishing stuttering events, time-out contingencies
7. Modifying contributing skills	Oral motor training
8. Generating fluency	Speaking under noise, speaking under delayed auditory feedback, stretched speech, rhythmic speech, hypnotic commands
9. Modifying body neurochemistry	Dopamine blocking medications

that, as we suggested previously, in actual practice some clinicians have narrowed their therapies to a single technique representing a single major approach, such as exclusive reliance on metronome-paced speech. Others have employed several techniques, all representing the same approach, whereas still others have devised complex programs composed of specific techniques representing several different major approaches. For example, Van Riper's (1972) traditional program for adults combines techniques borrowed from the general approach of modifying emotional reactions with those representing stuttering modification. Keeping this nine-approach scheme in mind, clinicians should have a better understanding of the essence of various therapies in the field and of what they currently practice. Similarly, this scheme can be helpful to clinicians who want to assemble their own programs. As we discuss in Chapter 13, for early childhood stuttering, when past and current specific therapeutic techniques are considered, all but Approach 2, modifying evaluative sets, and Approach 9, modifying body neurochemistry, have been applied.

Theoretical Bases

Scholars in the field of speech pathology, as in all scientific fields, are educated with the traditional view that research should be theory driven. The theory provides a frame of reference, the rationale for the research, specific current directions, and long-term perspectives. The findings of such research may support and strengthen the theory, add new dimensions or modify certain aspects of it, and point to logical questions for the next research activity. Or, the findings may fail to support the theory, forcing a reexamination of one's view of the nature of the phenomenon under investigation. This is the scientific method that we endorse. Although natural curiosity and the urge to make sense of our world as a motive for research is typically embraced in modern Western societies, it is also true that, for the most part, when such curiosity is unguided, unripe, and undisciplined, it is not welcomed by the established scientific community. It appears that, unlike natural or instinctive curiosity, the scientific method and the development of theoretical models have to be learned.

In a similar vein, we share the view that treatment of disorders, including treatment of stuttering, should emanate logically and clearly from theory—the clinician's belief about the cause and factors that influence development of stuttering (Guitar, 1998). It would make no sense to assume that stuttering is a symptom of psychological origin but then proceed with a treatment that focuses on improving oral motor skills. As in the case of research, a theory-driven therapy provides clinicians with a frame of reference about the nature of the disorder, and thus with the rationale for the therapeutic approach, as well as an understanding of why specific procedures are applied. The therapy is based on good reasoning rather than on authoritative opinions of experts advocating specific procedures or programs. New theories also affect new methods of treatment, at times in ways that were not imagined before (Siegel, 1998). For example, treating the child's stuttering directly was not very popular, and to many clinicians in the United States, virtually unthinkable, until the operant conditioning theory penetrated the field of stuttering. A therapy–theory connection also allows for sensible alternatives, rather than a haphazard trial-and-error search, if the client fails to improve. On the other hand, repeated failures might indicate the need to reexamine the theory and take a new approach with a given client.

Although adherence to the principle of theory-driven therapy is generally an attractive proposition, we also should be aware of, and watch for, possible negatives. Whereas theories can be helpful in guiding therapeutic strategies, they have a tendency to create blind adherence and thus shut the mind or even create active resistance to new ideas. Such influences can be seen in past theories, such as Johnson et al.'s (1959) diagnosogenic theory, that relied on the idea that stuttering develops out of normal disfluency, a concept that led to the clinical philosophy that the very onset of stuttering could actually be prevented. Furthermore, sometimes theories not only interfere with progress but also may have an undesirable, if not painful, clinical impact. For example, among other consequences of the cerebral dominance theory, clinicians discouraged clients who stuttered from engaging in activities that required bimanual tasks, such as playing the piano (Van Riper, 1958). Interpretations of the diagnosogenic theory have affected many millions of parents who may have been unjustifiably instilled with guilt feelings by speech pathologists' insinuations that the parents were to blame for their child's stuttering.

So we ask the question: Has there been a logical relationship between a theory of the cause or nature of stuttering and the kind of treatment that is being delivered? As pointed out by Sheehan (1970), the history of stuttering treatment serves as a good example illustrating the relationship between theory of stuttering and therapeutic regimen. One 18th-century idea was that an oversized tongue, a condition that interferes with normal movement, causes stuttering. At the time, in view of the theory, the logical solution was to reduce the tongue's size by cutting small pieces from it. Others thought that the tongue was too weak or too lazy and, quite logically for those times, applied hot spices to stimulate more movement of that poor organ.

Early in the 20th century, the psychoanalytic theory presented a cohesive frame of reference that had clear and logical implications for treatment. If stuttering is a symptom of a deep psychoneurosis, then psychoanalysis is indicated to resolve the unconscious conflicts that cause the symptoms by bringing them to the conscious level. Also, there is an additional interesting illustration. In the 1930s, a well-known view was that forcing left-handed children to use their right hand caused diminished cerebral dominance, which, in turn, resulted in stuttering. Following are several citations taken from an article of one person representing this view:

The matter of heredity is of some importance in connection with stuttering.... This does not mean that stuttering itself is inherited. It means, rather, that a particular type of body make-up is inherited.... In the stutterer, the two sides of the brain appear to be relatively equal in development. As a result, the two sides of the speech mechanism move independently of each other, and when this happens we see the muscle spasm which is the primary symptom of stuttering.... *This means that at its bottom stuttering has a physical basis* [emphasis added].

It is a popular opinion that various psychological factors may cause stuttering. Overindulgence or excessive sternness on the part of the child's parents, excessive timidity in the child, and the child's tendency to imitate the stuttering of other children are frequently mentioned in this connection. These factors, are *not* to be regarded as primary causes of stuttering.... The more important causes of stuttering are physical in nature. It appears that abnormal birth conditions are among these; at any rate, a much larger proportion of stutterers report unusual birth conditions than do normal speakers. Among these conditions are prolonged and difficult labor, improper presentation (as birth of a child feet first), cyanosis (blueness of the body), difficulty in initiating breathing, and abnormal formation of the head at birth. Illnesses and injuries, especially head injuries, are important causes of stuttering. Poor nutrition in infancy is important in this connection. Prolonged high fever appears to have a weakening effect on the higher brain levels and is sometimes followed by stuttering.... Perhaps the most important single cause of stuttering is interference with the development of the child's natural handedness.

If you have guessed that this quote was taken from the writings of Lee Travis, you are wrong. The author was none other than Wendell Johnson (1934, pp. 2–6). Johnson (1934) went on with several therapeutic suggestions, saying that

The parent should allow the child to develop his own natural handedness. Without question, much stuttering could be prevented altogether in this way. Certainly it is often possible to eliminate stuttering in its early stages by proper attention to the child's handedness. (pp. 7–8)

Indeed, as a logical consequence, at the University of Iowa Speech Clinic, the right arms of children and adults who stuttered were tied to their bodies, forcing them to use their left arms and hands. Because left-side movements are controlled by the right hemisphere of the brain, it was assumed that having the individual engaged in extra left-hand movement would create increased right-brain activity, and thus help reestablish the natural right cerebral dominance for that individual (D. E. Williams, personal communication, 1968).

Nevertheless, in the past as well as in the present, specific therapeutic techniques or complex programs have been employed without grounding in any particular theory other than the principle that if the treatment works, it does not matter why (e.g., Van Riper, 1972). This can result in a collection of therapeutic strategies that may originate from very different, or even conflicting, models. Such an eclectic, pragmatic approach may be appreciated by clients who seek effective help and by clinicians who wish to provide it. However, if therapeutic approaches originating from conflicting models are indeed effective, then the models must be changed or modified to account for this. In other words, a theoretical basis must account for the success of clinical strategies—optimal treatment and accurate models have to match up somehow. More important, a well-defined theoretical basis can foster development of new therapeutic strategies tailored to each client.

We do not mean to say that an eclectic program cannot be well supported through scientific studies of its various components or its overall level of success. A prominent example of an eclectic therapy for preschool-age children who stutter is the Lidcombe Program, which targets the speech signs of stuttering rather than its cause (Onslow, Packman, & Harrison, 2001). One problem with eclectic programs is that clinicians may end up delivering treatment that they do not understand or cannot explain why it works. Such "soft" theoretical standing may interfere in therapy because, as a rule, the rationale presented to the client greatly influences the therapeutic process. When identical procedures are presented to the client with different rationales, the result is different understanding, responses, and learning. When a person who stutters is told to speak slowly so that (a) he can better attend to and analyze what he does in speaking, or (b) he can better cope with neurological spasms, or (c) he can better control his hostile reaction to the listener, very different learning takes place.

Even when there is a logical theory–therapy relationship, however, it is often minimal. Typically, there appear to be large gaps between theory and practice where significant elements of the treatment do not emanate from the theory. Perhaps one reason is that the narrow scope of many stuttering theories, especially those that attempt to explain the dynamics of stuttering events, limits their clinical implications. The covert repair hypothesis (Postma & Kolk, 1993) is one example. The theory asserts that disfluencies result from problems in premotor phonological encoding wherein the speaker attempts to correct speech errors before they are uttered. Except perhaps for providing some rationale for therapies that emphasize slower speaking rate, the theory offers little guidance for clinicians when the grand scope of the disorder of stuttering is considered. Parent counseling also presents good examples of gaps between theory and practice. Although the general method of working with parents is grounded in several theories, much specific advice given, such as instructing parents to model slow speech to their stuttering children and to use short phrases and simple vocabulary, has no clear connection to these theoretical positions. Similarly, it is difficult to identify the theoretical background for the procedure of "cancellation" of stuttering in certain operant conditioning programs (e.g., Ryan, 1970).

The weak theory–therapy connection in stuttering during the past 25 years possibly could be explained by the absence of a dominant theory that is widely accepted by scientists and is also popular with the general public—an observation made by Siegel (1998). Whereas in the past, the cerebral dominance theory, the diagnosogenic theory, and the operant conditioning model each dominated the field of stuttering for a good number of years, they were replaced by several newer theories or models that are limited in scope and clinical applicability. Our discussion, however, does not intend to minimize the value of eclectic treatment. One has to realize that researchers and clinicians have different social responsibilities. Whereas researchers should defer a final conclusion until the evidence is in, clinicians must deal with the pressures of the moment. They cannot withhold therapy until the time when complete knowledge about stuttering is gathered. They have to respond to the client's immediate needs and demand for help and have the responsibility to apply the best knowledge *currently* available to them. Still, regardless of our lack of confirmation of any given theory, whenever someone makes clinical decisions, they are based on assumptions about the nature of the disorder. Therefore, a clinician must at least recognize what assumptions he or she is making that are the basis of his or her decisions regarding whether to intervene and regarding the intervention approaches to be employed. Clinicians, therefore, should strive to keep abreast of new developments in theories and basic knowledge of stuttering and look for a logical connection between them and the clinical strategies that they pursue.

Therapeutic Issues Regarding Early Childhood Stuttering

Can Stuttering Be Prevented?

The literature on childhood stuttering is filled with expressions and discussions of the idea that stuttering can be prevented. In its classical and most pervasive version, this belief rests on the premise that stuttering arises from normal disfluency that is allowed to develop and grow to become abnormal. If this belief is valid, one may infer that there must be an intermediate process between the "incubation" period of stuttering and the full flare-up of the disease. Taking the idea a step further, the implication is that something can be done to stop this pathological process from taking hold. In other words, stuttering is conceptualized as if it were a virus-caused epidemic that can be controlled, or prevented, with antibodies developed to kill the virus so it would not cause the disease.

In Chapter 4, a convincing body of evidence was presented, much of which was reported by us, indicating that early stuttering differs significantly from normal disfluency along the frequency, type, length, and acoustic dimensions (e.g., Ambrose & Yairi, 1999; Hubbard & Yairi, 1988; Throneburg & Yairi, 1994; Yairi & Lewis, 1984). We have shown that overlap with normal disfluency is rather minimal and concluded that stuttering does *not* arise from normal disfluency. This being the case, we agree with Hamre (1992) that the notion that normal disfluency must be prevented from turning into stuttering does not hold up. We also agree that in the great majority of clinical cases, identification of early stuttering is not too difficult and does not routinely present a practical clinical problem. Rarely has there been a disagreement between the parents and us regarding the presence of stuttering. Although listeners and parents may disagree on the categorization of specific disfluency events, whether or not a child exhibits a stuttering disorder appears to be easily determined, and consensus can be achieved. By the time children are brought to the clinic, their stuttering already exists, making prevention a moot alternative (Hamre, 1992).

Another notion of prevention has surfaced, however, that gives it an entirely different meaning. The idea is that once stuttering exists, secondary and tertiary prevention should be pursued (Starkweather, Gottwald, & Halfond, 1990). The intention is to prevent aggravation of the stuttering condition and the development of counterproductive responses, such as tensing the speech mechanism harder when a child feels "stuck" or preventing the negative attitude toward stuttering that leads to avoiding words and speaking opportunities. We also disagree with the underlying philosophical concept of secondary and tertiary prevention. Actually, what is done is not prevention but straight treatment. From a clinical point of view, the concepts and models that clinicians visualize, and the language they use, greatly influence the therapeutic objectives, the rationales, the kinds of influence and change that they hope to enact, and ideas transmitted to parents. Those who maintain that conceptual issues should matter to theorists but not to clinicians (Starkweather et al., 1990) seem to overlook the remarkable influence of stuttering theory on clinical practice that we have witnessed over a period of 40 years. We maintain that theoretical aspects are highly relevant to clinicians. Conceptual orientations are at the heart of the answer to the following question: In working with a preschool-age child who stutters, do we (a) prevent the further progress of the disorder, (b) eliminate the symptoms without eradicating the cause, (c) eradicate whatever is its cause, or (d) facilitate its progress toward eventual recovery in the many cases where recovery can be expected, while attempting to bring the disorder under control in cases that are apt to persist? We favor the fourth point of view. Our reservations about the concept of prevention, however, do not mean that parent counseling and early intervention are not called for. What we suggest is a different point of view about the objectives and rationale for intervention.

Should Early Childhood Stuttering Be Treated?

It is a bit odd in a chapter devoted to treatment of stuttering to raise the question of whether or not childhood stuttering is a disorder that should be treated. However, not all human diseases and ailments are always purposefully treated by either laypersons or professionals. Many people do not bother with restorative intervention methods when they sustain superficial cuts, bruises, headaches, stomach or muscle aches, colds, and other ailments of this nature. Even more serious conditions such as painful herniated lumbar discs are often left to heal on their own, as was the personal experience of one of us (approximately 70% of herniated discs heal without treatment). Similarly, we do not intervene in the case of communication deficits when they are expected to resolve on their own. For example, in the case of children who display phonological processes or language deficits, if the mature phonological or linguistic forms are emerging or the error patterns are expected to resolve based on generalization from other learning experiences, then precious time typically is not wasted addressing these targets with costly therapy. For some people, a certain vocal quality might represent a concern for treatment, but other people (and not only some TV or movie personalities) would utterly reject even considering remediation of that same vocal quality. Many adults who stutter have never sought treatment and, in our extensive experience, many parents of children who stutter prefer waiting a while before seeking professional advice. Furthermore, they often prefer to delay available optional treatments to a later time, or until the child displays a readiness for response to intervention activities. Clinicians in Sweden also have reported parents' preference for waiting (Lundstrom & Garsten, 2000).

In general, the reasons for inaction in regard to clinical intervention vary. Untreated health problems include situations in which (a) the disease is terminal, leaving no hope for survival; (b) the afflicted individual does not suffer; (c) the individual suffers but he or she (or a parent) is not sufficiently disturbed; (d) the client's choice is considered, as the treatment is more bothersome than the damage or the discomfort inflicted by the disorder; (e) the treatment is dangerous; (f) the individual desires help but for some reason hesitates to seek it; (g) services or treatment are not available; (h) services are not affordable; (i) the condition is expected to improve or expire of its own accord sooner or later; and (j) an effective cure is not known. As can be seen, these constitute a good mix of objective reasons with subjective motives.

Speech pathologists eager to treat every child who stutters should carefully consider available information about the developmental course of the disorder, its objective status at the time of the examination, and the child's and parents' attitudes. At times, some stuttering is quite tolerable. Our own data show that a good number of affected children exhibit only mild or moderate stuttering, many seem to be unaware of or not bothered by it, and quite a few parents are not interested in an immediate intervention. Furthermore, in the majority of children, stuttering will subside and disappear on its own accord. Thus, in view of the reasons listed above why patients or clients opt for inaction on their problems, and in view of the facts about the disorder just summarized, the question of whether or not early childhood stuttering should be treated is a legitimate one for serious discussion. The fact is that the answer to the big question of whether early childhood stuttering should be treated has been seesawing within the professional circle for a long time.

The Changing Approach and Models of Treatment

Only 25 to 30 years ago, the prevailing view in the United States was that therapy should not be administered to young children who had been diagnosed as exhibiting stuttering, at least until they grew older and entered school (Jameson, 1955). The main reason for this was the clinicians' belief that by increasing self-awareness of stuttering, thus triggering emotional reactions that may lead to more severe stuttering, therapy with very young children may be more harmful than beneficial. It is instructive to notice that parents held similar attitudes. The extensive body of data from parent interviews accumulated by Johnson et al. (1959) shows that many parents did not seek help for their young stuttering children for long periods, if at all.

A major change in philosophy took place during the past three decades when a growing number of speech–language clinicians began to voice a sharply different view, namely, that *all* children showing signs of early stuttering should immediately be directed toward an intervention program (e.g., Bernstein Ratner, 1997; Costello, 1983; Starkweather et al., 1990). There appears to be a widespread belief that treatment of younger children requires fewer hours of therapy than treatment of older children, and that fluency improvements resulting from treatment typically generalize better and last longer for younger children than for older children and adults (e.g., Gregory & Hill, 1980; Onslow, Andrews, & Lincoln, 1994). We summarize this philosophy in a unitary model shown in Figure 12.1. Accordingly, stuttering is considered to be a relatively uniform disorder, with all cases behaving the same way. Thus, all children should be treated, and a very high percentage of those will recover. Postponement of treatment, or no treatment at all, results in a high persistence rate and eventually leads to a steadily worsening problem, becoming more difficult to treat.

This "therapy for all and at all times" philosophy, however, did not last long before the next turn: a growing disagreement among experts about the necessity of treating every child who stutters as soon after onset as possible and about the real risks involved if treatment is postponed (Andrews, 1984; Curlee, 1993b; Curlee & Yairi, 1997; Yairi, 1997a). According to

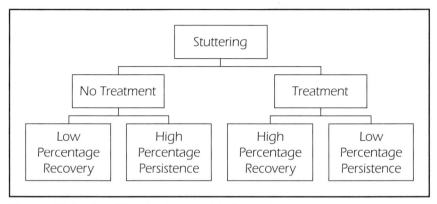

Figure 12.1. A traditional unitary model of stuttering treatment.

Curlee and Yairi (1997), clinicians advocating that children and their parents receive treatment as soon as possible after the onset of stuttering often argue that (a) the real rate of natural recovery is substantially lower than 75%, (b) fewer than half of the children who stop stuttering do so without having received some form of intervention, (c) most who do stop without formal therapy were assisted by parental intervention, (d) delaying intervention may actually lead to chronic stuttering, (e) clinical treatment for preschool-age children who stutter is effective, and (f) early treatment does no harm.

The key areas of disagreement involve different views of the natural course of stuttering (i.e., changes over time that are free of environmental interventions), what constitutes treatment or intervention, the risks of waiting to initiate treatment, the effectiveness of current therapies, the underlying philosophy about the justification for treatment, and economic realities. Specifically, those who prefer to systematically monitor a child's stuttering prior to recommending treatment believe that (a) the majority of children stop stuttering of their own accord within the first year or two after onset, (b) additional natural remissions continue to occur at decreasing rates for a number of years, (c) recovered and persistent stuttering have a genetic basis, (d) there is no credible evidence that either parental "comments" or formal treatment programs are indeed effective, and (e) there is no credible evidence that waiting a year or more to intervene will make treatment goals more difficult to achieve, increase the amount of treatment needed, or result in less satisfactory treatment outcomes. We support this position and offer three additional important arguments to boost it. First,

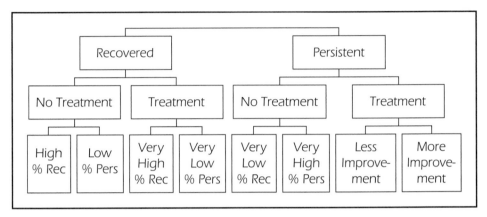

Figure 12.2. A double-type model of stuttering treatment. Rec = recovery; Pers = persistence.

the available research data concerning the effectiveness of modern treatment methods are not satisfactory; second, therapy should be given because it helps, not because it does not hurt; and third, clinicians are increasingly faced with the reality that resources are insufficient and too expensive for treating everyone.

This moderate approach can be depicted with a different, double-type model, as presented in Figure 12.2—one that assumes diversity in the developmental path of stuttering with or without treatment. Its underlying assumption is the presence of a strong genetic underpinning to naturally recovering stuttering and persistent stuttering. Children with a predisposition to recover may do so without treatment, whereas those with a predisposition to continue stuttering may do so in spite of treatment. As can be seen, the model conveys our hope that treatment may prove to hasten natural recovery or weaken and minimize reactions and symptoms, as well as maximize adjustment for continuing stuttering.

Ethics

We strongly disagree with the view that the examining clinician is unethical in withholding treatment if a child who has just begun stuttering is not immediately referred for treatment. Taking this a step further, we dare to say that, in fact, the charge may be reversed: That is, we should candidly entertain the proposition that it might be ethically inappropriate to categorically direct all cases of early childhood stuttering for treatment, as has been advocated by other clinicians. It seems that, intentionally or unintentionally, clinicians do tend to scare parents into submitting their child to treatment by presenting a bleak picture of what might happen to the child and his or her speech if therapy is not immediately initiated. Typically, they press the point that, if left untreated, stuttering will grow in severity and will acquire many additional unpleasant characteristics, such as strong fears of talking and social withdrawal. Statistically, however, the reverse is true. Clearly, the information given to or withheld from parents influences their decision. We posit that clinicians should refrain from sweeping, emotionally charged statements about what is and is not ethical in the treatment of childhood stuttering. Personal conviction should not blind the beholder and prevent the clinician from carefully and objectively examining the data of each case and making a fair presentation of competing views and alternative actions.

In summary, we return to the original question: Should stuttering be treated? The answer is yes in a good number of cases. Should every case of stuttering be treated? The answer is no, especially during the very early stage of the disorder. There are, at times, a variety of conditions and reasons, both personal and professional, that do not speak in favor of intervention. We are inclined to believe that recommending treatment for early childhood stuttering is one of several alternatives. A thorough diagnostic evaluation of each child soon after onset is always recommended. Indeed, most treatment programs emphasize the initial evaluation as their first phase (e.g., Costello, 1983; Pindzola, 1987).

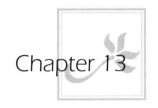

Chapter 13

Treatment of Early Childhood Stuttering

Application

Having discussed the theory–therapy connection, differentiated the major approaches to the treatment of stuttering in general, and coped with several fundamental questions concerning therapy for early childhood stuttering in particular, we are now prepared to take a closer look at the more practical aspects: the various ideas, techniques, and programs that have been offered for treating stuttering in very young children and related clinical issues. To this end, we begin with a brief historical review of stuttering therapies aimed at young children, which reveals cycles of interest in direct and in indirect approaches. Often, new techniques actually represent a rebirth of past practices. We then proceed to present a good number of current programs. The review identifies several categories of therapies, many employing combinations of different approaches. Although the list is not inclusive, it does reflect several variations of popular major directions. As the reader will see, what is current is not necessarily new. We then examine the questions of who should receive therapy and when it should begin, and end with a discussion of treatment outcome research.

Study Questions

1. *What was the main European approach employed for early direct therapies for childhood stuttering? Provide examples that illustrate the approach.*

2. *What were the bases of the rise of the indirect approach in the United States?*

3. *What were the reasons for the more recent emergence of the direct approach in the United States?*

4. *What are the different categories of current therapies? Provide at least one example for each.*

Brief History of Treatment
of Early Childhood Stuttering

Changing Trends

A search of the literature shows that in spite of constraints imposed by children's young ages, clinicians have employed diverse treatments. Although many contemporary clinicians are inclined to believe that indirect intervention has been used forever, in fact, over the years, most major approaches to stuttering therapy, with some vacillations in popularity, also have been employed in the treatment of early stuttering but using different procedures. Modern ideas and new techniques often represent rebirth of those expressed or practiced in the past but are now offered using different terminology and updated technologies. For example, the idea that stuttering is related to laryngeal malfunction, a focus of research during the 1970s and 1980s, was already expressed more than 150 years earlier by Arnott (1828). Certainly, vocal exercises for stuttering are not new; they were described by quite a few 19th-century speech clinicians (see review by Sheehan, 1970) and were experienced by one of us much later. More than 50 years ago, an old physician pioneering speech therapy in Israel instructed me (Yairi) to gradually increase my voice from a whisper to loud phonation using a conspicuous sirenlike pattern. We suspect that current popular techniques of gentle voice onset (e.g., Webster, 1980) have their roots in these old concepts about the role of the larynx in stuttering. Similarly, a complete cycle has occurred in the treatment of early childhood stuttering. Direct therapies aimed particularly at enhancing speech fluency were dominant during the 19th century and much of the first third or so of the 20th century. During the middle three to four decades of the 20th century, they were replaced by indirect therapies aimed at modifying parents' behavior. In the past 25 years, those, in turn, gave way to renewed popularity of direct therapies that focus on the child's speech. Recently, however, we witness once again a growing interest in certain indirect modes of intervention.

Early Direct Therapies

There have been ample descriptions of direct treatments in the literature from the beginning of the 20th century and even from the 19th century. In Europe, this was the dominant approach for a long time. Typically, European clinicians were not particularly interested in punishing or modifying stuttering but concentrated on eliciting, practicing, and reinforcing fluent speech. Considerable activities in this area took place in Russia. According to Pay and Sirotkina (1955), children as young as 2 years old were placed in residential programs and provided with direct speech lessons aimed at practicing fluency. The program included formal drills for memorizing sentences, repeating sentences, telling picture stories, rehearsing questions and answers, and drilling rhythmic activities. Another program was more focused on developing speech breathing, starting with short vowels, then progressing to prolonged vowels, followed by practice on words and short sentences. Dancing and singing, believed to enhance the child's sense of rhythm, have been quite popular in the Russian speech therapy programs for children. The inclusion of music and rhythm also was demonstrated to one of us during a visit to the (then) All Soviet Union Speech Pathology Center in Moscow (Yairi, 1990).

Also in Russia, Vlasova (1962) described therapy programs that began in the 1920s and were geared specifically to 2- to 4-year-olds who stutter. The treatment, developed primarily for working with groups, involved elements of environment modification, relaxation, modification of emotional reaction, and fluency enhancement. This program, practiced in special day-hospitals, placed the child in a new environment for much of the day. It included systemic tonic and sedative treatment for relaxation, and psychotherapeutic, as well as logopedic and logorhythmic exercises. Of special interest was the practice of coordinating speech utterances with body movements and music to facilitate rhythm and fluency. Reflecting the clinicians' view of stuttering as a disorder of both speech and language, the treatment was aimed not only at teaching the children to speak fluently but also at enriching their vocabulary and expressive language. Physical therapy and a regimen of rest and sleep to minimize exaggerated excitement and fatigue also were included.

Therapists in other countries also used direct therapies. Systematic speech exercises for enriching receptive and expressive language resources in the young child who stutters were employed by Daskalov (1962) in Bulgaria. In England, however, the techniques were quite different. Although Emil-Behnke (1947) thought that stuttering was a symptom of nervousness, her therapy emphasized teaching the young child how to coordinate breathing with speech and talking slowly. Kingdon-Ward (1941) had children practice talking in unison with the clinician, emphasizing vocal expression, whereas Marland (1957) used shadowing techniques to work with young children who stutter. The last two techniques appear to reflect the influence of the belief that stuttering may be the result of auditory feedback difficulties. In France, according to Van Riper (1972), Pichon and Borel-Maissonney (1937) drilled young children who stuttered in combining words into phrases. The exercises were accompanied by rhythmic body movement and performed while speaking in unison with the clinician. Finally, in the United States, and probably unknown to many experts, Wendell Johnson (1934) advocated direct nonspeech physical treatment, stating that "certainly it is often possible to eliminate stuttering in its early stages by proper attention to the child's handedness" (p. 8). E. Young and Hawk (1955), believing that the disorder was due to conflicting muscle movement in speech production, applied the motokinesthetic approach to preschoolers who stuttered. The treatment involved stimulation of speech muscles, directing them in the desired position, and practicing correct sequences of movement. Dunlap (1944), opting for a completely different treatment, recommended placing the child on "a rather full meat diet.... The meats advised are red meats: pork, beef, mutton, lamb; not cooked beyond the 'medium' stage. Fowl and fish do not seem to serve the purpose" (p. 190).

Indirect Therapies

A sharp contrast to the early direct therapies emerged in the United States from the early 1940s to the middle 1970s, and continues today. Beginning in the 1940s, clinicians leaned heavily on a general approach of modifying the child's home environment—namely, treating the family members with particular focus on parents. The clinical tendency toward indirect treatment of early childhood stuttering and the primacy placed on the home environments of young stuttering children are reflected in the inordinately large number of references in professional and mainstream literature. Its essence was captured in Schuell's (1949) statement, cited in Chapter 11, that "it is impossible to escape the need for working with the parents of the young child who stutters" (p. 251).

In Chapter 11, we suggested that the therapeutic focus on the child's home environment can be explained by influences from five widely different sources. The first emanated from the psychogenic view of stuttering, relating the disorder to *neurotic parental personalities.* Thus, it was parents who were thought to be the ones in need of treatment. (e.g., Glauber, 1958). A second source was the *diagnosogenic theory* (Johnson, 1942), with its emphasis on parental pressure as a major etiological factor. This source also singled out parents as the prime target for intervention, but treatment was aimed at modifying their pressure-inclined attitudes, not their morbid personalities. This influence was reinforced by yet another source: the large amount of *research findings* regarding families of children who stutter. Generally, the findings were interpreted as indicating that children who stutter were subject to more adverse parental pressures and negative attitudes than normally fluent controls (e.g., Despert, 1946; Moncur, 1951, 1952). Fourth was the idea that the child's *awareness* of his or her stuttering is critical in the development of the disorder (Bluemel, 1932). To prevent awareness, so went the considerations, the child should be kept out of therapy while (by default) treatment is limited to parent counseling (Van Riper, 1939). The fifth source was the influence of the idea that the high percentage of spontaneous recovery is not really "spontaneous" but is mediated through informal parental intervention (R. J. Ingham, 1976). This point of view has encouraged clinicians to employ parents more systematically in the treatment process.

Later Direct Therapies

In spite of the dominant "hands off the child" philosophy in the United States, a few clinicians focused their treatment on the child all along. Others experimented with various techniques that had the child in the therapy room but tackled his or her speech using what we call the "soft approach." Still others, influenced by the psychogenic perspectives of stuttering, held parents partly responsible, but also assigned portions of the stuttering problem to the child's neurotic reactions, sufficiently so as to target the child as a second focus of therapy. Thus, diverse therapeutic programs, especially play therapies, characterized by psychodynamic orientations, were applied to children who stutter either in individual or in group settings. An account of a treatment for a 3-year-old girl who stuttered and received 41 hours of psycho-play therapy from a psychiatrist inspired by traditional psychoanalytic concepts was provided by Harle (1946). A large systematic program was presented in detail by Murphy and Fitzsimons (1960): Convinced that stuttering was a symptom of deep-seated personal difficulties, their therapy was designed to help the child externalize and project his or her deeper feelings. Because very young children cannot or will not verbalize their feelings, the children were encouraged to express their inner world to an understanding adult through the highly symbolic nonverbal medium of play. Therapy was based on the theory that, through play, the clinician submits the child's wide range of emotions to conscious awareness that leads to relearning and differentiation, while the clinician acts as a "new parent" that accepts the child with impunity.

Whereas direct psychodynamic play therapy for children who stutter remained in limited use even after speech pathology took over stuttering treatment, speech-oriented techniques that stop short of being all-out direct speech modification were experimented with more aggressively during the period when the indirect method was still dominant. Excellent examples of these can be seen in Van Riper's work, summarized in his 1973 book. Procedures were designed to increase the child's interest in talking and his or her verbal output through associating speech with pleasure. Supposedly, this objective was achieved through planned "fun" activities that encouraged verbal output. The thought was that the more talking elicited while the child enjoys the situation, the better. The important underlying motivation was prevention of future avoidance of speech as the child grew aware of his or her stuttering and developed negative reactions to speaking. Less known is the fact that, in addition to his procedures used to reinforce fluent speech output and promote positive attitudes toward speech, Van Riper (1973) was among those who pioneered the application of operant conditioning techniques to childhood stuttering, employing procedures aimed at both reinforcing fluency and removing reinforcements of stuttering. In his own words,

> by intermittently and casually showing more attention and appreciation of the child's fluent communication but only ordinary acceptance of his stuttering speech, we have been able to get marked gain in fluency by this simple procedure and without the child's conscious awareness of the contingency. (p. 409)

Similarly, Bar in 1971 had already described a program in which parents of 59 stuttering preschool-age children were trained in reinforcing fluent utterances with verbal contingencies such as "I like the way you said this word."

To further facilitate fluency, Van Riper's (1973) therapy program emphasized modeling of simple utterances, so popular in present-day therapy. During play and other informal activities, the clinician began using single-word utterances in interactions with the child, progressing to short, simplified phrases and sentences while maintaining natural tempo. Plenty of pauses and silent periods were interjected. The progression was also from clinician solo talking to parallel talking (verbalizing what the child may be thinking or feeling) to communicative interaction, including fluency-enhancing speaking in unison. More direct attempts to influence the speaking patterns were employed using rhythmic timers. The clinician would tap a finger or foot with each syllable or word, and the child would then follow. A variety of timers were employed. Many other related activities, such as practicing rhymes, speaking while performing body motions, speaking while strongly chewing, and speaking while making loud noises, were among a large regimen of fluency-enhancing techniques.

Operant conditioning received further attention in the treatment of early childhood stuttering after Van Riper's initial experimentation. Whereas Shames and Sherrick (1963) used the theoretical model to explain the formation of stuttering via gradual shaping of normal disfluency, several clinicians made no theoretical assumptions about the cause of stuttering but applied operant methodology to modify the child's speech, fluent or disfluent. Actually, experimentations with operant-based stuttering therapy flourished in the 1960s. Particularly influential were the clinical programs developed by Ryan (1971). The well-known small, but controlled experiment reported by Martin, Kuhl, and Haroldson in 1972, however, provided research-based evidence that helped advance the application of operant procedures to the treatment of stuttering in preschool children. They had 2 preschool-age children converse with a lighted puppet. Employing time-out contingencies, the puppet stopped talking and the light was turned off for 10 seconds each time that the child stuttered. At the end of the program, stuttering was reduced in the clinic and the improvement was generalized to the home situation. (However, no controls were used, and long-term effects at home were not assessed.) In summary, as one may expect, many of the elements seen in the wide range of current therapies to be described next, including play therapy, direct speech modification, operant conditioning, parental involvement, individual and group parent counseling, and others, are founded on the ideas and work of past clinicians. We believe that some familiarization with past clinical work in stuttering should help clinicians better understand, appreciate, and analyze current clinical methods.

Current Therapies

The brief historical review shows that, alongside indirect treatment prevailing in this country from the 1940s to the 1970s with a focus on changing the child's home environment, direct therapies that emphasize fluency enhancement and/or modifying the child's emotional reactions also were practiced by a few clinicians. These paved the way for the next era in the clinical management of early childhood stuttering. A significant change occurred during the last two decades of the 20th century or even a few years earlier, when there began to be greater, and more widespread, inclusion of direct intervention in various forms. Six groups of therapeutic programs have emerged as available alternatives from which clinicians may choose. Of these, five rely primarily on one of the major approaches to stuttering therapy listed in Chapter 12 (see Table 12.1). First are programs anchored in the approach of generating fluency through alteration of speaking patterns. Second are programs that are based on reinforcing fluency and extinguishing stuttering. Third are therapies that attempt to improve the speaking apparatus. Fourth are therapies that focus on modifying emotional reactions, and fifth are family-oriented therapies geared toward the traditional approach of modifying the home environment. The sixth group is charcterized by a substantial mixture of these approaches. The following review of a sample of treatments is organized according to the five main approaches. They vary in level of experimental support, and their inclusion here does not indicate our endorsement. We have attempted, however, to provide significant presentation of therapies employed in countries outside of the United States.

Generating and Shaping Fluency Through Speech Pattern Modifications

In this section, four therapy programs are presented that share the general approach of instating fluent speech by forcing an unusual, exaggerated speech pattern (Approach 8 as listed in Table 12.1). Characteristically, no particular attempts are made to modify instances of stuttering or to incorporate systematic work on affective reactions. Note that although the techniques are very different, the principle is the same.

Rhythmic Speech

Metronomic-paced speech training that introduces both rhythmic speech and highly controlled speaking rate is an unmistakable example of direct speech treatment, although it has been applied primarily to adults who stutter (e.g., Brady, 1971; Wohl, 1968). Starting with a desktop metronome at very low rhythmic rates in the clinical environment, the client then would practice at home and gradually increase the rhythmic pace as well as the size of the speech units on which the pacing occurred. Next, the person would be switched to a miniature earpiece metronome (Meyer & Mair, 1963) carried into many everyday situations. Finally, the metronome would be used intermittently and then terminated altogether.

Although clinicians have used other forms of rhythmic speech, such as practicing rhymes, application of systematic metronome-paced speech programs for children has been limited. One published experiment with school-age children (Andrews & Harris, 1964) yielded rather impressive results, and we conducted one with preschool children (Coppola & Yairi, 1982). Our rationale at the time was that rhythmic speech should help the child cope with difficulties of coordinating ongoing speech movement while simultaneously planning following speech sequences. In our study, the child first repeated compound words (e.g., *baseball, hotdog*) along with the metronome pacing and clinician's modeling, progressing in small steps from 80 to 120 beats per minute. Next, the same was done with two-syllable words. After six sessions, the most comfortable rate, typically between 104 and 112 beats per minute, was determined according to each child's preference. Maintaining this rate through the rest of the program, the children practiced short phrases and sentences, then questions and answers, and eventually progressed to storytelling and conversational speech. The children were phased out of metronome use in the last three sessions. All in all, we showed that children as young as 2 years of age can master the principle and adhere to a rather boring practice regimen if special care is taken to prepare and interest them in the activities. The moderate success reported in decreasing the number of disfluencies and the reported generalization at home would appear to warrant further experimentation, which, so far, has not materialized. At the same period, we developed another fluency-enhancing therapy that relied on slow "stretched" speech, which we describe later in this chapter. Rhythmic speech, however, is still occasionally employed with some children. Since 1982, we have instituted other fluency-enhancing techniques with preschool-age children but occasionally employed metronomic speech in conjunction with them.

Easy Speaking Voice

Shine (1980) developed a program based on the assumption that exaggeration of physiological aspects and aerodynamic variables of speech production, such as high vocal pitch, vocal fold tension, hard glottal attacks, and airflow rate, is incompatible with fluency and should be altered in the young child who stutters if fluent speech is to be restored. The program employs very direct procedures to modify speaking patterns with a stated objective "to get the child to understand the concept of an 'easy speaking voice'" (p. 345). Thus, considerable emphasis is placed on soft voicing, with some attention also given to a slower speaking rate.

Therapy begins with establishing fluency in the clinic by having the child name preselected pictures by using whispered voice or prolonged speech in short utterances of single-syllable words that the child can speak fluently. Starting with an extremely soft voice, the child is gradually guided to use a more normal speaking voice. Activities are highly structured to minimize stuttered conversational speech; whispering is encouraged. Next, fluency is established in longer speech segments at the level of conversation. When fluency is achieved (0.5 or fewer stuttered words per minute) at each level, generalization is enhanced by bringing a significant person, typically a parent, into the therapy room. Three other activities are pursued in each session, all aimed at achieving fluency using soft voice: Language Lotto that allows for asking and responding to questions, as well as Story Book and Surprise Box that allow for practicing standard phrases. When generalization is achieved at conversations, the two weekly sessions are gradually diminished over a period of a 1-year maintenance schedule.

Stuttering Intervention Program
Pindzola (1987) presented an adaptation for young children of principles and procedures of fluency enhancing originally used with adults by Perkins and Curlee (1969) and by Webster (1980). The program incorporates extensive direct practice on three universal speech patterns (fluency targets) assumed to elicit fluent speech. First, the children are drilled in slow, stretched speech, beginning with monosyllabic words, then progressing to combined monosyllabic words, to polysyllables where the first syllable is stretched, to longer utterances, and eventually to spontaneous speech. Second, they practice soft speaking voice by lowering the overall voice loudness and by using extra-soft voice on the first syllable of an utterance. Smooth flow of speech, the third principle, is the blending of words within a breath group. It is facilitated by the child manipulating his or her index finger "from crest to crest" (Pindzola, 1987, p.130) while talking. This pac-

ing is initially done on a syllable-to-syllable basis, then for segmenting longer words wherever appropriate. Linguistic manipulation is included by allowing only short, simple utterances that are gradually lengthened when other fluency targets have been mastered. The three fluency targets are practiced both in the clinic and at home until they become habitual.

Reinforcing Fluency and Extinguishing Stuttering

Four therapies described in this section share elements representing Approach 6 as listed in Chapter 12 (see Table 12.1). Fluency is achieved through applying operant conditioning techniques, that is, either by reinforcing existing fluency or by eliminating stuttering through punishment. Modification of stuttering or affective reactions is not intended as part of the programs. In general, the degree of similarity among them is greater than that of therapies described in the previous section. Note, however, that some programs contain procedures that reflect elements of other approaches.

The Monterey Fluency Program

Roots of the Monterey Fluency Program can be traced back to earlier experimentation by Ryan and Van Kirk with the application of operant conditioning principles to childhood stuttering in the 1960s, with initial procedures and results published by Ryan in 1971. In further applications to preschool-age children, Ryan (1974, 2001b) and Ryan and Van Kirk (1999) employed the Gradual Increase in Length and Complexity of Utterance (GILCU) program.

Starting with the Establishment Phase, children who utter single words fluently in monologue and conversation are verbally reinforced in the clinical setting and at home. The children gradually progress to longer utterances within longer blocks of time, eventually reaching the level of 5-minute fluent monologues and 5-minute conversations with zero stuttered words per minute. In the second phase, Transference, fluency is generalized to other environments, such as the home. Again, being reinforced for fluency in gradually increasing steps, the child is led to eventually speak fluently in conversation for 3 minutes at the level of zero stuttered words per minute. This is followed by a Maintenance stage, a gradually diminished clinical contact schedule in which the child performs at a fluency level of no more than 1 stuttered word per minute.

Extended Length of Utterance

The Extended Length of Utterance (ELU) program was developed by Janis Costello Ingham (Costello, 1983), who later elaborated on it (J. C. Ingham, 1999). Although similar in principles and procedures to the GILCU program in the use of positive reinforcement of fluency and punishment of stuttering, it contains more detail and finer features. After the child satisfies criteria for success on the first step—10 consecutive fluent one-syllable responses—he or she moves to the next step, the production of two-syllable fluent responses that might include meaningless sequences ("house– red"), bisyllabic words, and meaningful two-word responses. As an example from the middle of the program, Step 9 requires the child to produce 10-second fluent, connected speech monologues. In Step 20, the final step, the requirement is for zero stuttered words in 5-minute conversations with the clinician, the criterion for passing being six consecutive fluent conversations.

Progress through the ELU program appears faster than using GILCU because steps may be skipped. For each of the 20 steps, the clinician presents five probes to determine whether the required response is already within the child's level of ability. If the child responds without stuttering, probes for the next level are presented. The 20 stages are designed to reach the goals of spontaneous and automatic stutter-free speech in all settings, in conversations with a variety of partners. Thus, children are encouraged to create spontaneous utterances rather than imitate models. Clinicians are to give regular positive and negative feedback, which is gradually faded as the child progresses through the stages. Generalization is facilitated through a self-management component in which children select materials and reinforcers to be used in therapy and self-monitor their progress. Parents' administration of the treatment at home helps transfer the child's fluency.

The Stocker Probe

The Stocker Probe (Stocker, 1976; Stocker & Goldfarb, 1995) was developed as a diagnostic tool to examine stuttering behavior across a range of linguistic complexity levels and to guide treatment. The underlying assumption is that communicative demands are elevated as speakers produce messages that are increasingly more complex. When children who stutter communicate ideas of heightened novelty, their speech is expected to become more disfluent. For diagnostic purposes, by systematically increasing the linguistic complexity of the message, it is possible to identify the level of linguistic demand at which disfluency occurs. For therapy purposes, the program can be used to establish fluency in a hierarchy of linguistic difficulty.

The Stocker program uses five levels of communication demands. Level I requires a forced-choice response (e.g., "Is it round or square?"); Level II, a single-word response (e.g., "What is it?"); Level III, a response to a more open-ended question (e.g., "What can you use it for?"); Level IV, a detailed description (e.g., "Tell me all about it"); and Level V, formulation of novel content (e.g., "Make up your own story about it"). The child is shown 10 objects, one at a time, and questions are presented to elicit verbal responses at all five levels. Responses containing disfluency of any kind or no responses (e.g., "I don't know") indicate that the child is susceptible to that level of demand.

When applied in therapy, the program combines reinforcement of fluency with linguistic manipulation. The child is given repeated opportunities to practice responding to questions and inquiries about novel objects. He or she is rewarded for periods of fluency above the baseline until the child has achieved fluent speech of 60 seconds on three consecutive occasions. Of course, the clinician aims at achieving fluency at progressively higher levels of linguistic demand, as the child successfully demonstrates fluent speech at a given level. Stocker suggests, however, that her procedures are secondary to other fluency treatment programs that are suited to the child's age, interests, and individual needs. A minimum of two 25-minute sessions of weekly therapy for children ages 3 to 5 is recommended.

Parents are counseled to reduce the levels of linguistic demands outside the clinic. The child's fluency is evaluated weekly using a shorter version of the Stocker Probe to help the clinician determine the level at which the following week's therapy may begin. Reevaluation takes place after approximately 25 weeks of therapy using the same version of the Stocker Probe as the initial evaluation. If progress is not indicated, other techniques are considered.

The Lidcombe Program

The Lidcombe Program (Onslow, Costa, & Rue, 1990; Onslow, Packman, & Harrison, 2001) is a behavioral treatment with a two-pronged method of applying response-contingent stimulation: The clinician reinforces the child's fluent speech and, in strict operant conditioning terms, also "punishes" stuttering events. Both types of stimuli are in the form of contingent verbal reactions. Fluent utterances are praised with expressions such as "good talking" or "smooth speech" or "no bumps," whereas stuttering events are responded to with expressions such as "that was bumpy speech," "that was a stuck word," and so forth. Sometimes self-evaluation is requested (e.g., "Was that smooth?"). The program, however, includes important additional elements that seem to be outside a strict operant program. Often the child's stuttering is actively corrected by the clinician, who models for the child how to produce the word fluently and asks the child to repeat it fluently. Furthermore, the child is to repeat the fluent word several times. Also, quite deliberately, the cardinal operant procedure of reinforcement and punishment lacks in program specifications, such as schedule of reinforcement, intermediate stages, and criteria of progress during the therapy phase.

Although the treatment is not a set of programmed, predetermined procedures, and it allows for many variations to suit each child, typically therapy begins in the clinical setting and is initially conducted by an experienced clinician. Parental involvement, however, is a critical feature. First, parents attend weekly sessions with the child, learning to implement the verbal contingencies correctly in carefully structured conversations. As parents become more proficient, they begin to apply contingencies in unstructured conversations. After observing and being trained, they are empowered to continue the program at home. Initially, the parent-administered home therapy consists of brief structured sessions. Gradually, formal home sessions are replaced by online feedback in everyday situations.

Desirable but nonessential targets in the Lidcombe Program are spontaneous self-evaluation and spontaneous self-correction of stuttering by the child. The program's objective is to achieve near-zero stuttering in the treatment phase. During the maintenance phase, increasingly spaced visits to the clinic and close monitoring of the child's stuttering take place. Necessary adjustment to parents' handling of the stuttering is made, and scheduled visits may be altered to ensure that treatment gains are maintained for the long term. The median treatment consists of 11 clinic visits. This program has generated an appreciable amount of rather encouraging research-based data concerning its effectiveness.

Modifying Contributing Skills

The single therapy described here, the Speech Motor Training (SMT) program, is characterized by its focus on developing specific oral motor skills without dealing directly with stuttering or other aspects of the disorder. G. D. Riley and Riley (1985, 1999) proposed a direct therapy protocol that, unlike many other programs for preschool-age children, is not aimed at either changing overt stuttering or enhancing certain speech patterns. Rather, it seeks to develop basic speech movement skills, specifically to improve syllable production characteristics. It is a speech oral motor sequencing therapy, *not* a fluency-shaping program. The target is uninterrupted production of multiple iterations of nonsense syllable sequences with as fast a rate as the client can achieve while maintaining accuracy.

The SMT program was developed from a theoretical framework that emphasizes feed-forward motor planning in speech production. Motivated by data from various studies interpreted to show that children who stutter exhibit reduced integration of the speech motor system, the treatment strives to improve speech motor control as a means of generating fluency. The behavioral goal is to have the child produce complex sets of syllables with correct airflow, voicing, sequencing, and rate. In a systematic program of 14 stages, the child is instructed to practice production of meaningless syllables, such as /vami/, to minimize cognitive self-monitoring. Gradually, there is an increase in the number of syllables (1 to 4), speaking rate (1 to 3 syllables per second), and unvoiced consonants (0 to 2). Additionally, the complexity of the syllable sets is increased as they are changed from consonant–vowel (CV) to longer patterns, such as VCCV, and the location of stress is altered. For example, practice could begin at Level 1 with the short syllable /mou/ and progress to /mi tan gu aet/ (CVCVCCVVC) at Level 14. At each level of complexity, the rate varies systematically. Practice begins with the clinician providing a model but not an explanation.

Modifying Emotional Reactions

As discussed earlier, in spite of the surge in treatment oriented toward modification of overt stuttering in preschool-age children, there remains interest in improving fluency through resolving deep emotional conflicts, as well as through increasing self-confidence and general personal interaction skills. The two therapies presented below reflect this approach.

Child-Centered Play Therapy

Current applications of psychotherapeutic play to the general population of preschool-age children who stutter can be found in many countries from Europe to the Far East. In Japan, Wakaba (1983, 1992, 1999) has maintained that many preschool children who stutter have experienced insufficient maternal attachment in infancy. To resolve the problem, she has employed a treatment program that reflects strong influences of Axline's (1947) child-centered play therapy. It is used when initial assessment indicates that the mother is unable to understand or appreciate her child's emotions and desires. Typically, the program is administered individually to one child, but children judged to also exhibit delayed social maturation are placed in a small group. Visit frequency varies greatly from once a week to once in 4 weeks, depending on the child's condition. Whereas two or three sessions may suffice for a child exhibiting mild stuttering, severe cases may require several years of treatment.

In therapy, the clinician concentrates on identifying the child's feelings and thinking, and on accepting his or her expressions of thoughts, inner feelings, emotions, and aggressive behaviors. Another focus is on understanding the child's stuttering in relation to his or her stress experience by analyzing the interaction between (a) stress sources and (b) reactions and changes in the child's behavior. The child is permitted to act without restriction as the clinician accepts his or her stuttering. According to Wakaba (1999), the stuttering fluctuates after the child expresses aggression either in the play therapy session or at home. When the child–mother relations are improved, the child is capable of expressing emotions, feelings, and desires. At the same time, the mother is able to accept them.

The therapy process progresses in the following sequence: emotional expression, expression of aggressive behavior, fluctuation in stuttering, decrease in stuttering, and disappearance of stuttering. Usually parents receive counseling separately by another clinician but do not participate in the play therapy activities. Every weekend, parents are told to record the child's stuttering characteristics, positive social behavior, aggressive behaviors, temporary regression to a younger developmental stage (e.g., using baby speech or seeking continual attachment to or attention from the mother or clinician), and mother–child and father–child relations. Parents discuss these with the clinician.

Tale Acting

In Italy, Tomaiuoli, Del Gado, Lucchini, Lattuca, and Spinetti (2001) developed a rather different approach to play therapy that uses known children's stories for treating stuttering in preschoolers. The authors view stuttering as a disorder that results from both predisposing endogenous factors and an environmental trigger factor—that is, a speech disorder as well as an interpersonal relation problem. The treatment, however, is geared toward the latter aspect, with the intention to stimulate positive attitudes toward interpersonal relations and communication, reduce fear, increase self-awareness, and optimize verbal experience.

The 6-month Tale Acting program requires two weekly sessions and is conducted on a play stage with changeable colorful panels showing the setting where the tale (e.g., "The Jungle Book" or "Winnie the Pooh") takes place. Using the tale, it is possible to "insert" people and problems that reflect the real world. Every scene has a precise title and objective and includes examples. The advantage is that complicated issues can be simplified by imposing them on clearer and more popular characters. For example:

Title	Objective
"Jack Panther and the Woodland Friends"	Interpersonal relations or assertiveness training
"Skittle the Baby Elephant"	Reducing fear of others' judgment

In the first scene, Jack, who lives in the forest, loses all his friends who escaped a fire. Moving to a new forest, he has to make new friends and be accepted into a new group. He has to experiment with various approaches, including performing roles he does not like, in order to finally succeed. In the last scene, Skittle, the baby elephant, experiences difficulties with precise movement because of his size, and is often clumsy in the presence of friends. He is subjected to negative judgments by the others, making him shy and producing feelings of inferiority. To change the situation, he will try to show other aspects of his personality, as well as overcome his handicap, transforming it to a point of strength. In this way the child finds himself in a near-real world, but a less fearful one, because of the stage pretense.

Every scene is preceded by a short explanation from the speech clinician. The child is instructed to act in different roles within the same tale. The clinician also actively participates, playing a role that either facilitates or hinders communication, and acts as an external destabilizing voice. Additionally, family members become involved. For tales that are acted early in the program, parents serve primarily as spectators. Later they become active participants, taking roles that allow assertiveness training. In this phase, the clinician becomes an important verbal and behavioral model for the parents.

According to Tomaiuoli et al. (2001), the different tales allow the child to play and interact with different personalities, and through these he or she realizes what the optimal behavior is, including assertiveness, to achieve the objective. The child also realizes the importance of nonverbal communication, learns to identify basic elements of verbal communication (voice tone, accentuation, rhythm, and pauses), and experiences the reinforcement of communication (handshakes, cheers, embraces). Thus, although the program does not attempt to deal directly with stuttered speech, it is aimed at helping the child cope better with the stuttering problem, improve self-awareness, adjust, and function well in school and society. Such gains eventually also result in a significant reduction in disfluency.

Modifying Environment

Over the years, the growing tendency to incorporate direct therapy in the treatment of early childhood stuttering has significantly eroded the long dominance of the indirect method aimed at changing home environment (Approach 5 listed in Chapter 12, Table 12.1). Nevertheless, the belief continues to be strong that, regardless of the cause of the disorder, the child's immediate environment, particularly parents, exerts enormous influence on the severity, complexity, and course of stuttering, as well as on the child's overall coping with the disorder and his or her emotional adjustment. This can be seen in the appreciable number of different programs that focus on the family—children and parents—of which three are reviewed here. The degree of emphasis varies considerably, with several programs combining the goals of modifying environment with those of generating fluency or modifying stuttering. Important components of parental involvement, such as analyzing parent–child interaction, parents' group therapy, and training parents to help their children, can be traced to earlier programs reviewed in Chapter 11.

Interaction Therapy

The therapeutic approaches advocated by a group of clinicians from Britain (Rustin, 1987b; Rustin, Botterill, & Kelman, 1996; Rustin, Cook, & Spence, 1995) are based on a multifactorial view of stuttering in which physiological, linguistic, psychological, and environmental factors determine each child's patterns of disfluency. The parent–child interaction emphasizes the environmental and psychological aspects of the problem, addressing the behavioral (speech) aspects only if it becomes necessary. The therapy is directed toward actively involving the parents with their child in the process of recognizing and making small changes in their interaction styles within the child's communicative environment. The goals are to restore the parents' confidence in working with the child and help them find better ways of communicating that promote their child's fluency.

Early on, the focus is on the parents' verbal and nonverbal behavior, assuming that children have a natural tendency to model their speech and language on that used by their immediate family members. For example, it is much harder for a child to talk at a pace that is appropriate for his needs if parents and siblings are talking very rapidly. Thus, the nature of the interactions between the parents and the child is explored. A "talking time" task is established in which each parent makes an individual commitment to spend 5 minutes, three to six times per week, playing and talking with the child. During these periods, the parents are encouraged to play with the child, avoiding commenting on his or her speech but listening carefully to what is being said, rather than how it is said. When parents have established the routine of talking time (usually within 1 week), they return for therapy sessions, which typically begin with the parent and child being video recorded during talking time. The clinician and parents then resort to a powerful technique of viewing the video together as a way of helping parents to take a step back and consider how they could make small alterations in their interpersonal communication with the child. This program seems to be influenced by Gregory and Hill's (1980) therapy.

During weekly sessions, the clinician encourages the parents to identify a small change that may facilitate the child's fluency, which they then practice in the clinic before trying it at home within the designated talking times. The fluency-disrupting factors that are most prevalent during parent–child interaction are rapid speech rate, poor listening, inadequate turn-taking, interruptions, repeated questioning, adult response time latency, and syntactic/semantic complexity of parents' speech. This process continues once a week for approximately 6 weeks, after which there is a six-week consolidation period in which these previously targeted goals are addressed through continued talking time tasks at home. The clinician monitors progress through weekly feedback sheets written by the parents. The consolidation period is followed by one session to evaluate the child's progress, followed by another progress review 3 months later. All children are monitored for at least 1 year, and the talking time tasks should be maintained for at least 6 months. When children get older and continue to stutter, these authors advocate a Family Communication Skills approach

(Rustin, 1987a, 1987b) that involves the active participation of parents as well as siblings. In addition to helping families provide a communicative environment that facilitates fluency, the child receives instruction in developing a variety of strategies for managing speech more successfully.

Parent–Child Groups

In Conture's (2001; Conture & Melnick, 1999) parent–child therapy group program, the overall objective is to facilitate communication rather than to achieve perfect fluency. There are three major foci: (a) communication interaction, (b) speech production behavior, and (c) child and parent attitudes toward speech. The program extends over a 12-week block of once-a-week sessions. Therapy is conducted in small, age-limited groups of children (e.g., 3- to 5-year-olds) and focuses on developing communication interaction skills. Through modeling and direct instruction, children are taught to listen when another person speaks, wait their turn, and not talk when someone else is talking. Occasionally, depending on the child's progress (or lack of progress) and the characteristics of his or her stuttering, direct speech therapy is administered with the aim of modifying stuttering events. Through modeling, instructions, and various concrete illustrations, the children learn to change tense stuttering to easy stuttering.

To facilitate extensive adult-level discussions, the parents of the children meet separately as a group. In procedures similar to those of Wyatt & Herzan (1962) and Egolf, Shames, Johnson, & Kasprisin-Burrelli (1972), parents are taught, also through modeling and direct instruction, that frequent interruptions, talking for the child, long complex utterances, excessively rapid speaking rate, and frequent correction of disfluencies do not facilitate their child's fluency. Additionally, the parents either observe part of the child's sessions or participate in them.

Multiple Approaches

Although none of the current therapy programs (except for the motor speech training program) reviewed in this chapter thus far can be regarded as representing exclusively one of the five general approaches, each is strongly based in one of them. Nevertheless, a good number of current programs appear to us to have a substantial mix of the objectives embedded and the procedures employed in those approaches. For example, a therapy may emphasize the objective of altering parents' behavior, as well as include a good deal of either fluency shaping or modification of stuttering techniques, and aim to change emotional reactions. Perhaps somewhat arbitrarily, we present five programs as a single group.

An Integrated Approach

Fluency shaping, modification of emotional reactions, and stuttering modification techniques are integrated in the therapy regimen suggested by Guitar (1998). Administered in either programmed instruction or informal game-oriented formats, it begins by establishing fluency in single words using the clinician to model normal, relaxed, slow speech. The child's fluent productions are reinforced, and the target length of fluent utterances is gradually increased to sentences and conversation through 13 steps. At each step, the clinician and parent take turns as the leading speaking partner and model in facilitate generalization. Typically, the success criterion at each level is set at 95% fluent production. As the length of utterances increases, (a) direct modeling is replaced by indirect modeling (the child does not repeat words identical to those uttered by the clinicians), (b) the modeling is faded altogether, (c) the speaking rate is returned to normal, and (d) fluency is generalized to the child's home. The second phase in the program is desensitization. The child is informed that the clinician is about to introduce fluency disruptors and that the child is to continue to use his or her smooth fluent speech. Disruptors are gradually increased in magnitude. The third stage is limited to those children who continue to exhibit tensed disfluencies. In addition to previous procedures, the children also learn to make their stuttering easier by contrasting "easy speech" with "hard speech," a technique with some resemblance to the popular inblock modifications used with adults who stutter (Van Riper, 1973). Guitar states that the program is designed for children 2 to 8 years of age. It is quite obvious, however, that the desensitization and modification procedures are not likely to be applicable to 3- or 4-year-olds.

A Swedish Program

Speech clinicians at the Helsingborg Hospital in Sweden developed a flexible intervention program for stuttering in preschoolers (Lundstrom & Garsten, 2000). Because most of the children are referred to the program within a year of stuttering onset, maximal flexibility in treatment choice is offered. Thus, the program presents alternatives to the view that advocates immediate intervention for all children who begin stuttering, as well as to the view that prefers an initial waiting period with active monitoring. The model's origin is a consultative method that does not necessarily have the premise of recovery but strives to reduce manifestations of stuttering and parental stress. It consists of six parts:

1. Parent consultation—The parents relate information about familial stuttering history, onset of the problem, and the child's reactions to the stuttering. In turn, the clinician provides information about childhood stuttering.
2. Assessment of the child's speech and language.
3. Support groups for parents and play groups for children who stutter.
4. Individual follow-up after completion of the group activity.
5. Individual or group therapy, followed by contact with the parents.
6. Intensive therapy for stuttering children and their parents.

The play group for children is based on a nonavoidance perspective, aiming to show the child that communication can continue smoothly even if he or she stutters. An important advantage is the opportunity to meet other children who stutter and play together in a nondemanding environment. This, in and of itself, has a significant psychological value and must not be underestimated in the therapeutic process. In the intensive therapy with parents, the child, together with one parent, spends three 1-week camp sessions with daily group and individual therapy for the children while the parent joins a parent support group. Clinicians talk openly about stuttering even with the young children. They explain to the children why they attend the camp and what their parents do in their group—that is, get education about stuttering. Children are asked if they know anything about stuttering. The children in each group determine the detail and depth of the open discussion. The clinician also does limited analyses of stuttering, as well as direct modification using a play modality (e.g., playing with toy animals that talk in different ways, or analyzing different kinds of stuttering in the clinician's speech). Because in Sweden children start school at age 7, the preschool range includes 6-year-olds. Therefore, all attempts are made to form homogeneous groups within the age range, a factor that influences the level of activities.

Parents could choose any or all of the six programs. It is interesting, however, that in a follow-up survey of 88 children seen in the hospital clinic from 1995 through 1997, in which parents responded to a questionnaire,

84% chose only the first option of the therapy model: inital consultation. The rest of the parents chose consultation with parents and a combination of other therapeutic options. The authors maintain that parent counseling reduced stress and worry and established a contact for initiating future treatment if needed.

Differential Strategies

The differential strategies approach to stuttering treatment (Gregory, 1999a; Gregory & Hill, 1980) is based on the theory that stuttering is a product of the interaction between environmental variables and the individual characteristics of the child. It uses three treatment strategies designed to meet the individual needs of the parent and child. In the main, the selection of a strategy is based on the child's fluency patterns. The first one, preventive parent counseling, is used when the clinician judges the child to have disfluencies typical of normally speaking children. The objectives are to provide information about normal speech development and styles of communication and interaction that may increase or decrease disfluency. The program consists of one or two sessions of counseling and a follow-up period of monthly telephone contacts.

The second treatment strategy is prescriptive parent counseling and brief therapy of four to six sessions, two per week, with the child. The treatment is aimed primarily at children with 2% to 3% atypically disfluent speech. It includes the parent counseling described in the first strategy, and the clinician also teaches the parent how to identify and chart different types of stuttering behavior in the child. Parent counseling sessions are based on daily charts, on which the parent describes the disfluent episode, the type of disfluency, the child's awareness, and the listener's reaction. The sessions also focus on modeling of easy, relaxed speech, first by the clinician and then by the parent.

The third treatment strategy is the comprehensive therapy program, designed for the child whose speech contains disfluencies typical of stuttered speech or some atypical disfluencies with concomitant disorders in speech, language, or behavior. This program includes the counseling and charting techniques employed in the first two strategies. Therapy is specific to the individual child, who is seen two to four times each week for approximately 6 to 12 months. The parents are counseled weekly. Therapy consists of a variety of techniques designed to meet the needs of the parents and child. These include desensitization; modeling of slow, easy, fluent speech; gaining fluency first in shorter, simpler syntactic structures; and treating concomitant speech and language disorders. Generalization is achieved by having the parent participate in therapy with the child.

A Danish Program

In Denmark, Bøstrup and Møller (1990) designed a 12-session group therapy program for preschool children who stutter and their parents. For the children, the purposes are to learn to stutter without struggle and to reduce their anxiety. The goals for parents are to reduce their own anxiety and to improve communication with the child. Therapy is conducted by two speech–language clinicians with groups of 4 children and their parents. In a typical session, each child receives individual therapy for 30 minutes, followed by 1-hour group therapy in which all 4 children and their parents participate.

The individual therapy focuses on modeling easy nonfluent speech adapted to each child. The parents are involved in the session practicing the new speaking pattern, and are asked to use their adapted speech at home. Depending on the child's age and stuttering characteristics, the clinician employs more direct therapy, for example, identification of soft and hard stuttering, as well as modification of stuttering. The group therapy usually begins with free play using toys and games. Parents participate and again are educated by watching the clinician's desired speech models. After a while, children and parents are separated into groups. The child group is engaged mostly in modeling easy speech but also in voluntary stuttering. The parent group receives information about stuttering and is counseled in coping with stuttering at home. Some follow-up for individual children and parents is a planned part of the program.

Our Therapy

For the past 25 years, our own therapy has emphasized intensive stimulation and practice with slow speech. It was initially developed under the influence of findings about the phenomenon of coarticulation and Van Riper's (1971, 1982) ideas relating stuttering to motor mistiming and discoordination. When we started, we believed that stuttering involves difficulties in planning ahead for upcoming movement sequences resulting in respiratory, phonatory, and articulatory lags. During the period of rapid speech and language expansion, ages 2 and 3, such difficulties are intensified and result in relatively tense disruptions of speech. We reasoned that slow-paced speech should help the child cope with the difficulty by allowing more time for speech planning and movement coordination while also executing smaller amounts of ongoing speech. Thus, in addition to experimenting with metronome-paced speech, described earlier, we later developed a 14-session program (Yairi, 1985) that used slow, stretched speech that eventually became our preferred method. (Since our initial experimentation with slow speech, our theoretical background has been expanded as presented in Chapter 14.)

In general, the clinician begins with constant modeling of slow speech at 50% to 70% slower than habitual rate while interacting with the child in unstructured activities. Part of the session is devoted to direct practice on single words; the clinician presents stimulus pictures, says one word at a time, and asks the child to repeat the word several times in a similar fashion. Eventually the child repeats without the clinician model, responding only to the visual stimulation. Gradually, the therapist increases the length of the speech segments practiced. Parents are invited to sit in the therapy room and then participate in the session under proper instruction, learning to speak slowly while interacting with the child in the clinic and at home. The range of speaking activities increases to play activity, then short stories, and finally conversations. The speaking rate is gradually increased, but we suggest keeping it perceptibly slower than normal. Parent counseling is provided individually as needed. Data for several children are presented later in this chapter.

Comments on Past and Current Therapies

At the beginning of the previous chapter, 16 stuttering treatments that were personally received by one of us (Yairi) were listed. Historically, however, only one or two treatments on this list of specific procedures have been employed with preschoolers. One reason is that not all therapies that are applicable to adults or older children can be reasonably applied to preschoolers. There seem to be two factors that constrain the repertoire of stuttering therapies appropriate for this group. First is the age per se. There are intellectual, cognitive, and emotional limitations in children 2 to 5 years of age. They are not likely to have the capacity to talk about their stuttering, or the ability to understand or execute instructions to identify, analyze, or modify stuttering events that are common skills of older clients. Typically, they are incapable of discussing complex emotions, using masking noise devices, taking on home assignments, and so on. Second, there are differences between the characteristics of the stuttering disorder in preschoolers and those in older people, and these influence treatment. Thus, whereas secondary characteristics are present (Conture & Kelly, 1991) in young children, they tend to be less pronounced and do not require specific attention. Although a significant number of 2- to 4-year-olds are aware of their stuttering, many are only vaguely aware. Even if aware and appearing to be bothered, they show no apparent anticipation or fear of stuttering. Only a minority of children indicate avoidance and revert to word substitution or strategies such as whispering. Negative reactions from normally speaking peers are rare. Therefore, although the child may have various emotions that need attention, work on desensitization is not commonly needed.

Several major approaches to stuttering therapy in older groups also have been applied to preschool children, but it has been necessary to adopt suitable procedures to achieve the objectives. For example, many adults who stutter are quite willing to discuss their feelings and frustrations in individual therapy or group situations. As just mentioned, however, most 3-year-olds are unable to do this successfully. Therefore, play therapy and other means have been devised to help children vent their feelings. Similarly, because in many cases children are unlikely to comprehend or follow direct instruction to modify their speaking patterns, there has been heavy emphasis on clinician and parent modeling of speech.

In spite of the constraints, the review of many past and current therapies offered to preschool-age children continues to reveal a very broad range. In other words, the many years of stuttering research seem to have done little to create a better consensus on how stuttering should be treated in this age group. It should be interesting to clinicians, however, that in our analysis, the current therapies seem to cluster around four major approaches according to the classification system presented in Chapter 12. These are modification of environment, modification of emotional reactions, generating fluency, and extinction of stuttering. Although each of the therapy programs and each individual clinician emphasizes a particular direction, stripped down to essentials, the overall picture suggests a collective recognition of the need for a multidimensional treatment that reflects multifactorial views of stuttering (e.g., A. Smith & Kelly, 1997). If the "wisdom of the field" is to be used as a guide, then clinicians may wish to consider or develop programs that provide the child with intensive systematic training in fluent speech skills, regardless of the specific way of achieving it, while simultaneously attending to creating a home environment that facilitates maintenance of fluency, as well as attending to the child's emotional status. A word of caution, however: The wisdom of the field is not a substitute for good controlled research that documents clinical outcomes using the scientific method. In this regard, much remains to be done.

Issues and Controversies

Who Should Receive Therapy?

As was already pointed out, between the earlier extreme of no direct therapy for early childhood stuttering and the more recent view that everyone should receive it, a few clinicians (Andrews, 1984; Curlee, 1993b; Curlee & Yairi, 1997; Ryan, 2001; Yairi & Curlee, 1997) have advocated a middle-ground position that some children should receive immediate therapy but that it is not necessary for every child. We do not oppose intervention, but assert that all clinical decisions should be based on three major research tracks that examine (a) the nature and evolution of childhood stuttering, (b) risk factors, and (c) efficacy of early intervention. Inasmuch as treatment is proven effective, it is warranted on a selective basis for individual cases carefully screened through analyses of risk factors and considerations of pertinent alternatives. Prior to formulation of unrealistic policies (e.g., therapy for all), one must consider costs, economic differences among people and communities, and competing demand for qualified services.

Although it is clear from scientific and practical points of view that early intervention with *every* child who begins to stutter is neither necessary nor possible, the information needed to predict which children will stop stuttering without treatment, and which will not, is still being acquired and refined. Current knowledge is too limited to make an accurate prognosis for each child. Hence, we are talking about estimating the *chance* of risk. Such clinical intervention decisions should be made in consideration of epidemiological information, overt manifestation of stuttering, associated characteristics, and home environment dynamics. More detailed discussion of possible prognostic criteria was presented in Chapter 10 on the initial evaluation. Suffice it to say at this point that, for example, a boy age 5 or older, coming from a family with a history of chronic stuttering, whose stuttering has not declined for more than a year, and who exhibits a substantial proportion of disrhythmic phonations, would appear to represent the highest risk. Hence, he should be at the top of the waiting list for treatment, assuming treatment is indeed effective. For example, even the limited prognostic information currently available to us should be quite useful for triage purposes at the Michael Palin Center for Stammering in London, where potential clients often have to wait 6 months prior to initiation of therapy.

Epidemiology and Therapy

Several scholars (e.g., Packman & Onslow, 1998) have expressed doubts about the clinical usefulness of the epidemiological findings on childhood stuttering that we have reported, positing that because data of the Illinois studies were representative of the population at large, they are not quite relevant to clinical populations. They claim that most children who stutter who are treated in clinics are first seen there after "much longer" stuttering histories than those of children in the Illinois studies. Unfortunately, whether intentional or not, this position pointedly seeks to divorce clinical decisions from the mainstream scientific database. In our opinion, our samples, being less restrictive in their ascertainment of subjects than any clinical population, yield more valid information about that population. Whether the children in our studies were identified through various sources, not only concerned parents, is not relevant to the question of who should or should not receive early intervention in light of the knowledge of the course of stuttering.

Another argument against delaying treatment for preschool children who stutter was put forward by R. J. Ingham and Cordes (1998) who attributed lower therapeutic success rates in older children to long waiting periods prior to initiation of therapy. This is another example of explanations that, by overlooking the epidemiological facts of natural recovery, lead to erroneous clinical conclusions. School-age children who stutter represent but a small minority of the original stuttering population because most children stop stuttering at earlier ages. Thus, school-age children who stutter are those with the strongest genetic-based tendencies for persistent stuttering (Ambrose, Cox, & Yairi, 1997), a fact that reduces their chances for therapeutic success. They may require more therapy primarily because they have a more resistant type of stuttering. A longer waiting period could allow for negative patterns to be reinforced, but the underlying nature of the stuttering remains, with or without treatment. Incidentally, arguments that school-age children require more therapy is also contradicted by present data. Packman and Onslow (1998) stated that their therapy is effective with school-age children. This group required approximately one visit more than did preschool-age children. Such small differences should not cloud the issue. Thus, claims by R. J. Ingham and Cordes (1998) and Packman and Onslow (1998) that there are significant dangers in delaying treatment for young preschoolers do not have convincing empirical support.

When Should Therapy Begin?

The question of when therapy should begin is raised primarily in relation to children who have just started stuttering or have been stuttering for only a few weeks or months. For most of these children, we recommend some waiting period. Even proponents of early intervention suggest waiting at times. For example, R. J. Ingham and Cordes (1998) wrote, "it certainly does make sense for clinicians to consider waiting perhaps from 3 to 6 months from the time of stuttering onset before initiating intervention" (p. 15), and Packman and Onslow (1999) suggested flexibility in regard to when treatment should begin. Furthermore, Jones, Onslow, Harrison, and Packman (2000), in a study conducted in Australia, found no statistically significant relationship between longer onset-to-treatment interval and longer treatment time. Also, Kingston, Huber, Onslow, Jones, and Packman (2003) reported a British study of 66 stuttering children showing that delaying intervention with the Lidcombe Program for 1 year after onset, within the preschool years, is unlikely to jeopardize responsiveness to treatment.

It would appear, therefore, that in spite of the controversy on this issue, the gap among opinions is not as wide as it first seemed. Given that some children will be designated for immediate intervention, what remains open for the majority of them is not the wisdom of waiting but the precise length of the waiting period. Consequently, clinicians are left to operate with the time-tested notion that each client is a unique case; that is, the decision about intervention timing is based on each child's combination of personal strengths, needs, and risk factors, as well as unique circumstances.

Thus, there is no definite answer to the question of when intervention should begin. It is too complicated for formulation of standing rules.

Yaruss, LaSalle, and Conture (1998) attempted to base such decisions regarding intervention timing primarily on several measures of disfluency. Their guidelines suggest that total disfluency of 10% and a sound prolongation index of 30% are good pointers. In our opinion, this is insufficient information that disregards developmental and epidemiological information. Our data clearly show that the frequency of stuttering-like disfluencies at the very early stage of the disorder has no prediction power for the risk for chronic stuttering. The problem with using fixed disfluency figures as criteria is that they do not take into account what preceded them—that is, the client's recent disfluency profile history. A total of 10% disfluent syllables measured at a given time but preceded by 20% disfluent syllables measured a month or two earlier is *not* convincing evidence for initiating therapy. To the contrary, it may be taken as an encouraging sign that recovery processes are operating. It has a very different meaning than a measure of 10% disfluent syllables that was preceded by a similar amount in speech samples taken during the preceding month or two, indicating lack of improvement. Whereas the data on the development of stuttering and its natural recovery presented in Chapter 5 would seem to indicate that 1 year postonset is a reasonable cutoff point, actually it is a rather "soft" one. The reason is that only 9% of the children completely recover by that time. Of the children who continue to stutter at 1 year after onset, 77% (70% of the original group) still have a good chance of recovery without intervention during the next 2 to 4 years. Although they continue to stutter, if signs of improvement, such as a substantial decline in disfluencies, or little or no disrhythmic phonation, are seen, additional improvement is quite probable, and considerations for further waiting are warranted. Declining disfluency, however, is not the only factor. Age, awareness, and the child's or others' reactions enter into the overall picture and decision-making process. On the other hand, children who have stuttered for 1 year and have not shown reasonable declines in the amount of disfluency that they exhibit are less likely to recover. For these children, initiation of treatment after 1 year postonset might be indicated. Simply waiting for the 1-year postonset mark, however, is not wise. For those who have stuttered for a few or several months, and either they or their parents manifest extreme reactions, some form of counseling or intervention is called for, at least to reduce stress. Additional discussion on this topic was presented in Chapter 10 on the initial evaluation.

Clinical Treatment Research

Early Research

Many of the published clinical activities and innovations pertaining to treatment of stuttering in preschool-age children are still waiting to be tested with well-controlled efficacy research. In an early account of the clinical research concerning this age group (Yairi, 1993), only six published studies were identified. They employed conventional operant conditioning (Martin et al., 1972; Reed & Godden, 1977), parent-administered responses (Onslow et al., 1990), metronome-paced speech (Coppola & Yairi, 1982), electromyographic (EMG) biofeedback–induced relaxation (St. Louis, Clausell, Thompson, & Rife, 1982), and play therapy (Wakaba, 1983). The total number of subjects in these six studies was a mere 14. A study by Stocker and Gerstman (1983), comparing the Stocker Probe technique with "conventional" methods, used primarily older children. In Europe, Derazne (1966) reported successful experiments with several thousand children on the effects of bromides and calcium chlorides. Little information, however, is available about this project. Particularly disappointing is the fact that controlled studies of parent counseling, the most commonly used therapeutic method, were not published by that time.

In general, these early attempts suffered from one or more of several problems. These included lack of consecutive baseline measures during a period of several months preceding the therapy program, insufficient or no follow-ups, lack of clear definitions of stuttering, unspecified speech sample size, insufficient measures (e.g., no speech measures in one study), inadequate attention to gender distribution, age range, time elapsed from the onset of stuttering, few participants, and lack of control groups.

Recent Research

Since the beginning of the 1990s, several treatment programs for young children have appeared or reappeared, a good number of them without experimental support. Furthermore, several clinicians have made unsubstantiated claims of extremely high levels of therapeutic success. Starkweather, Gottwald, and Halfond (1990), for example, reported 100% success for 29 children who completed their program and presented normal disfluency 2 years later. No data were provided to support the claim. It is also worthwhile noting that an almost equal number of children seen by these clinicians were not treated, withdrew from therapy, or continued to stutter. Similarly, in 1993, Fosnot reported on 33 preschool stuttering children who received direct fluency precision treatment. On average, 30 therapy sessions were administered in weekly 2-hour blocks. The author stated that 30 participants (91%) achieved normal fluency and maintained it at the end of a 5-year follow-up. Actual data, however, were presented for only a single child. The general status of a good number of current therapies is reflected in a 1995 publication edited by Fosnot in which seven different presentations on stuttering therapy for children were presented. None was backed by quantitative data. In commenting on this publication, Ingham and Cordes (1999) suggested that several authors went on to advocate techniques that were shown in past research as ineffective.

Although reports from several countries reflect growing activities in treatment research, they are often characterized by inadequate data and control procedures. In Japan, Wakaba (1999) reported treatment results of her play therapy program for 19 preschoolers representing the entire range of stuttering severity, all of whom began stuttering at age 2 years. She claimed that 90% of the group recovered in response to the treatment. Progress was assessed by three observers employing the *Scale for Severity of Stuttering* (Johnson, Darley, & Spriestersbach, 1963) for each therapy session, as well as at home by the child's mother. No control groups were included. In England, Matthews, Williams, and Pring (1997) conducted a case study with a single preschool-age child to evaluate interaction therapy (Rustin et al., 1995). The design included a 5-week base period, 6 weeks of active parent instruction, and 5 weeks of consolidation (i.e., home practice without advice). A significant reduction in stuttering that occurred after therapy was sustained during the consolidation period.

In Italy, Tomaiuoli et al. (2001), whose Tale Acting program was described earlier, reported results for 10 preschool children without histories of treatment who completed the entire Tale Acting program. Statistically significant reduction in typical and atypical speech disfluency was reported for several speaking situations. Using results from the *Child Behavior Checklist* (Achenbach, 1991), the researchers documented improvement in the children's problem-solving capacity, reduced withdrawal behavior, and a greater interest in new things and activities. Reduction of anxiety and more positive attitudes were indicated for the parents. In Sweden, Lundstrom and Garsten (2000) reported a follow-up survey of 88 preschoolers seen for early intervention, mostly in the form of parent counseling only.

The overall rate of recovery in the entire group was 54%, with 5% of the children who still stuttered exhibiting severe stuttering. Most of the parents (97%) expressed satisfaction with the counseling.

In the United States, initial efficacy data for a single preschool child trained with the GILCU program and for a second child using slow speaking rate for parents and child were reported by Ryan (2001b). Although both children showed considerable improvement, the report is clouded in that therapy lasted 2 to 3 years, was composed of more than one treatment program, and was delivered by several clinicians. G. D. Riley and Ingham (1995) reported the success of the ELU program in reducing the frequency of stuttering through informal clinical observations and through one formal study of 5 children with various levels of stuttering severity. Stuttering was decreased by more than 60% over 20 hours of treatment. G. D. Riley and Riley (1999) reported that 24 sessions of their speech motor training program reduced stuttering frequency by 49% and severity by 46% in 6 children. They concluded that changes in speech motor production may contribute to long-term maintenance of treatment gains because overlearned motor skills tend to remain stable.

The same period also has witnessed a growing number of more systematic clinical treatment effectiveness studies, as well as larger samples of participants. A good example is the contribution of J. C. Ingham and Riley (1998), who proposed several criteria for documenting treatment efficacy for young children who stutter: demonstration of outcome in speech data, use of several dependent variables (e.g., stuttering frequency and speech naturalness ratings), adequate description of the treatment, and evidence that the applied treatment, not other factors, is responsible for the changes reported. Session-by-session data illustrated the success of the speech motor training program described earlier. A substantial body of data also was reported by Conture (2001) for his team's parent–child therapy group program applied to 26 children ages 3 to 8 over a period of 3 months. The mean frequency of the group's stuttering, averaged for the first four sessions, was reduced from 10 to 7 per 100 words, with 65% of the participants following the declining trend. Conture also illustrated the difficulties of distinguishing between treatment effect and spontaneous recovery for some children and provided examples of children who did not follow the group tendency to decrease stuttering (Conture, 2001, p. 176).

Our own slow speech program also has generated some organized results. Some data for 6 children who persisted in stuttering at the time they were enrolled in treatment, from 13 to 29 months after onset, are presented in Table 13.1. Variations in the frequency of Stuttering-Like Disfluencies for two testing periods prior to therapy and four follow-up periods are shown. Overall, for this group of relatively older children, all exhibiting moderate to severe stuttering, we show mixed results in spite of the intensive treatment.

By far, the bulk of the recent treatment effectiveness research is credited to an Australia-based group under the leadership of Mark Onslow. As described earlier, this group experimented with the Lidcombe program, in which the goal is to train parents in contingency management of stuttering: punishing stuttering events while reinforcing fluent utterances. In 1990, Onslow et al. published preliminary data for 4 preschool children who had received from 5 to 8 clinical treatment hours. Based on speech samples and parent reports, none of the children exhibited stuttering 9 months after termination of therapy. In a second study with 13 children, Onslow, Andrews, and Lincoln (1994) again reported encouraging results. Speech samples from 12 months posttreatment indicated a median of only 1% stuttering, and responses from five parents confirmed low-level stuttering. In 1997, Lincoln and Onslow provided new data, this time for a larger group of 43 stuttering children, ages 2 to 5. Speech recorded by parents from 2 to 7 years posttreatment indicated that near-zero stuttering was maintained. Undoubtedly, these investigators have provided important initiatives in treatment outcome research and have remained in the forefront of this effort. Nevertheless, a close inspection of their procedures reveals several weaknesses, especially lack of control for natural recovery, although the data clearly indicate that such recovery processes (descending base rates) were in progress in at least a number of subjects. Fortunately, to our knowledge, in their present ongoing studies, this group appears to be correcting some of the problems.

A different direction in the effect of treatment research was taken by G. D. Riley and Ingham (2000). They measured selected acoustic durations before and after two therapies, Speech Motor Training (SMT) and Extended Length of Utterance (ELU). Both treatments reduced stuttering. Vowel durations were lengthened and intervocalic intervals were shortened by SMT; ELU did not alter these durations. To the extent that acoustic measures reflect motor speech performance, these findings imply that motor speech changes provided at least part of the mechanism for stuttering reduction.

Table 13.1

Individual Data for Frequency of Stuttering-Like Disfluencies (SLD)
Pre- and Posttreatment Using Slow Speech

Child	SLD 2 mos. Pre-treatment	SLD Immediately Pre-treatment	SLD Immediately Post-treatment	SLD 1 mo. Post-treatment	SLD 3 mos. Post-treatment	SLD 6 mos. Post-treatment
1	3.36	4.97	5.72	6.05	7.69	3.88
2	15.27	20.69	9.02	14.05	31.22	16.34
3	14.39	11.14	2.86	2.00	4.24	1.32
4	13.20	11.34	5.79	6.61	3.48	21.22
5	3.12	3.13	4.57	3.82	9.23	2.58
6	9.90	7.08	4.82	8.33	9.85	2.66

Related Research

Inasmuch as a number of therapies and parent counseling programs involving preschool children who stutter have emphasized the need for parents to speak more slowly to foster slower speaking rate and, thus, more fluent speech in the children, it is worthwhile to briefly comment on the relevant research. Three studies (Guitar, Kopff Schaefer, Donahue-Killburg, & Bond, 1992; Starkweather & Gottwald, 1984; Stephanson-Opsal & Bernstein Ratner, 1988), with a total of 13 mother–child pairs, reported that when mothers slowed down their speaking rate, the children's fluency improved. Nevertheless, the stuttering children's speaking rate was not lowered. Because of experimental difficulties in measuring rate in people who stutter, Bernstein Ratner (1992) studied a group of 20 normally speaking children and their mothers and found that, as a group, there was little effect of parental slowing on the children's speaking rate. The length of the exposure to slow speech, however, was short and there were individual variations. Similar findings with 5 parent–child dyads were reported by Zebrowski, Weiss, Savelkoul, and Hammer (1996), although in their study there was a uniform trend toward reduction in the children's rate. Most recently, Guitar and Marchinkoski (2001) studied 6 mother–child dyads, employing improved procedures that included a substantially reduced (50%) parent speech rate. These investigators were the first to report statistically significantly reduced rate in 5 children. Clearly, much more research of this critical issue is required, paying attention to the length of exposure and the specific speaking rate required of parents.

Weakness of Clinical Efficacy Research

In spite of the heightened level of research activities concerning treatment of early childhood stuttering and the encouraging refinement of procedures, the scientific credibility of clinical treatment studies is still questioned. We have yet to see random assignment of subjects to various treatment groups, independent data collection, independent data analyses, and comparisons of various treatments, employing adequate control groups, all incorporated into the same study. These standard features of many health treatment studies have yet to be widely adopted in the field of communication disorders. Deficiencies in experimental controls are indeed a major roadblock that has hampered research in the treatment of early childhood stuttering. In view of the increasing body of data that affirms the presence of a strong natural recovery factor, the failure to set up adequate control groups is perhaps the most glaring weakness of treatment efficacy claims involving preschool-age children who stutter. Good illustrations of the difficulties arising in interpreting the data from both past and more recent research can be found in Reed and Godden's (1977) study, in which the length of the stuttering history of the participating subjects was from 1 to 3 months, and in the experimental studies with the Lidcombe methods, in which quite a few children began treatment a relatively short time after stuttering onset. Developmental data (Ryan, 2001a; Yairi & Ambrose, 1999a; Yairi, Ambrose, & Niermann, 1993), however, clearly show that considerable amelioration of stuttering or complete natural recovery, even from severe forms of the disorder, may take place within weeks to several months postonset, up to about 4 years after onset. Such cases are predictably common. Claims of high rates of successful therapy, therefore, are suspect for contamination by failing to separate the effect of the treatment from the effect of natural processes. In our opinion, information about the natural developmental course of stuttering in young children is more robust than information about the results of its treatment. Conture (2001) acknowledged the problem in discussing the results of one of his subjects who began treatment only 3 months after onset. We admit, however, that controlling for natural recovery in such research is not a simple matter, from both experimental design and ethical perspectives. Another related epidemiological factor is the type of familial history of stuttering. Children coming from families with histories of recovered stuttering also tend to recover, whereas those who come from families with histories of persistent stuttering also tend to persist (Ambrose et al., 1997). Clinical researchers should be encouraged to carefully document the family history of stuttering for the children who participate in treatment studies.

An additional feature that raises questions about the meaning of the findings of clinical treatment research has been the multiple-aspect characteristics of therapies. The Lidcombe Program, for example, includes six different aspects: treatment in the clinic, treatment by parents at home, reinforcement of fluency, disapproval of stuttering, direct modification of stuttering, and self-evaluation. It is impossible, therefore, from current data, to determine which procedure contributed to the observed progress. In particular, it is difficult to experimentally control home-administered therapy or the speech samples recorded by parents. Likewise, although

Conture (2001) estimated that his parent–child therapy group program has yielded approximately 65% recovery, in addition to the question of whether improvement was effected by the treatment, it is not feasible to determine what part of it was responsible for the progress: the parent group, the children's group, or the direct speech therapy. One way of improving future research is to narrow the scope of therapy by studying a single treatment program, or to select only one procedure from a complex program. Examples of such narrow treatments include Speech Motor Training (G. D. Riley & Riley, 1999) and metronome-paced speech (Coppola & Yairi, 1982). On the other hand, current research has been too narrow in terms of parameters of improvement included. Certainly, the level of fluency is paramount; however, parents' perceptions, child's behaviors and interactions, speech naturalness, and other parameters also should be included.

Conclusions Regarding Clinical Efficacy Research

All health fields recognize that the body of epidemiological information about factors that influence the incidence and prevalence of a disorder, its natural course of becoming chronic or remitting, characteristic changes in symptomatology during its course, and its subtypes, forms an essential database for conducting basic and applied research in a clinical population and for developing effective clinical management strategies. It is such information that eventually guides differential diagnoses, the execution of prevention programs, and the selection of appropriate treatments. Attempts to downplay the importance of current information concerning the development of stuttering (e.g., Ingham & Bothe, 2001; Onslow & Packman, 1999), especially the apparent high rate of natural recovery, have been regrettable. Overlooking this information has yielded, and will continue to yield, treatment efficacy data that are not scientifically credible. We are encouraged, however, that more recent work by some of these colleagues has indicated a move toward recognition of current epidemiological findings.

Although progress has been made in the approach to clinical treatment research concerned with early childhood stuttering, work in this area is still in its infancy. Bloodstein (1987, pp. 400–406) suggested the following common standards in controlled clinical trials research:

> The method must be shown to be effective with an ample and representative group of stutterers.

Suitable control groups and control conditions must be used to
show that reductions in stuttering are the result of treatment.
The success of a program of therapy should not be inflated by
dropouts.
The method must be shown to be effective in the hands of essentially any qualified clinician, including those without unusual
status, prestige, or force of personality.

Additionally, as noted earlier, random assignment of subjects to various
treatment groups, independent data collection, independent data analyses,
and comparisons of various treatments will move research in this field
into desired levels of quality. Encouraging progress toward these aims was
recently reported by a team of investigators and clinicians from the
Netherlands (Franken, Kielstra-van der Schalk, & Boelens, 2003). They
compared two stuttering treatment therapies, the Lidcombe Program,
described earlier, and one based on the demands and capacities model as
described by Starkweather et al. (1990). The 32 children who stuttered, all
under age 6, were randomly assigned to one of the two treatments and received 12 therapy sessions. Results indicated that, in general, there were
not substantial differences in immediate treatment effects of the two therapies as measured by the frequency of stuttering, severity of stuttering, and
parents' evaluation of the methods.

We believe that much more scientific evidence is needed to support
treatment decisions and the procedures used with childhood stuttering. To
a significant extent, additional progress depends on sound longitudinal
clinical treatment studies of early childhood stuttering, as well as longitudinal studies regarding the disorder's natural patterns of progression and
remission that provide the basis for clinical efficacy of early and later treatment interventions (Curlee & Yairi, 1998).

Future Directions

Investigators at the University of Illinois Stuttering Research Program and
cooperating laboratories in other universities are exploring epidemiology,
genetics, neuroanatomy, neurophysiology, temperament, and language aspects of stuttering. These research activities, in parallel with advances in understanding human genetics, brain structures, brain chemistry, and neural
functions in general, will undoubtedly result in better knowledge about the

etiology and subtypes of the disorder. As visualized by Curlee (2000), with more research results, and with the invention of revolutionary technologies that modify the expression of genes and neural functions of the brain, drastic changes will be seen in the treatment of human disease, syndromes, and disabilities in unimaginable ways within the next few decades, including treatments for stuttering. We should not be surprised to witness the introduction of drugs, such as dopamine blocking medications, designed to modify the biochemical environment of the brain, applied to the treatment of stuttering (Costa & Kroll, 2000; Maguire, Riley, Franklin, & Gottschalk, 2000). So far, however, there has been very limited experimentation with very young children. Furthermore, inasmuch as brain structure abnormalities are involved (Foundas, Bollich, Corey, Hurley, & Heilman, 2001), it is tempting to support Curlee's (2000) vision that stem cell transplants that are able to become any other type of human cell, even neurons, will replace those structures to allow production of fluent and natural-sounding speech. Curlee also suggested the possible application of transcranial magnetic stimulation (TMS) applied to the skull, making established neural pathways in the brain more malleable to change when accompanied by the new neural activity. Tasks performed concurrently with TMS are "learned" and "remembered" with less practice. Techniques that have yielded promising results with psychiatric conditions, as well as Parkinsonism, also may be applicable to fluency-enhancing behaviors. Thus, even in these medically related developments, speech–language clinicians will still be involved. Also, as more information on subtypes of stuttering is accumulated, speech–language clinicians will continue their vital role on the diagnostic team.

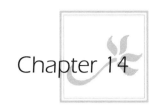

Chapter 14

Theoretical Considerations and Conclusions[1]

This brief chapter begins with a review of major shifts that have occurred during the past 30 years in five aspects of stuttering, ranging from etiology to treatment. Based on these observations, our own findings, and the conclusions of our findings, we offer three principles that provide the essential groundwork for a working theoretical model of early stuttering. Guarded speculations about the nature of stuttering in the domains of biology, personality, language processes, and motor functioning are offered.

Study Questions

1. What are the main significant changes that have occurred in stuttering research and treatment during the past three decades? Briefly state and explain each one.

2. What are the three principles that provide the essential groundwork for a model of stuttering development in children? Explain.

3. What biological bases are speculated to explain the basis for persistent and recovered stuttering?

---

[1] Ruth Watkins also contributed to this chapter.

Gradually occurring changes are often overlooked in the context of daily routines. When watching oneself daily in the mirror, one hardly notices changes in facial features, even over a period of a few years. On the other hand, comparing one's photos taken 10 years apart (e.g., when a new passport is issued) leaves no doubt as to the striking differences. Similarly, researchers and clinicians who routinely work in the area of stuttering may not quite realize the full extent of progress that has taken place in the knowledge about and treatment of stuttering during the last two or three decades. Again, however, when current scientific and other professional literature pertaining to research and clinical work in stuttering is placed side by side with that available 20 or 30 years ago, major changes are readily apparent. Our views of the most significant shifts in conceptions about early childhood stuttering, many of which have been catalyzed by findings of the University of Illinois Stuttering Research Program, are summarized in this chapter. In addition, we offer an initial integration of our key findings into a working model of stuttering in young children.

Significant Shifts in Understanding Early Childhood Stuttering

Etiology

Conceptions regarding possible causes of stuttering have shifted focus from learning perspectives to that of multiple etiologies grounded in biological underpinnings. The notion that stuttering is caused by children's responses to environmental factors has been, by and large, discredited. Strong evidence for the presence of genes underlying stuttering has emerged, and scientists are within reach of identifying them. In fact, even current knowledge concerning the genetic contributions to stuttering, limited as it is, already allows clinicians to use the information for clinical purposes.

Epidemiology

Major developments have occurred in regard to the etiology of stuttering. On the whole, there has been a shift from conceptions of uniformity of onset to those of significant diversity. Regarding the natural course of the disorder, although some children who persist progress to more severe stuttering, on the whole, views of a progressively ascending disorder have been replaced with views of one that typically is progressively descending in severity over time. Whereas additional information about the event of onset is needed for it to become clinically useful, current data about the developmental course of stuttering have reached the point of serving practical clinical purposes in predicting risk chances for chronicity. Additionally, the view of stuttering as a homogeneous disorder has been gradually changing with an eye toward subtype differentiation. We have begun with the distinction between children who persist and those who recover. As research progresses and extends to various developmental domains (e.g., language skills, motoric abilities, and personality development), a full subtype differentiation is anticipated.

Symptomatology

Three different shifts have occurred in the domain of symptomatology. The first reflects expansion. Characterizations of early stuttering as mainly effortless repetitions were replaced by a considerably richer, more complex symptomatology of speech, physical, cognitive, and affective elements. Associated physical tension, awareness of stuttering, and emotional reactions, once listed as advanced characteristics of the disorder, are now recognized as part of its early symptomatology. The second trend reflects contraction. It has been shown that the large number of speech disfluency features traditionally used in quantifying stuttering can be reduced to only three essential, relevant features: part-word repetition, single-syllable word repetition, and disrhythmic phonation. Third, traditional concepts of extensive overlap between stuttering and normal disfluency have given way to a much sharper distinction based on the frequency–type distribution of disfluency, length of disfluency, and temporal features of disfluency production.

Skills in Related Domains

There has been growing attention to the association between stuttering and development in related domains, especially language and phonology. Although this possible association continues to present many challenges, long-held assumptions that children who stutter possess lower linguistic skills than typically developing peers have been largely dispelled. Counter to expectations based on previous research and discussions, participants in the University of Illinois Stuttering Research Program, as well as in other recent investigations, have demonstrated expressive language skills at or above normative expectations. This pattern held for both those children whose stuttering persisted and those whose stuttering abated. In contrast, in the area of phonology, our participants who persisted in stuttering demonstrated slower phonological development than peers who would later recover. Thus, an important outcome of the current project is the suggestion of varied patterns of strength and limitation in the communication skills of young children who stutter.

Neural Base of Stuttering

In the past, the neurological focus was on peripheral neuromuscular organization that characterizes stuttered as well as fluent speech. Activation of speech muscles, articulator motility, fine adjustment and control of movement, as well as the function and coordination of nonspeech musculature, were investigated using electromyography, kinematic and acoustic analysis, and other methods. Slowness in movement or reaction time was explained in several ways, including neural innervation, heightened tension of antagonistic muscles, and reflex bombardment of the speech muscles. There has been a shift to examine the origination of disfluent speech in a much larger context, by including the roles of central processes of language formulation and of speech planning and execution. It is not simply that people who stutter have slower motor reaction times, or articulators that struggle to carry out an intended plan, but that the speech production system as a whole is less stable and more easily perturbed, leading to speech breakdown that is realized as stuttering. We note, however, that little neurological research has been done so far with very young children who stutter.

Clinical Management

As stated at the outset of this book, the long-term objective of all the research that has been done is to facilitate the clinical management of stuttering. In clinical management for adults who stutter, treatment has shifted from the major approach aimed at modifying stuttering and emotional reactions to the approach of generating fluency. For preschool-age children, our main interest in this book, the approach to treatment has changed from emphasizing *indirect* modes of modifying the child's home environment to *direct* speech modification.

Integrating Shifts: Developing a Working Model of Early Childhood Stuttering

Considered together, what do research findings suggest about the mechanisms underlying stuttering in young children? Our own work does not yet permit development of a full model or theory of early childhood stuttering. Nevertheless, our findings suggest at least three principles that provide the essential groundwork for a model of stuttering development in children.

▶ 1. **Stuttering is a unique disorder.** We do *not* view stuttering as an exaggeration of normal behavior, placed somewhere along a disfluency continuum that is normal at its low end and gradually becoming stuttering toward the upper end. In the vast majority of cases, stuttering begins as a definite, identifiable event *after* a period when the child's speech was regarded as normally fluent. It is marked with a loss of an existing function (fluency) and the appearance of new, unusual speech characteristics. Furthermore, it is recognized by parents either immediately or within a relatively short period of either days or a few weeks. There is strong evidence that the speech interruptions of children at stuttering onset are abnormal and, from the very beginning, differ substantially in several dimensions from disfluency exhibited by nonstuttering children. Were a trained expert to be present at the time of stuttering onset, considering current knowledge, he or she should be able to diagnose it, even in milder forms.

▶ 2. **Stuttering is biologically based.** Genetic factors are necessary, with few exceptions, but are not sufficient to cause stuttering. Genes transmit a susceptibility to stuttering but may be realized only with the addition of environmental components (by this we do *not* mean home environment). Additionally, although only a few genes probably underlie stuttering, resulting perhaps in a relatively straightforward anatomical–physiological abnormality, these genes no doubt interact with other genes. In fact, our own data indicate that there is one gene involved in all familial stuttering, and subtype diversity is due to additional genetic and environmental contributions (Ambrose, Cox, & Yairi, 1997).

▶ 3. **Stuttering is complex, multifaceted, and varied** in its developmental course and expression; is subject to environmental influences; and is inextricably intertwined with development in related domains. Regardless of genetic and environmental factors underlying the initial cause of stuttering, environment always plays a role in the further development of the disorder. From the time that stuttering emerges, its course is influenced by environmental factors, including not only situations, but also internal states of the individual, including illness or disease. Therefore, although stuttering is a unique single disorder, our view of stuttering emphasizes its variants. Furthermore, the genetics–environmental complex involved in the cause and progression of stuttering in young children is related to dynamic systems involving speech, language, motor, and personality–temperament aspects. By "dynamic" we mean that the timing and degree of influence of these domains or factors varies considerably, so that the disorder is nonlinear; it does not progress or change systematically from simple to more complex forms along a steadily escalating path. Differences in genetic loading, environmental factors, speech and language processes, motor function, and psychosocial behaviors would be reflected among individuals in the form of different subtypes, and vary within the individual over time because of considerable fluidity—that is, a change of balance across domains.

Some Speculations

Biological Perspectives

As stated previously, biological bases must be considered in developing a model or theory of stuttering. Although our own work does not yet permit development of a full model or theory of early childhood stuttering, we would like at this point to offer some speculations in this regard. What kind(s) of anatomical or physiological changes or abnormalities occur that might cause stuttering? What is the role of genetics in these changes? How can natural recovery be understood accordingly? Why does stuttering begin after a child has been speaking fluently, representing a breakdown in a previously normal skill? We propose that eventually it will be possible to explain stuttering within the context of structural and functional neurological development within the brain that underlies processes responsible for speech, also taking sensorimotor skills and personality into account.

Not only does stuttering mysteriously begin in a normally fluent child, stuttering also temporarily disappears, or is greatly reduced, under a number of conditions. These are documented back to the time of the Greek philosopher Demosthenes, who spoke with pebbles in his mouth to suppress his stuttering. Stuttering also can be virtually eliminated by speaking in a novel fashion, receiving noise or delayed auditory feedback through headphones, singing, speaking in unison with another person, and talking with a metronome. Also of interest, when normally fluent speakers receive delayed auditory feedback, many exhibit some disfluencies. Although questions about why these situations occur cannot yet be answered definitively, these situations provide intriguing hints about the nature of stuttering.

With the advent of new imaging capabilities, such as PET (positron emission tomography) and fMRI (functional magnetic resonance imaging), it has become possible to view brain activity in adults who stutter. Despite inconsistent findings, some appear robust. Converging findings based on functional imaging (fMRI and PET) indicate that, compared with normally fluent speakers, people who stutter show increased activity in a number of areas in the right hemisphere during speech and language activities, creating decreased asymmetry of the hemispheres. Many locations in both hemispheres of the brain are implicated, notably posterior and anterior sensorimotor speech areas in the left hemisphere. In addition to activation patterns in areas in the temporal and frontal cortex, differences also have been shown in other cortical and subcortical areas, as well as in the cerebellum (see R. Ingham, 2001, for a review). Thus, although stuttering is not reflected in abnormal brain activity in any single specific region, these findings provide strong evidence for a physiological basis for stuttering.

All of the biological studies mentioned have involved adults. Many techniques are not appropriate for young children; therefore, because stuttering begins in young children, we are unable to view brain functions that are involved in causing stuttering, rather than those that may develop as a result of stuttering. We can, however, apply knowledge of neurological development in normal children to evidence from adults who stutter.

In the normally developing child, proliferation of synapses through axon and dendrite growth begins before birth and continues at a rapid pace during early childhood (for a review, see Webb, Monk, & Nelson, 2001). This process is basically governed by genetics. As neural pathways are repeatedly utilized, based on the child's internal and external environment, they become stronger, more efficient, and more heavily myelinated, whereas connections that are not stimulated become nonfunctional and are pruned. Perhaps such pruning may increase efficiency and reduce disorganized neural impulses. This means that the young child's brain is quite plastic and primed for reception of stimuli and experience, such as that provided by speech and language. It is during this time frame that stuttering onset typically occurs.

As the child grows, synaptic connections continue to be selectively reinforced and organized. Looking at Broca's area in the left hemisphere and its homologue in the right hemisphere (oral motor skill), the density of connections are at first greater in the right; by age 2, the left hemisphere catches up; and by age 6, Broca's area in the left hemisphere has attained greater density (Kent, 1999). It is quite possible that this process may occur differently in children who stutter. Perhaps parts of the left hemisphere necessary for speech fail to fully develop, leaving the right hemisphere to compensate, or both hemispheres develop with involvement in language. Such defects could be genetically orchestrated and manifest in early childhood.

We know that a great majority of children who stutter recover naturally by school age, and some persist. How can we account for this? Could it be that, in early years, many children who begin to stutter have slightly delayed neural development in the speech and language areas? With time, perhaps, they complete the maturational processes, eventually forming efficient neural pathways needed to regain fluent speech. In children who persist in stuttering, is it possible that the normal pruning of neural connections that reduces disorganized neural impulses is incomplete? Or, is it possible that, rather than a delay in maturation, the left hemisphere fails to ever achieve the expected greater neural development than the right, as described above? Thus, the old ideas of difficulty with cerebral dominance, as presented in the Orton–Travis theory (Travis, 1931), have resurfaced in a new light.

With abnormalities in the neural system supporting speech, what might happen? The stuttering speaker knows what he or she wants to say, has no problem identifying the semantic item or its correct grammatical form, and has no problem with syntactic structure or with correct phoneme choice, but has difficulty with the flow of instructions; in other words, planning and implementation of the motor plan are somehow disturbed. It may take longer to set up a motor plan, and conditions such as slow speech may give the system more time. The use of externally imposed rhythm and slowing articulation rates, such as in singing, talking with a metronome, or choral reading, may possibly also reduce stress on the system. If the sensorimotor speech system is "corrected" or "normalized" by such phenomena, when no additional load from language complexity or situational factors is present, fluent speech can occur.

The neural abnormality, stemming from genetic sources, is the basis of the disorder, with other factors being secondary. Thus, for people who stutter, one or more parts (subsystems) of the complex multilevel system responsible for the planning and orderly execution of fluent speech are fragile and easily perturbed. Perhaps these subsystems are not sufficiently insulated from interferences of concurrent cognitive activities in the multilevel system (Bosshardt, 2002), causing fluctuations or variability in the output. The speech generating system, however, can operate normally, but only within a narrow range of variability. In other words, the greater variability produced by a malfunctioning system may exceed the threshold for fluent speech.

Language Perspectives

Clearly, even as a biological source for early childhood stuttering is implicated, an underlying organic difficulty must play out in specific ways as speech and language are formulated and produced. It is in the process of planning utterances, selecting sounds and words, and formulating sentences that stuttering behavior is observed. By what mechanisms, then, might a biologically based, genetically transmitted limitation interface with phonological, semantic, and syntactic aspects of language? How do we reconcile the findings reported thus far from the University of Illinois Stuttering Research Program, namely, (a) a proposed genetic foundation of the disorder, (b) some initial slowing in phonological development for those whose stuttering persists, and (c) relatively strong and perhaps even advanced semantic and syntactic skills in this same population?

One working view that we are exploring is the extent to which asynchronies in ability across developmental domains may be linked to difficulties in the production of fluent speech. For example, whereas many youngsters in the University of Illinois Stuttering Research Program demonstrated expressive language skills at or above expectations for age, phonological skills tended to lag behind age expectations in the same population. Such asynchrony across developmental domains may pose challenges in the production of fluent speech; as one aspect of communication development pushes forward, other areas may lag behind and the children's overall speech–language formulation and production system may be unable to "keep up" with demands created by a system that is out of sync. This working hypothesis is related to other current models, such as the demand and capacity model, which suggests generally that demand in one area may exceed capacity in another—that is, the demand created by a complex semantic and syntactic system may exceed a child's ability to produce speech fluently (see Bernstein Ratner, 1997, for further discussion). Our own exploration of these issues is quite tentative, but some findings to date are intriguing and warrant further investigation. In future studies, we plan to evaluate developmental levels and proficiencies across a wider range of domains, including motoric abilities and social–emotional development, as well as linguistic skills.

Personality Perspectives

Many years ago, one of the authors (Yairi) frequently drew the ire of his fellow graduate students at the University of Iowa by suggesting, half jokingly, that the world population can be divided into two: those who stutter and those who are insensitive. Interestingly, although past theories suggesting the disorder of stuttering is deeply rooted in unconscious psychological conflicts have been discarded for lack of scientific support, several current theoretical models assert that some personality factors, especially children's temperaments (e.g., sensitivity), might be involved. Indeed, past and more recent research that (unfortunately) focused on personality factors in adults or school-age children who stutter, has provided indications of heightened sensitivity, introversion, feelings of helplessness and dependence. Speech–language clinicians have been shown to perceive school-age children who stutter as highly sensitive, shy, tense, introverted, and inhibited (e.g., Yairi & Williams, 1970). Recent research with mothers of preschool-age children (Anderson, Pellowski, Conture, & Kelly, 2003) suggests that mothers of preschoolers who stutter perceive their children, when compared with control children, as more apt to exhibit temperamental profiles consistent with hypervigilance (i.e., less distractibility), nonadaptability to change, and irregular biological functions. Conture (2001) and Guitar (1998) hypothesized that children who stutter are born with sensitive temperaments that persist over time and are heightened by the experience of chronic stuttering. Likewise, it has been concluded that, as a group, children who stutter are more likely to be raised in families that are pressure-creating, less harmonious, and more socially withdrawn than those of nonstuttering children (Yairi, 1997a).

Currently, we venture to guess that personality and temperament indeed play a significant role in the ways that preschool children respond to and cope with their stuttering, and thus influence its eventual course. Furthermore, we venture to guess that, inasmuch as subtypes of stuttering are identified, personality and temperament factors play a role in such variants of the disorder. Is it possible that brain processes involved in stuttering are influenced by emotions or temperament characteristics such as oversensitivity? Interestingly, in a recent review of twin studies, Goldsmith, Buss, and Lemery (1997) concluded that heredity accounted for a significant proportion of toddlers' temperament characteristics. Perhaps the biological foundations of stuttering and of temperament interact at some level. So far, however, it has been difficult to discern if the perceived characteristics of children who stutter and their parents are related to inherent personality differences, a consequence of stuttering, or an interaction of such diverse influences.

Motor Perspectives

Speech output represents the end product of all the factors that contribute to verbal communication. Thus, regardless of its etiology and both linguistic and personality influences, stuttering manifests itself as a breakdown in speech motor control. In spite of the equivocal findings of rich research concerned with motor speech (as well as other motor functions) of people who stutter, on balance, it would appear that, compared with normally fluent individuals, they are somewhat different—that is, they are slightly slower (Zimmermann, 1980), are discoordinated (Alfonso, Watson, & Baer, 1987), exhibit movement mistiming (Kent, 1984), and have slower reaction times (Bishop, Williams, & Cooper, 1991). Although relatively little in our research has dealt with this aspect (except our studies regarding second formant transition, fundamental frequency, and speaking rate, as reported in Chapter 8), we have suggested that inconsistent findings may be partially attributed to population heterogeneity. Furthermore, the great majority of studies have examined adults who stutter. Inasmuch as differences in motor functions exist between children who stutter and those who do not, they appear to be subtle and require further research and substantiation.

It is important to recognize that researchers do not yet agree on the mechanisms that underlie stuttering. Some believe that the difficulty lies in the assembly of the motor plan (e.g., Postma & Kolk, 1993); others espouse that the problem is at the level of the motor execution stage (Peters, Hulstijn, & Van Lieshout, 2000). In either case, delay and disruption in the ongoing planning and execution processes across language and speech modalities necessary to produce running speech, surface at the overt speech level and are reflected in aberrant speech movements (e.g., Van Lieshout, Hulstijn, & Peters, 1996). The abnormality seen and heard at the level of the articulators is not itself the origin of the problem, but is the end result of the chain involving speech production that acts to lower thresholds for speech perturbations. One can imagine a domino effect that leads to further increase the degree of speech aberrancy (i.e., stuttering-like disfluencies), which leads to abnormal kinesthetic and auditory feedback, leading to problems in planning and execution of speech, and so on. Many factors, including cognition, language formulation, and language complexity, as well as situational pressures, can interfere and push the system to exceed its limits for fluent speech (e.g., see Bernstein Ratner, 1998; Bosshardt, 2002). The motor plan is assembled and delivered to be executed by the articulators, which provide feedback to the motor assembly plan. It is difficult to pinpoint exactly where derailment occurs in stuttered speech. In fact, differences in motor performance have been illustrated in fluent as well as disfluent speech of stutterers.

The findings of motor studies and the development of increasingly sophisticated brain imaging techniques are beginning to allow researchers to view a larger picture. When researchers are able to identify the effects of increasing demands in brain scans and measure them through muscle activity (as well as brain waves), the picture of stuttering will come into much sharper focus. This investigation may also provide more insight into the reported, though not firmly established, co-occurrence of stuttering and phonological delay in young children. Could the specific extent or nature of the abnormality explain why some children who stutter also exhibit phonological difficulties whereas others do not? Research shows that severity of stuttering does not seem to be related to the presence or degree of phonological impairment. Would it become possible to use speech motor data in early differentiation between children who would persist and those who would recover? Could the smaller change in the second formant frequency transition reflect restricted movement of the articulators on a spatial plane, and thus create difficulties with transitions and coarticulation across sounds? In other words, could the anticipated articulatory plan require adjustments for coarticulation that exceed the system's threshold for fluent speech?

The brain abnormalities alluded to above affect speech planning and production in ways that might delay parallel planning processes across language and speech modalities that are necessary to produce continuous fluent speech. Our working hypothesis, then, is that if a child (a) has a slightly inferior motor system with low thresholds, (b) uses a rapid speaking rate and complex linguistic patterns, and (c) is highly sensitive to communicative pressure, stuttering events occur. In sum, for better understanding of the role of biological, language, personality, and motor factors in the pathogenesis of stuttering and its developmental course, close and simultaneous examination of multiple potentially relevant variables is necessary beginning from close to the onset of the stuttering and continuing over time.

Theory-Based Therapy

Stuttering results from strong genetic components in interaction with environmental factors. As theorized in the previous section, whatever is being inherited probably has to do with brain structure and functions that cause delays or other interferences in the complex parallel planning processes across the language and speech modalities necessary to produce running speech. These are reflected on the surface at the motor level. When one has a vulnerable speech planning system causing problems in motor execution to begin with, the addition of possible asynchrony across developmental speech and language domains poses increased challenges for the production of fluent speech. High physiologic reactivity further lowers the threshold of vulnerability. We must also keep in mind the high chances for natural recovery that are potentially operating in many children.

Therefore, treatment should address the child's speech production system, as well as his or her ability to deal with complex language and to cope with stress. Treatment should attempt to enhance slower speaking rate, which will minimize the chain of delays from top to bottom, and the out-of-phase planning and speech execution. This change can be achieved through either direct practice or modeling. Although long-term usage of simple language structure may interfere with normal language development, short-term implementation may be considered as a part of a treatment program. Additionally, aiming at the home environment through parent counseling and advising to promote potential natural recovery processes by creating a reasonably tolerant environment—reducing pressure on the one hand and enhancing slow speech on the other—is a logical avenue to pursue. Still, logical assumptions must be scientifically tested. Regardless of theory, every child who has begun stuttering should be evaluated and monitored until treatment is in progress or recovery has occurred. No child should be sent home with the message, "Don't worry, it's normal; it will go away on its own."

Conclusions

Robert Louis Stevenson (1886) wrote, "You start a question and it's like starting a stone. You sit quietly on the top of a hill; and away the stone goes, starting others." In our quest for answers, we began by collecting a few pebbles, and soon enough, we were shoulder to shoulder in boulders (and a lot more pebbles). In this text, we have summarized the general status of current thought in the discipline and reported what we have learned in our quest for answers to our questions about the development of stuttering in young children. Here, however, lies a constant danger of falling into a trap of our own bias and we have been mindful of George Santayana's (1923) quip that "the empiricist thinks he believes only what he sees, but he is much better at believing than at seeing." In this book, we have also offered some working hypotheses and speculations about the broader meaning of our most essential findings. We have attempted to recognize our own limitations, as well as point out those of past researchers. In this respect, we are keenly aware of Albert Einstein's comparison of stupidity with genius. He reflected that genius, unlike stupidity, has its limits. Hopefully, future generations will judge our ventured views and hypotheses mercifully. We provide this text as illumination on a path that hopefully leads to diminishing our ignorance and achieving more complete understanding of the development, trajectory, and treatment of stuttering in young children. Realizing that our efforts have raised nearly as many questions as they have answered, we look ahead with anticipation toward future discoveries. As Ludwig Wittgenstein (1922) observed, "What *can* be shown *cannot* be said."

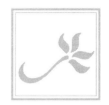

References

Abidin, R. R. (1986). *Parenting Stress Index* (2nd ed.). Charlottesville, VA: Pediatric Psychology.

Achenbach, T. M. (1991). *Manual for the Child Behavior Checklist: 4–18 and 1991 profile.* Burlington: University of Vermont, Department of Psychiatry.

Adams, M. R. (1977). A clinical strategy for differentiating the normally nonfluent child and the incipient stutterer. *Journal of Fluency Disorders, 2,* 141–148.

Adams, M. R. (1986, November). *Stuttering, disfluency, and fluency: A perspective overview.* Paper presented at the convention of the American Speech-Language-Hearing Association, Detroit, MI.

Adams, M. R. (1990). The demands and capacities model I: Theoretical elaborations. *Journal of Fluency Disorders, 15,* 135–141.

Adams, M. R. (1993). The home environment of children who stutter. *Seminars in Speech and Language, 14,* 185–192.

Adams, S. (1932). A study of the growth of language between two and four years. *Journal of Juvenile Research, 16,* 267–277.

Ainsworth, S., & Fraser-Gruss, J. (1977). *If your child stutters: A guide* (3rd ed.). Memphis, TN: Speech Foundation of America.

Ainsworth, S., & Fraser, J. (2002). *If your child stutters: A guide* (6th ed.). Memphis, TN: Speech Foundation of America.

Alfonso, P., Watson, B., & Baer, T. (1987). Measuring dynamical vocal tract characteristics by X-ray microbeam pellet tracking. In H. F. Peters & W. Hulstijn (Eds.), *Speech motor dynamics in stuttering* (pp. 141–150). New York: Springer Verglag Wien.

Al-Yagon, M., & Margalit, M. (2002). Relations between mother's sense of coherence, children's experience of loneliness and family climate profile among kindergarten at risk for developing learning disabilities. *Thalamus, 29*(1), 40–49.

Ambrose, N. G., Cox, N. J., & Yairi, E. (1997). The genetic basis of persistence and recovery in stuttering. *Journal of Speech, Language, and Hearing Research, 40,* 567–580.

Ambrose, N. G., & Yairi, E. (1994). The development of awareness of stuttering in preschool children. *Journal of Fluency Disorders, 19,* 229–245.

Ambrose, N. G., & Yairi, E. (1995). The role of repetition units in the differential diagnosis of early childhood incipient stuttering. *American Journal of Speech–Language Pathology, 4*(3), 82–88.

Ambrose, N. G., & Yairi, E. (1999). Normative disfluency data for early childhood stuttering. *Journal of Speech, Language, and Hearing Research, 42,* 895–909.

Ambrose, N. G., & Yairi, E. (2001). Perspectives on stuttering: Response to Onslow & Packman (2001). *Journal of Speech, Language, and Hearing Research, 44,* 595–597.

Ambrose, N., & Yairi, E. (2002). The Tudor study: Data and ethics. *American Journal of Speech–Language Pathology, 11*(2), 190–203.

Ambrose, N. G., Yairi, E., & Cox, N. (1993). Genetic aspects of early childhood stuttering. *Journal of Speech and Hearing Research, 36,* 701–706.

American Speech-Language Hearing Association Special Interest Division 4: Fluency and Fluency Disorders. (1999, March). Terminology pertaining to fluency and fluency disorders: Guidelines. *ASHA Leader, 41,* 29–36.

Amir, O., & Yairi, E. (2002). The effect of temporal manipulation on the perception of disfluencies as normal or stuttering. *Journal of Communication Disorders, 35,* 63–82.

Anderson, J. D., & Conture, E. G. (2000). Language abilities of children who stutter: A preliminary study. *Journal of Fluency Disorders, 25,* 283–304.

Anderson, J. D., Pellowski, M., & Conture, E. (2001, November). *Temperamental characteristics of children who stutter.* Paper presented at the convention of the American Speech-Language-Hearing Association, New Orleans.

Anderson, J., Pellowski, M., Conture, E., & Kelly, E. (2003). Temperament characteristics of young children who stutter. *Journal of Speech, Language and Hearing Research, 46,* 1221–1233.

Andrews, G. (1984). Epidemiology of stuttering. In R. F. Curlee & W. H. Perkins (Eds.), *Nature and treatment of stuttering: New directions* (2nd ed., pp. 1–12). San Diego, CA: College-Hill.

Andrews, G., Craig, A., Feyer, A., Hoddinott, S., Howie, P., & Neilson, M. (1983). Stuttering: A review of research findings and theories circa 1982. *Journal of Speech and Hearing Disorders, 48,* 226–246.

Andrews, G., Guitar, B., & Howie, P. (1980). Meta-analysis of the effects of stuttering treatment. *Journal of Speech and Hearing Disorders, 45,* 308–324.

Andrews, G., & Harris, M. (1964). *The syndrome of stuttering: Clinics in Developmental Medicine,* No. 17. London: Spastics Society Medical Education and Information Unit in association with Wm. Heinemann Medical Books.

Andrews, G., Morris-Yates, A., Howie, P., & Martin, N. G. (1991). Genetic factors in stuttering confirmed. *Archives of General Psychiatry, 48,* 1034–1035.

Andrews, J., & Andrews, M. (1986). A family-based systematic model for speech–language services. *Seminars in Speech and Language, 7,* 359–364.

Andronico, M., & Blake, I. (1974). The application of filial therapy to young children with stuttering problems. *Journal of Speech and Hearing Disorders, 36,* 377–381.

Arndt, J., & Healey, E. C. (2001). Concomitant disorders in school-age children who stutter. *Language, Speech, and Hearing Services in Schools, 32,* 68–78.

Arnott, N. (1828). *Elements of physics.* Edinburgh: Publisher unknown.

Arthur, G. (1952). *Arthur Adaptation of the Leiter International Performance Scale.* Los Angeles: Western Psychological Services.

Au-Yeung, J., Howell, P., & Pilgrim, L. (1998). Phonological words and stuttering on function words. *Journal of Speech, Language, and Hearing Research, 41,* 1019–1030.

Axline, V. M. (1947). *Play therapy.* London: Metbuen.

Bar, A. (1971). The shaping of fluency not the modification of stuttering. *Journal of Communication Disorders, 4,* 1–8.

Beitchman, J. H., Nair, R., Clegg, M., & Patel, P. G. (1986). Prevalence of speech and language disorders in 5-year-old kindergarten children in the Ottawa–Carleton Region. *Journal of Speech and Hearing Disorders, 51,* 98–110.

Bender, J. (1943). The prophylaxis of stuttering. *Nervous Child, 2,* 181–198.

Bernstein Ratner, N. (1992). Measurable outcomes of instructions to modify normal parent–child verbal interactions: Implications for indirect stuttering therapy. *Journal of Speech and Hearing Research, 35,* 14–20.

Bernstein Ratner, N. (1993). Parents, children, and stuttering. *Seminars in Speech and Language, 14,* 238–248.

Bernstein Ratner, N. (1997). Stuttering: A psycholinguistic perspective. In R. F. Curlee & G. M. Siegel (Eds.), *Nature and treatment of stuttering: New directions* (2nd ed., pp. 99–127). Boston: Allyn & Bacon.

Bernstein Ratner, N. (1998). Linguistic and perceptual characteristics of children at stuttering onset. In E. C. Healey & H. F. M. Peters (Eds.), *Proceedings of the Second World Congress on Fluency Disorders* (pp. 3–6). Nijmegen, The Netherlands: Nijmegen University.

Bernstein Ratner, N., & Sih, C. C. (1987). Effects of gradual increases in sentence length and complexity on children's disfluency. *Journal of Speech and Hearing Disorders, 52,* 278–287.

Berry, M. F. (1937). Twinning in stuttering families. *Human Biology, 9,* 329–346.

Berry, M. F. (1938). A common denominator in twinning and stuttering. *Journal of Speech Disorders, 3,* 51–57.

Bishop, J., Williams, H., & Cooper, W. (1991). Age and task complexity variables in motor performance of stuttering and nonstuttering children. *Journal of Fluency Disorders, 16,* 207–217.

Blood, G. W., & Seider, R. (1981). The concomitant problems of young stutterers. *Journal of Speech and Hearing Disorders, 46,* 31–33.

Blood, I. M., Wertz, H., Blood, G. W., Bennett, S., & Simpson, K. C. (1997). The effects of life stressors and daily stressors on stuttering. *Journal of Speech, Language, and Hearing Research, 40,* 134–143.

Bloodstein, O. (1944). Studies in the psychology of stuttering: XIX. The relationship between oral reading rate and severity of stuttering. *Journal of Speech Disorders, 9,* 161–173.

Bloodstein, O. (1958). Stuttering as anticipatory struggle reaction. In J. Eisenson (Ed.), *Stuttering: A Symposium.* New York: Harper & Row.

Bloodstein, O. (1960a). The development of stuttering: I. Changes in nine basic features. *Journal of Speech and Hearing Disorders, 25,* 219–237.

Bloodstein, O. (1960b). The development of stuttering: II. Developmental phases. *Journal of Speech and Hearing Disorders, 25,* 366–376.

Bloodstein, O. (1961). The development of stuttering: III. Theoretical and clinical implications. *Journal of Speech and Hearing Disorders, 26,* 67–82.

Bloodstein, O. (1970). Stuttering and normal disfluency: A continuity hypothesis. *British Journal of Disorders of Communication, 5,* 30–39.

Bloodstein, O. (1974). The rules of early stuttering. *Journal of Speech and Hearing Disorders, 39,* 379–394.

Bloodstein, O. (1981). *A handbook on stuttering* (3rd ed.). Chicago: National Easter Seal Society for Crippled Children and Adults.

Bloodstein, O. (1987). *A handbook on stuttering* (4th ed.). Chicago: National Easter Seal Society for Crippled Children and Adults.

Bloodstein, O. (1995). *A handbook on stuttering* (5th ed.). San Diego, CA: Singular.

Bloodstein, O., & Grossman, M. (1981). Early stutterings: Some aspects of their form and distribution. *Journal of Speech and Hearing Research, 24,* 298–302.

Bluemel, C. S. (1913). *Stammering and cognate defects of speech: Vol. 1.* New York: G. E. Stechert.

Bluemel, C. S. (1932). Primary and secondary stuttering. *Quarterly Journal of Speech, 18,* 187–200.

Bluemel, C. S. (1959). If a child stammers. *Mental Hygiene, 43,* 390–393.

Boada, K., & Meyers, S. (1990, November). *Verbal communicative patterns of stutters following intervention.* Presented at the convention of the American Speech-Language-Hearing Association, Seattle, WA.

Bosshardt, H. G. (2002). Effects of concurrent cognitive processing on the fluency of word repetition: Comparison between persons who do and do not stutter. *Journal of Fluency Disorders, 27,* 93–114.

Bøstrup, B., & Møller, B. (1990). Småbørnsstammegrupper. *Dansk Audiologopædi, 1,* 21–25.

Brady, J. P. (1971). Metronome-conditioned speech retraining for stuttering. *Behavioral Therapy, 2,* 129–150.

Brandenburg, G. (1915). The language of a three-year-old child. *Pedagological Seminary, 22,* 89–120.

Branscom, M. (1942). *The construction and statistical evaluation of a speech fluency test for young children.* Unpublished master's thesis, University of Iowa, Iowa City.

Branscom, M., Hughes, J., & Oxtoby, E. (1955). Studies of nonfluency in the speech of preschool. In W. Johnson & R. R. Leutenegger (Eds.), *Stuttering in children and adults: Thirty years of research at the University of Iowa* (pp. 157–180). Minneapolis: University of Minnesota.

Brill, A. (1923). Speech disturbances in nervous and mental diseases. *Quarterly Journal of Speech Education, 9,* 129–135.

Brown, R. (1973). *A first language.* Cambridge, MA: Harvard University.

Brown, S. (1938). A further study of stuttering in relation to various speech sounds. *Quarterly Journal of Speech, 24,* 390–397.

Brown, S. (1945). The loci of stutterings in the speech sequence. *Journal of Speech Disorders,* *10,* 181–192.

Brown, S. (1949). Advising parents of early stutterers. *Pediatrics, 4,* 170–175.

Brutten, G. J., & Dunham, S. L. (1989). The Communication Attitude Test: A normative study of grade school children. *Journal of Fluency Disorders, 14,* 371–377.

Brutten, G. J., & Shoemaker, D. (1967). *The modification of stuttering.* Englewood Cliffs, NJ: Prentice Hall.

Bryngelson, B. (1932). A photo–phonographic analysis of the vocal disturbances in stuttering. *Psychological Monograph, 43,* 1–30.

Bryngelson, B. (1938). Prognosis of stuttering. *Journal of Speech Disorders, 3,* 121–123.

Bryngelson, B., & Rutherford, B. (1937). A comparative study of laterality of stutterers and non-stutterers. *Journal of Speech Disorders, 2,* 15–16.

Buck, S., & Lees, R. (2000, July). How does family history of stuttering influence the onset and recovery from stuttering? In K. Baker (Ed.), *Proceedings of the Fifth Oxford Dysfluency Conference* (pp. 7–15), St. Catherine's College, Oxford, England.

Buck, S., Lees, R., & Cook, F. (2002). The influence of family history of stuttering on the onset of stuttering in young children. *Folia Phoniatrica et Logopaedica, 54,* 117–124.

Byrd, K., & Cooper, E. B. (1989a). Expressive and receptive language skills in stuttering children. *Journal of Fluency Disorders, 14,* 121–126.

Byrd, K., & Cooper, E. B. (1989b). Apraxic speech characteristics in stuttering, developmentally apraxic, and normal speaking children. *Journal of Fluency Disorders, 14,* 215–229.

Campbell, J., & Hill, D. (1987, November). *Systematic disfluency analysis: Accountability for differential evaluation and treatment.* Paper presented at the convention of the American Speech-Language-Hearing Association, New Orleans.

Canter, G. J. (1971). Observations on neurogenic stuttering: A contribution to differential diagnosis. *British Journal of Disordered Communication, 6,* 139–143.

Cantwell, D., & Baker, L. (1985). Psychiatric and learning disorders in children with speech and language disorders: A descriptive analysis. *Advances in Learning and Behavioral Disabilities, 2,* 29–47.

Caspi, A. (1998). Personality development across the life course. In N. Eisenberg & W. Damon (Eds.), *Handbook of child psychology: Vol. 4. Social, emotional, and personality development* (5th ed., pp. 311–388). New York: Wiley.

Cave, D. (1977). Assessment and treatment of stuttering in children. *Developmental Medicine and Child Neurology, 19,* 410–412.

Chevekeva, N. A. (1967). About methods of overcoming stuttering: A survey of the literature. *Spetsial Shkola, 3,* 9–15.

Clark, R., & Snyder, M. (1955). Group therapy for parents of preadolescent stutterers. *Group Psychology, 8,* 226–232.

Colburn, N. (1985). Clustering of disfluency in nonstuttering childrens' early utterances. *Journal of Fluency Disorders, 10,* 51–58.

Conture, E. G. (1982). *Stuttering* (1st ed.). Englewood Cliffs, NJ: Prentice Hall.

Conture, E. G. (1990). *Stuttering* (2nd ed.). Englewood Cliffs, NJ: Prentice Hall.

Conture, E. G. (1991). Young stutterers' speech production: A critical review. In H. F. M. Peters, W. Hulstijn, & C. W. Starkweather (Eds.), *Speech motor control and stuttering: Proceedings of the 2nd International Conference on Speech Motor Control and Stuttering* (pp. 365–384). New York: Elsevier.

Conture, E. G. (1999). Why does my child stutter? In J. Fraser (Ed.), *Stuttering and your child: Questions and answers* (pp. 9–18). Memphis, TN: Stuttering Foundation of America.

Conture, E. G. (2001). *Stuttering: Its nature, diagnosis, and treatment.* Boston: Allyn & Bacon.

Conture, E. G., & Brayton, E. R. (1975). The influence of noise on stutterers' different disfluency types. *Journal of Speech and Hearing Research, 18,* 381–384.

Conture, E. G., & Caruso, A. (1987). Assessment and diagnosis of childhood disfluency. In L. Rustin, H. Purser, & D. Rowley (Eds.), *Progress in the treatment of fluency disorders* (pp. 57–82). London: Taylor & Francis.

Conture, E. G., Colton, R. H., & Gleason, J. R. (1988). Selected temporal aspects of coordination during fluent speech of young stutterers. *Journal of Speech and Hearing Research, 31,* 640–653.

Conture, E. G., & Kelly, E. M. (1991). Young stutterers' nonspeech behaviors during stuttering. *Journal of Speech and Hearing Research, 34,* 1041–1056.

Conture, E. G., Louko, L. J., & Edwards, M. L. (1993). Simultaneously treating stuttering and disordered phonology in children: Experimental treatment, preliminary findings. *American Journal of Speech–Language Pathology, 2,* 72–81.

Conture, E. G., McCall, G. N., & Brewer, D. W. (1977). Laryngeal behavior during stuttering. *Journal of Speech and Hearing Research, 20,* 661–668.

Conture, E. G., & Melnick, K. (1999). Parent–child group approach to stuttering in preschool and school-age children. In M. Onslow & A. Packman (Eds.), *Early stuttering: A handbook of intervention strategies* (pp. 17–51). San Diego, CA: Singular.

Conture, E. G., Rothenberg, M., & Molitor, R. D. (1986). Electroglottographic observations of young stutterers' fluency. *Journal of Speech and Hearing Research, 29,* 384–393.

Cooper, E. (1979). *Understanding stuttering.* Chicago: National Easter Seal Society for Crippled Children and Adults.

Cooper, E., & Cooper, C. (1985). *Cooper personalized fluency control therapy* (revised). Allen, TX: DLM Teaching Resources.

Coppola, V. A., & Yairi, E. (1982). Rhythmic speech training with preschool stuttering children: An experimental study. *Journal of Fluency Disorders, 7,* 447–457.

Cordes, A. K., & Ingham, R. J. (1994). The reliability of observational data: II. Issues in the identification and measurement of stuttering events. *Journal of Speech and Hearing Research, 37,* 279–294.

Cordes, A., & Ingham, R. (1995). Stuttering includes both within-word and between-word disfluencies. *Journal of Speech and Hearing Research, 38,* 382–386.

Cordes, A. K., & Ingham, R. J. (1996). Disfluency types and stuttering measurement: A necessary connection? *Journal of Speech and Hearing Research, 39,* 404–405.

Coriat, I. (1943). The psychoanalytic conception of stammering. *Nervous Child, 2,* 167–171.

Costa, L., & Kroll, R. M. (2000). Stuttering: An update for physicians. *Canadian Medical Association Journal, 1621,* 1849–1855.

Costello, J. C. (1980). Operant conditioning and the treatment of stuttering. In W. H. Perkins (Ed.), *Strategies in stuttering therapy* (pp. 311–325). New York: Thieme.

Costello, J. C. (1999). Behavioral treatment of young children who stutter: An extended length of utterance method. In R. F. Curlee (Ed.), *Stuttering and related disorders of fluency* (2nd ed., pp. 80–109). New York: Thieme.

Costello, J. M. (1983). Current behavioral treatments for children. In D. Prins & R. Ingham (Eds.), *Treatment of stuttering in early childhood: Methods and issues* (pp. 69–112). San Diego, CA: College-Hill.

Costello, J. M., & Ingham, R. J. (1984). Stuttering as an operant disorder. In R. F. Curlee & W. H. Perkins (Eds.), *Nature and treatment of stuttering: New directions* (pp. 187–213). San Diego, CA: College-Hill.

Cox, N., Cook, E., Ambrose, N., Yairi, E., Rydmarker, S., Lundstrom, C., et al. (2000). *The Illinois–Sweden–Israel Genetics of Stuttering Project.* Paper presented at the Third World Congress on Fluency Disorders, Nyborg, Denmark.

Cox, N., & Kidd, K. K. (1983). Can recovery from stuttering be considered a genetically milder subtype of stuttering? *Behavior Genetics, 13,* 129–139.

Cox, N., Kramer, P., & Kidd, K. (1984). Segregation analyses of stuttering. *Genetic Epidemiology, 1,* 245–253.

Curlee, R. F. (1980). A case selection strategy for young disfluent children. *Seminars in Speech, Language, and Hearing, 1,* 277–287.

Curlee, R. F. (1981). Observer agreement on disfluency and stuttering. *Journal of Speech and Hearing Research, 24,* 595–600.

Curlee, R. F. (1993a). Evaluating treatment efficacy for adults: Assessment of stuttering disability. *Journal of Fluency Disorders, 18,* 319–331.

Curlee, R. F. (1993b). Identification and management of beginning stuttering. In R. F. Curlee (Ed.), *Stuttering and related disorders of fluency* (pp. 1–22). New York: Thieme.

Curlee, R. F. (1999a). Does my child stutter? In J. Fraser (Ed.), *Stuttering and your child: Questions and answers* (pp. 1–8). Memphis, TN: Stuttering Foundation of America.

Curlee, R. F. (1999b). Identification and case selection guidelines for early childhood stuttering. In R. F. Curlee (Ed.), *Stuttering and related disorders of fluency* (2nd ed., pp. 1–21). New York: Thieme.

Curlee, R. F. (2000, November). *The evolution of stuttering treatment: Future directions.* Paper presented at the convention of the American Speech-Language-Hearing Association, Washington, DC.

Curlee, R. F., & Yairi, E. (1997). Early intervention with early childhood stuttering: A critical examination of the data. *American Journal of Speech–Language Pathology, 6*(2), 8–18.

Curlee, R. F., & Yairi, E. (1998). Treatment of early childhood stuttering: Advances and research needs. *American Journal of Speech–Language Pathology, 7*(3), 20–26.

Curran, M. F., & Hood, S. B. (1977). Listener ratings of severity for specific disfluency types in children. *Journal of Fluency Disorders, 2,* 87–97.

Daley, D. (1981). Differentiating stuttering subgroups with Van Riper's developmental tracks: A preliminary study. *Journal of National Student Speech and Hearing Association, 11,* 89–101.

Darley, F. (1955). The relationship of parental attitudes and adjustment to the development of stuttering. In W. Johnson & R. R. Leutenegger (Eds.), *Stuttering in children and adults: Thirty years of research at the University of Iowa* (pp. 74–156). Minneapolis: University of Minnesota.

Darley, F. L., & Spriestersbach, D. C. (1978). *Diagnostic methods in speech pathology* (2nd ed.). New York: Harper & Row.

Daskalov, D. (1962). Kvoprosu ob osnovnikh printsipakh I metodakh preduprezhdenia lechenia zaikania. *Zh. Nevropatol. Psikhiat, 62,* 1047–1052.

Davis, D. M. (1939). The relation of repetitions in the speech of young children to certain measures of language maturity and situational factors: Part I. *Journal of Speech Disorders, 4,* 303–318.

De Ajuriaguerra, J., De Gobineau, D., Narlian, S., & Stambak, M. (1958). Stuttering. *Press Medicale Disorders, 48,* 171–177.

De Nil, L. F., & Brutten, G. J. (1990). Speech-associated attitudes: Stuttering, voice disordered, articulation disordered, and normal speaking children. *Journal of Fluency Disorders, 15,* 127–134.

De Nil, L. F., & Brutten, G. J. (1991). Speech-associated attitudes of stuttering and nonstuttering children. *Journal of Speech and Hearing Research, 34,* 60–68.

Dell, G. (1990). Effects of frequency and vocabulary type on phonological speech errors. *Language and Cognitive Processes, 5,* 313–349.

Dennis, M. (2000). Developmental plasticity in children: The role of biological risk, development, time, and reserve. *Journal of Communication Disorders, 33,* 321–332.

Derazne, J. (1966). Speech pathology in the U.S.S.R. In R. W. Rieber & R. S. Brubaker (Eds.), *Speech pathology* (pp. 611–618). Amsterdam: North Holland.

Despert, J. L. (1946). Psychosomatic study of fifty stuttering children: I. Social, physical, and psychiatric findings. *American Journal of Orthopsychiatry, 16,* 100–113.

Dickson, S. (1971). Incipient stuttering and spontaneous remission of stuttered speech. *Journal of Communication Disorders, 4,* 99–110.

Dollaghan, C., & Campbell, T. (1998). Nonword repetition and child language impairment. *Journal of Speech, Language, and Hearing Research, 41,* 1136–1146.

Douglass, E., & Quarrington, B. (1952). The differentiation of interiorized and exteriorized secondary stuttering. *Journal of Speech and Hearing Disorders, 17,* 377–385.

Drayna, D. T. (1997). Genetic linkage studies of stuttering: Ready for prime time? *Journal of Fluency Disorders, 22,* 237–241.

Drever, J. (1952). *A dictionary of psychology.* Harmondsworth, Middlesex: Penguin Books.

Dunlap, K. (1944). Stammering: Its nature, etiology, and therapy. *Journal of Comparative Psychology, 37,* 187–202.

Dunn, L., & Dunn, L. (1981). *Peabody Picture Vocabulary Test–Revised.* Circle Pines, MN: American Guidance Service.

Egolf, D. B., Shames, G. H., Johnson, P. R., & Kasprisin-Burrelli, A. (1972). The use of parent–child interaction patterns in therapy for young stutterers. *Journal of Speech and Hearing Disorders, 37,* 222–232.

Eisenson, J. (1958). A perseverative theory of stuttering. In J. Eisenson (Ed.), *Stuttering: A symposium* (pp. 223–271). New York: Harper & Row.

Eisenson, J., & Ogilvie, M. (1957). *Speech correction in the schools.* New York: Macmillan.

Eisenson, J., & Ogilvie, M. (1977). *Speech correction in the schools* (2nd ed.). New York: Macmillan.

Ekman, P., & Friesen, W. (1978). *Facial action coding system.* Palo Alto, CA: Consulting Psychologist.

Embrechts, M., Ebben, H., Franke, P., & van de Poel, C. (2000). Temperament: A comparison between children who stutter and children who do not stutter. In H. G. Bosshardt, J. S. Yaruss, & H. F. M. Peters (Eds.), *Proceedings of the Third World Congress on Fluency Disorders* (pp. 557–562). Nijmegen, The Netherlands: Nijmegen University.

Emil-Behnke, K. (1947). *Stammering: Its nature, causes, and treatment.* London: Williams & Norgate.

Ezrati-Vinacour, R., Platzky, R., & Yairi, E. (2001). The young child's awareness of stuttering-like disfluency. *Journal of Speech, Language, and Hearing Research, 44,* 368–380.

Falck, F. J., Lawler, P. S., & Yonovitz, A. (1985). Effects of stuttering on fundamental frequency. *Journal of Fluency Disorders, 10,* 123–135.

Fein, L. (1970, November). *Stuttering as a cue related to the precipitation of moments of stuttering.* Paper presented at the convention of the American Speech-Language-Hearing Association, New York.

Felsenfeld, S., McGue, M., & Broen, P. A. (1995). Familial aggregation of phonological disorders: Results from a 28-year follow-up. *Journal of Speech and Hearing Research, 38,* 1091–1107.

Fenichel, O. (1945). *The psychoanalytic theory of neurosis.* New York: Norton.

Finn, P., Ingham, R. J., Ambrose, N., & Yairi, E. (1997). Children recovered from stuttering without formal therapy: Perceptual assessment of speech normalcy. *Journal of Speech, Language, and Hearing Research, 40,* 867–876.

Fisher, M. (1932). Language patterns of preschool children. *Experimental Education, 1,* 70–85.

Fogerty, E. (1930). *Stammering.* New York: Dutton.

Fortier-Blanc, J., Labonte, S., Beauchemin, M., & Jutras, G. (1997, August). *Does indirect stuttering therapy produce effective changes in preschoolers?* Paper presented at the meeting of the Second World Congress on Fluency Disorders, San Francisco.

Fosnot, S. M. (1993). Research design for examining treatment efficacy in fluency disorders. *Journal of Fluency Disorders, 18,* 221–251.

Fosnot, S. M. (Ed.). (1995). Some contemporary approaches in treating fluency disorders in preschool-age children, and adolescent children [Special issue]. *Language, Speech, and Hearing Services in Schools, 26*(2).

Fosnot, S. M., & Woodford, L. L. (1992). *The fluency development system for young children.* Buffalo, NY: United Educational Services.

Foundas, A. L., Bollich, A. M., Corey, D. M., Hurley, M., & Heilman, K. M. (2001). Anomalous anatomy of speech–language areas in adults with persistent developmental stuttering. *Neurology, 57*(2), 207–215.

Franken, M., Kielstra-van der Schalk, C., & Boelens, H. (2003, August). *Treatment for early childhood stuttering: A randomised clinical pilot.* Paper presented at the 4th Congress of the International Fluency Association, Montreal.

Fritzell, B. (1976). The prognosis of stuttering in schoolchildren: A 10-year longitudinal study. In *Proceedings of the XVI Congress of the International Society of Logopedics and Phoniatrics* (pp. 186–187). Basel, Switzerland: Karger.

Froeschels, E. (1921). Beitrage zur symptomatologie des stotterns. *Monatsschrift fur Ohrenheilkunde, 55,* 1109–1112.

Froeschels, E. (1943). Pathology and therapy of stuttering. *Nervous Child, 2,* 148–161.

Froeschels, E. (1952). The significance of symptomatology for the understanding of the essence of stuttering. *Folia Phoniatrica, 4,* 217–230.

Froeschels, E. (1964). *Selected papers (1940–1964).* Amsterdam: North-Holland.

Gillis, J. S. (1980). *Child Anxiety Scale manual.* Champaign, IL: Institute for Personality and Ability Testing.

Gladstien, K. L., Seider, R. A., & Kidd, K. K. (1981). Analysis of the sibship patterns of stutterers. *Journal of Speech and Hearing Research, 24,* 460–462.

Glasner, P. J. (1947). Nature and treatment of stuttering. *American Journal of Diseased Children, 74,* 218–225.

Glasner, P. J. (1949). Personality characteristics and emotional problems in stutterers under the age of five. *Journal of Speech and Hearing Disorders, 14,* 135–138.

Glasner, P. J. (1962). Psychotherapy for the young stutterer. In D. Barbara (Ed.), *The psychotherapy of stuttering* (pp. 240–257). Springfield, IL: Thomas.

Glasner, P. J., & Rosenthal, D. (1957). Parental diagnosis of stuttering in young children. *Journal of Speech and Hearing Disorders, 22,* 288–295.

Glauber, P. J. (1958). Stuttering and personality dynamics. In J. Eisenson (Ed.), *Stuttering: A symposium* (pp. 71–120). New York: Harper & Row.

Glaze, L. E., Bless, D. M., Milenkovic, P., & Susser, R. D. (1988). Acoustic characteristics of children's voice. *Journal of Voice, 2,* 312–319.

Godai, U., Tatarelli, R., & Bonanni, G. (1976). Stuttering and tics in twins. *Acta Geneticae Medicae et Gemellologiae, 25,* 369–375.

Goldberg, S. A., & Culatta, R. (1991, November). *Differences between stutterers with and without family histories of stuttering.* Paper presented at the convention of the American Speech-Language-Hearing Association, Atlanta, GA.

Goldman, R., & Fristoe, M. (1972). *The Goldman–Fristoe Test of Articulation.* Circle Pines, MN: American Guidance Service.

Goldman, R., & Fristoe, M. (1986). *The Goldman–Fristoe Test of Articulation* (rev. ed.). Circle Pines, MN: American Guidance Service.

Goldsmith, H., Buss, K., & Lemery, K. (1997). Toddlers and childhood temperament. *Developmental Psychology, 33,* 891–905.

Golinkoff, R. M., & Hirsh-Pasek, K. (2000). *How babies talk: The magic and mystery of language in the first three years of life.* New York: Plume.

Gordon, P. A., & Luper, H. L. (1992). The early identification of beginning stuttering I: Protocols. *American Journal of Speech–Language Pathology, 1*(3), 43–53.

Graf, O. (1955). Incidence of stuttering among twins. In W. Johnson & R. Leutenegger (Eds.), *Stuttering in children and adults* (pp. 381–386). Minneapolis: University of Minnesota.

Green, J. (1924). Your child's speech. *Hygeia, 2,* 11–12.

Gregg, B. A., & Yairi, E. (2001, November). *The co-occurrence of stuttering and phonology: Looking in both directions.* Paper presented at the convention of the American Speech-Language-Hearing Association, New Orleans.

Gregory, H. (1999a). Developmental intervention: Differential strategies. In M. Onslow & A. Packman (Eds.), *The handbook of early stuttering intervention* (pp. 83–102). San Diego, CA: Singular.

Gregory, H. (1999b). What is involved in therapy? In J. Fraser (Ed.), *Stuttering and your child: Questions and answers.* Memphis: Stuttering Foundation of America.

Gregory, H., & Gregory, C. B. (1999). Counseling children who stutter and their parents. In R. F. Curlee (Ed.), *Stuttering and related disorders of fluency* (2nd ed., pp. 43–63). New York: Thieme.

Gregory, H., & Hill, D. (1980). Stuttering therapy for children. In W. H. Perkins (Ed.), *Stuttering disorders* (pp. 351–364). New York: Thieme-Stratton.

Guerney, B., Jr. (1964). Filial therapy: description and rationale. *Journal of Consulting Psychology, 28,* 303–310.

Guitar, B. (1998). *Stuttering: An integrated approach to its nature and treatment* (2nd ed.). Baltimore: Williams & Wilkins.

Guitar, B. (1999). What if my child continues to stutter? In J. Fraser (Ed.), *Stuttering and your child: Questions and answers* (pp. 51–58). Memphis, TN: Stuttering Foundation of America.

Guitar, B., Kopff Schaefer, H., Donahue-Kilburg, G., & Bond, L. (1992). Parental verbal interactions and speech rate: A case study in stuttering. *Journal of Speech and Hearing Research, 35,* 742–754.

Guitar, B., & Marchinkoski, L. (2001). Influence of mothers' slower speech on their children's speech rate. *Journal of Speech, Language, and Hearing Research, 44,* 853–861.

Gutzmann, H. (1894). *Das stottern.* Frankfurt am Main: J. Rosenheim.

Häge, A. (2001). Können kognitive und linguistische fähigkeiten zur velaufsprognose kindlichen stotterns beitragen? (Cognitive and linguistic abilities in young children: Are they able to predict the further development of stuttering?) *Sprache Stimme Gehör 25,* 20–24.

Hahn, E. F. (1942). A study of the relationship between stuttering occurrence and phonetic factors in oral reading. *Journal of Speech Disorders, 7,* 143–151.

Hall, K. D., Amir, O., & Yairi, E. (1999). A longitudinal investigation of speaking rate in preschool children who stutter. *Journal of Speech, Language, and Hearing Research, 42,* 1367–1377.

Hall, K. D., & Yairi, E. (1992). Fundamental frequency, jitter, and shimmer in preschoolers who stutter. *Journal of Speech, Language, and Hearing Research, 35,* 1002–1008.

Hall, N. E., Yamashita, T. S., & Aram, D. M. (1993). Relationship between language and fluency in children with developmental language disorders. *Journal of Speech and Hearing Research, 36,* 568–579.

Hamre, C. (1992). Stuttering prevention I: Primacy of identification. *Journal of Fluency Disorders, 17,* 3–24.

Harle, M. (1946). Dynamic interpretation and treatment of acute stuttering in a young child. *American Journal of Orthopsychiatry, 16,* 156–162.

Harrington, J. (1987). Acoustic cues for automatic recognition of English consonants. In M. A. Jack & J. Laver (Eds.), *Speech technology: A survey* (pp. 19–74). Edinburgh, Scotland: University Press.

Hegde, M. N., & Hartman, D. E. (1979a). Factors affecting judgments of fluency: I. Interjections. *Journal of Fluency Disorders, 4,* 1–11.

Hegde, M. N., & Hartman, D. E. (1979b). Factors affecting judgments of fluency: II. Word repetitions. *Journal of Fluency Disorders, 4,* 13–22.

Hinkle, W. (1971). *A study of subgroups within the stuttering population.* Unpublished doctoral dissertation, Purdue University, West Lafayette, IN.

Hodson, B. W. (1986). *The Assessment of Phonological Processes–Revised.* Austin, TX: PRO-ED.

Hodson, B. W. (1997). Disordered phonologies: What have we learned about assessment and treatment? In B. W. Hodson & M. L. Edwards (Eds.), *Perspectives in applied phonology* (pp. 197–224). Gaithersburg, MD: Aspen.

Hodson, B. W., & Paden, E. P. (1991). *Targeting intelligible speech* (2nd ed.). Austin, TX: PRO-ED.

Hoepfner, T. (1911–1912). Stottern als assoziative aphasie. *Zeitschrift fur Pathopsychologie, 1,* 448–552.

Howell, P., & Au-Yeung, J. (1995). The association between stuttering, Brown's factors, and phonological categories in child stutterers ranging in age between 2 and 12 years. *Journal of Fluency Disorders, 20,* 331–344.

Howell, P., Au-Yeung, J., & Sackin, S. (1999). Exchange of stuttering from function words to content words with age. *Journal of Speech, Language, and Hearing Research, 42,* 345–354.

Howell, P., Sackin, S., & Glenn, K. (1997). Development of a two-stage procedure for the automatic recognition of disfluencies in the speech of children who stutter: II. ANN recognition of repetitions and prolongations with supplied word segment markers. *Journal of Speech, Language, and Hearing Research, 40,* 1085–1096.

Howell, P., & Vause, L. (1986). Acoustic analysis and perception of vowels in stuttered speech. *Journal of the Acoustical Society of America, 79,* 1571–1579.

Howell, P., Williams, M., & Vause, L. (1987). Acoustic analysis of repetitions in stutterers' speech. In H. F. M. Peters & W. Hulstijn (Eds.), *Speech motor dynamics in stuttering* (pp. 371–380). New York: Springer Verglag Wien.

Howie, P. M. (1981a). Concordance for stuttering in monozygotic and dizygotic twin pairs. *Journal of Speech and Hearing Research, 24,* 317–321.

Howie, P. M. (1981b). Intrapair similarity in frequency of disfluency in monozygotic and dizygotic twin pairs containing stutterers. *Behavior Genetics, 11,* 227–238.

Hubbard, C. P. (1998). Reliability of judgments of stuttering and disfluency in young children's speech. *Journal of Communication Disorders, 31,* 245–260.

Hubbard, C. P., & Yairi, E. (1988). Clustering of disfluencies in the speech of stuttering and nonstuttering preschool children. *Journal of Speech and Hearing Research, 31,* 228–233.

Hughes, J. (1943). *A quantitative study of repetition in the speech of two-year-olds and four-year-olds.* Unpublished master's thesis, University of Iowa, Iowa City.

Hull, F., Mielke, P., Willeford, J., & Timmons, R. (1976). *National speech and hearing survey: Final Report* (Project No. 50987). Washington, DC: Office of Education, Department of Health, Education and Welfare.

Ingham, J. C. (1999). Behavioral treatment of young children who stutter: An extended length of utterance method. In R. F. Curlee (Ed.), *Stuttering and related disorders of fluency* (2nd ed., pp. 80–100). New York: Thieme.

Ingham, J. C., & Riley, G. (1998). Guidelines for documentation of treatment efficacy for young children who stutter. *Journal of Speech, Language, and Hearing Research, 41,* 753–770.

Ingham, R. (2001). Brain imaging studies of developmental stuttering. *Journal of Communication Disorders, 34,* 493–516.

Ingham, R. J. (1976). "Onset, prevalence, and recovery from stuttering": A reassessment of findings from the Andrews and Harris study. *Journal of Speech and Hearing Disorders, 41,* 280–281.

Ingham, R. J. (1983). Spontaneous remission of stuttering: When will the emperor realize he has no clothes on? In D. Prins & R. Ingham (Eds.), *Treatment of stuttering in early childhood: Methods and issues* (pp. 113–135). San Diego, CA: College-Hill.

Ingham, R. J., & Bothe, A. K. (2001). Recovery from early stuttering: Additional issues within the Onslow & Packman-Yairi & Ambrose (1999) exchange. *Journal of Speech, Language, and Hearing Research, 44,* 862–867.

Ingham, R. J., & Cordes, A. K. (1998). Treatment decisions for young children who stutter: Further concerns and complexities. *American Journal of Speech–Language Pathology, 7*(3), 10–19.

Ingham, R. J., & Cordes, A. K. (1999). On watching a discipline shoot itself in the foot: Some observations on current trends in stuttering treatment research. In N. Bernstein Ratner & C. Healey (Eds.), *Stuttering research and treatment: Bridging the gap* (pp. 211–230). Mahwah, NJ: Erlbaum.

Ingham, R. J., Cordes, A. K., & Gow, M. L. (1993). Time-interval measurement of stuttering: Modifying interjudge agreement. *Journal of Speech and Hearing Research, 36,* 503–515.

Irwin, A. (1980). *Successful treatment of stuttering.* New York: Walker.

Jameson, A. M. (1955). Stammering in children: Some factors in the prognosis. *Speech, 19,* 60–67.

Janssen, P., & Kraaimaat, F. (1980). Disfluency and anxiety in stuttering and nonstuttering adolescents. *Behavior Analysis and Modification, 4,* 116–126.

Janssen, P., Kraaimaat, F., & Brutten, G. (1990). Relationship between stutterers' genetic history and speech-associated variables. *Journal of Fluency Disorders, 15,* 39–48.

Johanssen, E. (1998). Design of the longitudinal study and influence of symptomatology, heredity, sex-ratio, and lateral dominance on the further development of stuttering. In E. C. Healey & H. M. F. Peters (Eds.), *Proceedings of the Second World Congress on Fluency Disorders* (pp. 114–118). Nijmegen, The Netherlands: Nijmegen University.

Johannsen, H. S. (2001). Der einfluss alter, geschlecht, symptomatologie, heredität und händigkeit auf den verlauf de stotterns im kindesalter. *Sprache Stimme Gehör, 25,* 14–19.

Johnson, B., Humphreys, K., Watkins, R., Ambrose, N., & Yairi, E. (2001, November). *The relationship between word frequency and stuttering in young children.* Paper presented at the convention of the American Speech-Language-Hearing Association, New Orleans.

Johnson, L. (1980). Facilitating parental involvement in therapy of disfluent child. In W. Perkins (Ed.), *Strategies in stuttering therapy* (pp. 301–310). New York: Thieme-Stratton.

Johnson, W. (1934). Stuttering in the preschool child. *Child Welfare Pamphlets No. 37,* University of Iowa: Iowa City.

Johnson, W. (1942). A study of the onset and development of stuttering. *Journal of Speech Disorders, 7,* 251–257.

Johnson, W. (1946). *People in quandaries: The semantics of personal adjustment.* New York: Harper & Row.

Johnson, W. (1948). Stuttering. In W. Johnson, S. Brown, J. Curtis, C. Edney, & J. Keaster (Eds.), *Speech handicapped school children* (pp. 179–257). New York: Harper & Row.

Johnson, W. (1949). An open letter to a mother of a stuttering child. *Journal of Speech and Hearing Disorders, 14,* 3–8.

Johnson, W. (1955). Explorations of experimental extinction and spontaneous recovery in stuttering. In W. Johnson & R. R. Leutenegger (Eds.), *Stuttering in children and adults* (pp. 226–231). Minneapolis: University of Minnesota.

Johnson, W. (1959). *Toward understanding stuttering*. Chicago: National Society for Crippled Children and Adults.

Johnson, W. (1961). *Stuttering and what you can do about it*. Minneapolis: University of Minnesota.

Johnson, W., & Associates. (1959). *The onset of stuttering: Research findings and implications.* Minneapolis: University of Minnesota.

Johnson, W., & Brown, S. (1935). Stuttering in relation to various speech sounds. *Quarterly Journal of Speech, 21,* 481–496.

Johnson, W., & Colley, W. H. (1945). The relationship between frequency and duration of moments of stuttering. *Journal of Speech Disorders, 10,* 35–38.

Johnson, W., Darley, F. L., & Spriestersbach, D. C. (1963). *Diagnostic methods in speech pathology.* New York: Harper & Row.

Jones, M., Onslow, M., Harrison, E., & Packman, A. (2000). Treating stuttering in young children: Predicting treatment time in the Lidcombe Program. *Journal of Speech, Language, and Hearing Research, 43,* 1440–1450.

Karniol, R. (1995). Stuttering, language, and cognition: A review and a model of stuttering as suprasegmental sentence plan alignment (SPA). *Psychological Bulletin, 117,* 104–124.

Katsovaskaia, I. (1962). The problems of children stuttering. *Deafness, Speech, and Hearing Abstracts, 2,* 296.

Kelly, E. M. (1994). Speech rates and turn-taking behaviors of children who stutter and their fathers. *Journal of Speech and Hearing Research, 37,* 1284–1294.

Kelly, E. M. (1999, November). *The effects of parental speech rate modification on the speech rates and fluency of children who stutter.* Paper presented at the convention of the American Speech-Language-Hearing Association, San Francisco.

Kelly, E. M., & Conture, E. G. (1992). Speaking rates, response time latencies, and interrupting behaviors of young stutterers, nonstutterers, and their mothers. *Journal of Speech and Hearing Research, 35,* 1256–1267.

Kent, R. D. (1984). Psychobiology of speech development: Coemergence of language and a movement system. *American Journal of Physiology, 246*(6, Pt. 2), 888–894.

Kent, R. D. (1999). Motor control: Neurophysiology and functional development. In A. Caruso & E. Strand (Eds.), *Clinical management of motor speech disorders in children* (pp. 46–62). New York: Thieme.

Kent, R. D. (2000). Research on speech motor control and its disorders: A review and prospective. *Journal of Communication Disorders, 33,* 391–428.

Kidd, K. K. (1977). A genetic perspective on stuttering. *Journal of Fluency Disorders, 2,* 259–269.

Kidd, K. K. (1980). Genetic models of stuttering. *Journal of Fluency Disorders, 5,* 187–201.

Kidd, K. K. (1984). Stuttering as a genetic disorder. In R. F. Curlee & W. H. Perkins (Eds.), *Nature and treatment of stuttering: New directions* (pp. 149–169). San Diego, CA: College-Hill.

Kidd, K. K., Heimbuch, R. C., & Records, M. A. (1981). Vertical transmission of susceptibility to stuttering with sex-modified expression. *Proceedings of the National Academy of Sciences, 78,* 606–610.

Kidd, K. K., Heimbuch, R. C., Records, M. A., Oehlert, G., & Webster, R. L. (1980). Familial stuttering patterns are not related to one measure of severity. *Journal of Speech and Hearing Research, 23,* 539–545.

Kidd, K. K., Kidd, J. R., & Records, M. A. (1978). The possible causes of the sex ratio in stuttering and its implications. *Journal of Fluency Disorders, 3,* 13–23.

Kidd, K. K., Reich, T., & Kessler, S. (1973). *Genetics, 74*(2, Pt. 2), S137.

Kingdon-Ward, W. (1941). *Stammering.* London: Hamilton.

Kingston, M., Huber, A., Onslow, M., Jones, M., & Packman, A. (2003). Predicting treatment time with the Lidcombe Program: Replication and meta-analysis. *International Journal of Language and Communication Disorders, 38,* 165–177.

Kloth, S. A. M., Janssen, P., Kraaimaat, F. W., & Brutten, G. J. (1995). Speech-motor and linguistic skills of young stutterers prior to onset. *Journal of Fluency Disorders, 20,* 157–170.

Kloth, S. A. M., Kraaimaat, F. W., Janssen, P., & Brutten, G. J. (1999). Persistence and remission of incipient stuttering among high-risk children. *Journal of Fluency Disorders, 24,* 253–265.

Kolk, H., Conture, E., Postma, A., & Louko, L. (1991, November). *The covert repair hypothesis and childhood stuttering.* Paper presented at the convention of the American Speech-Language-Hearing Association, Atlanta, GA.

Kolk, H., & Postma, A. (1997). Stuttering as a covert repair phenomenon. In R. F. Curlee & G. M. Siegel (Eds.), *Nature and treatment of stuttering: New directions* (2nd ed., pp. 182–203). Needham Heights, MA: Allyn & Bacon.

Lahey, M. (1988). *Language disorders and language development.* New York: Macmillan.

Lai, C., Fisher, S., Hurst, J., Vargha-Khadem, F., & Monaco, A. (2001). A forkhead-domain gene is mutated in a severe speech and language disorder. *Nature, 413,* 519–523.

LaSalle, L. R., & Conture, E. G. (1995). Disfluency clusters of children who stutter: Relation of stutterings to self-repairs. *Journal of Speech and Hearing Research, 38,* 965–977.

Levina, R. (1968). Study and treatment of stammering children. *Journal of Learning Disabilities, 1,* 26–29. [Original work published 1966]

Lewis, B. (1990). Familial phonological disorders: Four pedigrees. *Journal of Speech and Hearing Disorders, 55,* 160–170.

Lewis, B., & Thompson, L. (1992). A study of developmental speech and language disorders in twins. *Journal of Speech and Hearing Research, 35,* 1086–1094.

Lewis, R. (1949). The psychological approach to the preschool stutterer. *Canada Medical Association Journal, 60,* 497–500.

Lincoln, M., & Onslow, M. (1997). Long-term outcome of early intervention for stuttering. *American Journal of Speech–Language Pathology, 6,* 51–58.

Lingwall, J., & Bergstrand, G. (1979, November). *Perceptual boundaries for judgment of "normal," "abnormal," and "stuttered" prolongations.* Paper presented at the convention of the American Speech-Language-Hearing Association, Atlanta, GA.

Logan, K. J., & Conture, E. G. (1995). Length, grammatical complexity, and rate differences in stuttered and fluent conversational utterances of children who stutter. *Journal of Fluency Disorders, 20,* 35–61.

Louko, L. J., Edwards, M. L., & Conture, E. G. (1990). Phonological characteristics of young stutterers and their normally fluent peers: Preliminary observations. *Journal of Fluency Disorders, 15,* 191–210.

Luchsinger, R., & Arnold, G. (1965). *Voice–speech–language.* Belmont, CA: Wadsworth.

Lund, N., & Duchan, J. F. (1993). *Assessing children's language in naturalistic contexts* (3rd ed.). Englewood Cliffs, NJ: Prentice Hall.

Lundstrom, C., & Garsten, M. (2000). A model for intervention with childhood stuttering. In H. G. Bosshardt, J. S. Yaruss, & H. F. M. Peters (Eds.), *Proceedings of the Third World Congress of Fluency Disorders* (pp. 335–340). Nijmegen, The Netherlands: Nijmegen University.

Luper, H., & Mulder, R. (1964). *Stuttering therapy for children.* Englewood Cliffs, NJ: Prentice Hall.

Maguire, G., Riley, G., Franklin, D., & Gottschalk, L. (2000). Risperidone for the treatment of stuttering. *Journal of Clinical Psychopharmacology, 20,* 479–482.

Mahr, G., & Leith, W. (1992). Psychogenic stuttering of adult onset. *Journal of Speech and Hearing Research, 35,* 283–286.

Makuen, G. (1914). A study of 1,000 cases of stammering with special reference to the etiology and treatment of the affliction. *Therapeutic Gazette, 38,* 385–390.

Mallard, R. (1991). Using families to help the school age stutterer: A case study. In L. Rustin (Ed.), *Parents, families and the stuttering child* (pp. 72–87). San Diego, CA: Singular.

Manning, W. (1996). *Clinical decision making in fluency disorders.* Albany, NY: Delmar.

Manning, W. (2001). *Clinical decision making in fluency disorders* (2nd ed.). Albany, NY: Delmar.

Manning, W., & Shirkey, E. (1981). Fluency and the aging process. In D. S. Beasley & G. A. Davis (Eds.), *Aging: Communication processes and disorders* (pp. 175–189). New York: Grune & Stratton.

Mansson, H. (2000). Childhood stuttering: Incidence and development. *Journal of Fluency Disorders, 25,* 47–57.

Margalit, M. (2003). Resilience model among individuals with learning disabilities (LD): Proximal and distal influences. *Learning Disabilities Research & Practice, 18*(2), 82–86.

Margalit, M., Leyser, Y., Ankonina, D. B., & Avraham, Y. (1991). Community support in Israeli kibbutz and city families of disabled children: Family climate and parental coherence. *Journal of Special Education, 24,* 427–440.

Marland, P. M. (1957). Shadowing: A contribution to the treatment of stuttering. *Folia Phoniatrica, 9,* 242–245.

Martin, R. R., & Haroldson, S. K. (1981). Stuttering identification: Standard definition and moment of stuttering. *Journal of Speech and Hearing Research, 24,* 59–63.

Martin, R. R., Kuhl, P., & Haroldson, S. (1972). An experimental treatment with two preschool stuttering children. *Journal of Speech and Hearing Research, 15,* 743–752.

Martin, R. R., & Lindamood, L. (1986). Stuttering and spontaneous recovery: Implications for speech–language pathologists. *Language, Speech, and Hearing Services in Schools, 17,* 207–218.

Martyn, M., & Sheehan, J. (1968). Onset of stuttering and recovery. *Behavioral Research Therapy, 6,* 295–307.

Matthews, S., Williams, R., & Pring, T. (1997). Parent–child interaction therapy and dysfluency: A single case study. *European Journal of Disorders of Communication, 32,* 1244–1259.

McCarthy, D. (1930). *The language development of the preschool child.* Minneapolis: University of Minnesota.

McClean, M. (1997). Functional components of the motor system: An approach to understanding the mechanisms of speech disfluency. In W. Hulstijn, H. Peters, & P. Van Lieshout (Eds.), *Speech production: Motor control, brain research and fluency disorders* (pp. 99–118). Amsterdam, The Netherlands: Elsevier.

McDearmon, J. R. (1968). Primary stuttering at the onset of stuttering: A reexamination of data. *Journal of Speech and Hearing Research, 11,* 631–637.

McDowell, E. D. (1928). *Educational and emotional adjustment of stuttering children.* New York: Columbia Teachers College.

McLelland, J. K., & Cooper, E. B. (1978). Fluency-related behaviors and attitudes of 178 young stutterers. *Journal of Fluency Disorders, 3,* 253–263.

Meltzer, H. (1934). Personality differences between stuttering and nonstuttering children as indicated by the Rorschach Test. *Journal of Psychology, 17,* 39–59.

Meyer, V., & Mair, J. M. M. (1963). A new technique to control stammering: A preliminary report. *Behavioral Research Therapy, 1,* 251–254.

Meyers, S. (1986). Qualitative and quantitative differences and patterns of variability in disfluencies emitted by preschool stutterers and nonstutterers during dyadic conversation. *Journal of Fluency Disorders, 11,* 293–306.

Meyers, S. (1989). Nonfluencies of preschool stutterers and conversational partners: Observing reciprocal relationships. *Journal of Speech and Hearing Disorders, 54,* 106–112.

Meyers, S. (1990). Verbal behaviors of preschool stutterers and conversational partners: Observing reciprocal relationships. *Journal of Speech and Hearing Disorders, 4,* 706–712.

Meyers, S., & Freeman, F. (1985). Mother and child speech rate as a variable in stuttering and disfluency. *Journal of Speech and Hearing Research, 28,* 436–444.

Milenkovic, P. (1987). Least mean square measures of voice perturbation. *Journal of Speech and Hearing Research, 30,* 529–538.

Milenkovic, P. (1995). *CspeechSP quick reference manual.* Madison: University of Wisconsin Press.

Miles, S., & Bernstein Ratner, N. (2001). Parental language input to children at stuttering onset. *Journal of Speech, Language and Hearing Research, 44,* 1116–1130.

Milisen, R., & Johnson, W. (1936). A comparative study of stutterers, former stutterers, and normal speakers whose handedness has been changed. *Archives of Speech, 1,* 61–86.

Miller, J. F., & Chapman, R. (1996). *SALT: Systematic Analysis of Language Transcripts.* Madison: University of Wisconsin.

Miller, J. F., & Chapman, R. (1997). *Systematic Analysis of Language Transcripts* [Computer software]. Madison: University of Wisconsin.

Moncur, J. P. (1951). Environmental factors differentiating stuttering children from non-stuttering children. *Speech Monographs, 18,* 312–325.

Moncur, J. P. (1952). Parental domination in stuttering. *Journal of Speech and Hearing Disorders, 17,* 155–165.

Moos, R. (1976). *The human context: Environmental determinants of behavior.* New York: Wiley.

Morley, M. (1957). *The development and disorders of speech in childhood.* Edinburgh, Scotland: Livingston.

Mowrer, D. E. (1998). Analysis of the sudden onset and disappearance of disfluencies in the speech of a 2½-year-old boy. *Journal of Fluency Disorders, 23,* 103–118.

Murphy, A. (Ed.). (1962). *Stuttering: Its prevention.* Memphis, TN: Speech Foundation of America.

Murphy, A. T., & Fitzsimons, R. M. (1960). *Stuttering and personality dynamics: Play therapy, projective therapy, and counseling.* New York: Ronald.

Murray, H. L., & Reed, C. G. (1977). Language abilities of preschool stuttering children. *Journal of Fluency Disorders, 2,* 171–176.

Mysak, E. D. (1966). *Speech pathology and feedback theory.* Springfield, IL: Thomas.

National Institute of Health. (1981). *Stuttering through research.* Washington, DC: U.S. Department of Health and Human Services.

Nelson, L. (1999). How does our home life influence his stuttering? In J. Fraser (Ed.), *Stuttering and your child: Questions and answers.* Memphis, TN: Stuttering Foundation of America.

Nelson, S. F., Hunter, N., & Walter, M. (1945). Stuttering in twin types. *Journal of Speech Disorders, 10,* 335–343.

Newcomer, P., & Hammill, D. D. (1982). *Test of Language Development.* Austin, TX: PRO-ED.

Nice, M. (1920). Concerning all day conversations. *Pedagological Seminary, 27,* 166–177.

Nippold, M. A. (1990). Concomitant speech and language disorders in stuttering children: A critique of the literature. *Journal of Speech and Hearing Disorders, 55,* 51–60.

Nippold, M. A. (2002). Stuttering and phonology: Is there an interaction? *American Journal of Speech–Language Pathology, 11,* 99–110.

Nippold, M. A., & Rudzinski, M. (1995). Parents' speech and children's stuttering: A critique of the literature. *Journal of Speech and Hearing Research, 38,* 978–989.

Okasha, A., Bishry, Z., Kamel, M., & Hassan, A. (1974). Psychosocial study of stammering in Egyptian children. *British Journal of Psychiatry, 124,* 531–533.

Onslow, M., Andrews, C., & Lincoln, M. (1994). A control/experimental trial of an operant treatment for early stuttering. *Journal of Speech and Hearing Research, 37,* 1244–1259.

Onslow, M., Costa, L., & Rue, S. (1990). Direct early intervention with stuttering: Some preliminary data. *Journal of Speech and Hearing Disorders, 55,* 405–416.

Onslow, M., Gardner, K., Bryant, K. M., Stuckings, C. L., & Knight, T. (1992). Stuttered and normal speech events in early childhood: The validity of a behavioral data language. *Journal of Speech and Hearing Research, 35,* 79–87.

Onslow, M., & Packman, A. (1999). Treatment recovery and spontaneous recovery from early stuttering: The need for consistent methods in collecting and interpreting data. *Journal of Speech, Language, and Hearing Research, 42,* 398–402.

Onslow, M., & Packman, A. (2001). Ambiguity and algorithms in diagnosing early stuttering: Comments on Ambrose and Yairi (1999). *Journal of Speech, Language, and Hearing Research, 44,* 593–594.

Onslow, M., Packman, A., & Harrison, E. (2001). *The Lidcombe program of early stuttering intervention: A clinician's guide.* Austin, TX: PRO-ED.

Orton, S. (1937). *Reading, writing, and speech problems in children.* New York: Norton.

Otto, F., & Yairi, E. (1976). A disfluency analysis of Down's syndrome and normal subjects. *Journal of Fluency Disorders, 1,* 26–32.

Oxtoby, E. (1943). *A quantitative study of the repetition in the speech of three-year old children.* Unpublished master's thesis, University of Iowa, Iowa City.

Oyler, M. E. (1996, November). *Temperament: Stuttering and the behaviorally inhibited child.* Paper presented at the convention of the American Speech-Language-Hearing Association, Seattle, WA.

Oyler, M. E., & Ramig, P. (1995, November). *Vulnerability in stuttering children.* Paper presented at the convention of the American Speech-Language-Hearing Association, Orlando, FL.

Packman, A., & Onslow, M. (1998). What is the take-home message from Curlee and Yairi? *American Journal of Speech–Language Pathology, 7*(3), 5–9.

Packman, A., & Onslow, M. (1999). Issues in the treatment of early stuttering. In M. Onslow & A. Packman (Eds.), *The handbook of early stuttering intervention* (pp. 1–16). San Diego, CA: Singular.

Paden, E. P., Ambrose, N. G., & Yairi, E. (2002). Phonological progress during the first 2 years of stuttering. *Journal of Speech, Language, and Hearing Research, 45,* 256–267.

Paden, E. P., & Yairi, E. (1996). Phonological characteristics of children whose stuttering persisted or recovered. *Journal of Speech, Language, and Hearing Research, 39,* 981–990.

Paden, E. P., Yairi, E., & Ambrose, N. G. (1999). Early childhood stuttering II: Initial status of phonological abilities. *Journal of Speech, Language, and Hearing Research, 42,* 1113–1124.

Panelli, C. A., McFarlane, S. C., & Shipley, K. G. (1978). Implications of evaluating and intervening with incipient stutterers. *Journal of Fluency Disorders, 3,* 41–50.

Paterson, S. (1958). The stammering child. *The Practitioner, 180,* 428–433.

Pay, A., & Sirotkina, M. M. (1955). *My experience in logoped work.* Moscow: Academy of Education, Institute of Defectology.

Pellowski, M. W., & Conture, E. G. (2002). Characteristics of speech disfluency and stuttering behaviors in 3- and 4-year-old children. *Journal of Speech, Language, and Hearing Research, 45,* 20–34.

Perkins, W. H. (1973). Replacement of stuttering with normal speech: Clinical procedures. *Journal of Speech and Hearing Disorders, 38,* 295–303.

Perkins, W. H. (1990). What is stuttering? *Journal of Speech and Hearing Disorders, 55,* 370–382.

Perkins, W. H. (1999). Should we seek help? In J. Fraser (Ed.), *Stuttering and your child: Questions and answers* (pp. 59–63). Memphis, TN: Stuttering Foundation of America.

Perkins, W. H., & Curlee, R. F. (1969). Clinical impressions of portable masking unit effects in stuttering. *Journal of Speech and Hearing Disorders, 34,* 360–362.

Perkins, W. H., Kent, R. D., & Curlee, R. F. (1991). A theory of neuropsycholinguistic function in stuttering. *Journal of Speech and Hearing Research, 34,* 734–752.

Peters, H., Hulstijn, W., & Van Lieshout, P. (2000). Recent developments in speech motor research into stuttering. *Folia Phoniatrica et Logopaedica, 52,* 103–119.

Pichon, E., & Borel-Maissoney, S. (1937). *Le begaiment, sa nature, et son traitment.* Paris: Maisson.

Pindzola, R. H. (1987). *Stuttering intervention program: Age 3 to grade 3.* Austin, TX: PRO-ED.

Pindzola, R. H., & White, D. (1986). A protocol for differentiating the incipient stutterer. *Language, Speech, and Hearing Services in Schools, 17,* 2–11.

Porter, J. H., & Hodson, B. W. (2001). Collaborating to obtain phonological acquisition data for local schools. *Language, Speech, and Hearing Services in Schools, 32,* 165–171.

Postma, A., & Kolk, H. (1993). The covert repair hypothesis: Prearticulatory repair processes in normal and stuttered disfluencies. *Journal of Speech and Hearing Research, 36,* 472–487.

Poulos, M. G., & Webster, W. G. (1991). Family history as a basis for subgrouping people who stutter. *Journal of Speech and Hearing Research, 34,* 5–10.

Preus, A. (1981). *Identifying subgroups of stutterers.* Oslo, Norway: University of Oslo.

Prins, D. (1983). Issues and perspectives. In D. Prins & R. Ingham (Eds.), *Treatment of stuttering in early childhood: Methods and issues* (pp. 141–145). San Diego, CA: College-Hill.

Proctor, A., Duff, M., Patterson, A., & Yairi, E. (2001, November). *Stuttering in African American and European American preschoolers.* Paper presented at the convention of the American Speech-Language-Hearing Association, New Orleans.

Quarington, B. (1974). The parents of stuttering children: The literature re-examined. *Canadian Psychiatric Association Journal, 19,* 103–110.

Ramig, P. (1993). High reported spontaneous recovery rates: Fact or fiction? *Language, Speech, and Hearing Services in Schools, 24,* 156–160. ·

Reed, C. G., & Godden, A. L. (1977). An experimental treatment using verbal punishment with two preschool stutterers. *Journal of Fluency Disorders, 2,* 225–233.

Reynolds, C. R., & Richmond, B. O. (1994). *Revised Children's Manifest Anxiety Scale.* Los Angeles: Western Psychological Services.

Riley, G. D. (1972). Stuttering Severity Instrument for Children and Adults. *Journal of Speech and Hearing Disorders, 37,* 314–322.

Riley, G. D. (1980). *Stuttering Severity Instrument for Children and Adults* (rev. ed.). Austin, TX: PRO-ED.

Riley, G. D. (1981). *Stuttering Prediction Instrument for Young Children.* Austin, TX: PRO-ED.

Riley, G. D. (1994). *Stuttering Severity Instrument for Children and Adults* (3rd ed.). Tigard, OR: CC Publications.

Riley, G. D., & Ingham, J. C. (1995). Vocal response time changes associated with two types of treatment. In C. W. Starkweather & H. M. F. Peters (Eds.), *Stuttering: Proceedings of the First World Congress in Fluency Disorders* (pp. 470–474). New York: Elsevier.

Riley, G. D., & Ingham, J. C. (2000). Acoustic duration changes associated with two types of treatment for children who stutter. *Journal of Speech, Language, and Hearing Research, 43,* 965–978.

Riley, G. D., & Riley, J. (1979). A component model for diagnosing and treating children who stutter. *Journal of Fluency Disorders, 4,* 279–293.

Riley, G. D., & Riley, J. (1985). *Oral motor assessment and treatment: Improving syllable production.* Austin, TX: PRO-ED.

Riley, G., & Riley, J. (1986). *Oral motor assessment and treatment.* Tigard, OR: CC Publications.

Riley, G. D., & Riley, J. (1999). Speech motor training. In M. Onslow & A. Packman (Eds.), *The handbook of early stuttering intervention* (pp. 139–158). San Diego, CA: Singular.

Riley, G. D., & Riley, J. (2000). A revised component model for diagnosing and treating children who stutter. *Contemporary Issues in Communication Sciences and Disorders, 27,* 188–199.

Riley, J. (1999). Clinician/researcher: A way of thinking. In N. Bernstein Ratner & C. Healey (Eds.), *Stuttering research and treatment: Bridging the gap* (pp. 103–114). Mahwah, NJ: Erlbaum.

Robb, M., & Blomgren, M. (1997). Analysis of F2 transitions in the speech of stutterers and nonstutterers. *Journal of Fluency Disorders, 22,* 1–16.

Robinson, F. (1964). *Introduction to stuttering.* Englewood Cliffs, NJ: Prentice Hall.

Rodgers, R., & Hammerstein, O. (1956). *The King and I* (Motion picture). Twentieth Century Fox.

Roman, G. A. (1972). *An investigation of the disfluent speech behavior of parents of stuttering and parents of nonstuttering children.* Unpublished master's thesis, Texas Tech University, Lubbock.

Rommel, D., Häge, A., Kalehne, P., & Johannsen, H. (2000). Developmental, maintenance, and recovery of childhood stuttering: Prospective longitudinal data 3 years after first contact. In K. Baker, L. Rustin, & K. Baker (Eds.), *Proceedings of the Fifth Oxford Disfluency Conference* (pp. 168–182). Chappell Gardner, UK: Windsor, Berkshire.

Rosenbek, J., Messert, B., Collins, M., & Wertz, R. T. (1978). Stuttering following brain damage. *Brain and Language, 6,* 82–96.

Rosenfield, D., McCarthy, M., McKinney, K., Viswanath, N., & Nudelman, H. (1994). Stuttering induced by theophylline. *Ear Nose Throat Journal, 73,* 914–920.

Roth, C. R., Aronson, A. E., & Davis, L. J. (1989). Clinical studies in psychogenic stuttering of adult onset. *Journal of Speech and Hearing Disorders, 54,* 634–646.

Rustin, L. (1987a). *Assessment and therapy programme for dysfluent children.* Windsor, Ontario, Canada: NFER-Nelson.

Rustin, L. (1987b). The treatment of childhood dysfluency through active parental involvement. In L. Rustin, H. Purser, & D. Rowley (Eds.), *Progress in the treatment of fluency disorders* (pp. 166–180). London: Taylor & Francis.

Rustin, L., Botterill, W., & Kelman, E. (1996). *Assessment and therapy for young disfluent children: Family interaction.* London: Whurr.

Rustin, L., Cook, F., & Spence, R. (1995). *The management of stuttering in adolescence: A communicative skills approach.* London: Whurr.

Rustin, L., & Pursure, H. (1991). Child development, families, and the problem of stuttering. In L. Rustin (Ed.), *Parents, families, and the stuttering child* (pp. 1–24). San Diego, CA: Singular.

Ryan, B. P. (1970). An illustration of operant conditioning therapy for stuttering. In M. Fraser (Ed.), *Conditioning in stuttering therapy* (pp. 58–76). Memphis, TN: Speech Foundation of America.

Ryan, B. P. (1971). Operant procedures applied to stuttering therapy for children. *Journal of Speech and Hearing Disorders, 36,* 264–280.

Ryan, B. P. (1974). *Programmed therapy for stuttering in children and adults.* Springfield, IL: Thomas.

Ryan, B. P. (1992). Articulation, language, rate, and fluency characteristics of stuttering and nonstuttering preschool children. *Journal of Speech and Hearing Research, 35,* 333–342.

Ryan, B. P. (2001a). A longitudinal study of articulation, language, rate, and fluency of 22 preschool children who stutter. *Journal of Fluency Disorders, 26,* 107–127.

Ryan, B. P. (2001b). *Programmed therapy for stuttering in children and adults* (2nd ed.). Springfield, IL: Thomas.

Ryan, B. P., & Van Kirk, B. (1999). The Monterey fluency program. In M. Onslow & A. Packman (Eds.), *The handbook of early stuttering intervention* (pp. 170–188). San Diego, CA: Singular.

Sacco, P. R., & Metz, D. E. (1989). Comparison of period-by-period fundamental frequency of stutterers and nonstutterers over repeated utterances. *Journal of Speech and Hearing Research, 32,* 439–444.

Sambrookes, L. J. (1999). *A study of specific errors on consonant clusters among children who would persist in or recover from stuttering.* Unpublished senior honors thesis, University of Illinois, Urbana-Champaign.

Sander, E. (1959). Counseling parents of stuttering children. *Journal of Speech and Hearing Disorders, 24,* 262–271.

Sander, E. K. (1963). Frequency of syllable repetition and "stutter" judgments. *Journal of Speech and Hearing Disorders, 28,* 19–30.

Santayana, G. (1923). *Scepticism and animal faith: Introduction to a system of philosophy.* New York: Charles Scribner & Sons.

Sawyer, J., & Yairi, E. (2003). *The effect of sample size on the assessment of stuttering severity.* Paper presented at the convention of the American Speech-Language-Hearing Association, Chicago.

Schaefer, M. (1965). A configurational analysis of children's reports of parent behavior. *Journal of Consulting Psychology, 29,* 552–557.

Schilling, A., & Goler, D. (1961). Zur frage der monotonie-untersuchung beim stottern. *Folia Phoniatrica, 13,* 202–218.

Schindler, M. A. (1955). A study of educational adjustments of stuttering and nonstuttering children. In W. Johnson & R. R. Leutenegger (Eds.), *Stuttering in children and adults* (pp. 348–357). Minneapolis: University of Minnesota.

Schuell, H. (1946). Sex differences in relation to stuttering: Part I. *Journal of Speech Disorders, 11,* 277–298.

Schuell, H. (1947). Sex differences in relation to stuttering: Part II. *Journal of Speech Disorders, 12,* 23–38.

Schuell, H. (1949). Working with parents of stuttering children. *Journal of Speech and Hearing Disorders, 14,* 251–254.

Schultze, H. (1991). Time pressure variables in the verbal parent–child interaction patterns of fathers and mothers of stuttering, phonologically disordered and normal preschool children. In H. F. M. Peters & W. H. Hulstijn (Eds.), *Speech motor control and stuttering* (pp. 441–452). New York: Exerpta Medica.

Schwartz, H. D., & Conture, E. G. (1988). Subgrouping young stutterers: Preliminary behavioral observations. *Journal of Speech and Hearing Research, 31,* 62–71.

Schwartz, H. D., Zebrowski, P. M., & Conture, E. G. (1990). Behaviors at the onset of stuttering. *Journal of Fluency Disorders, 15,* 77–86.

Schwartz, M. (1976). *Stuttering solved.* New York: McGraw-Hill.

Schwartz, M. (1979). *Is somebody in your family showing signs of stuttering?* New York: National Center for Stuttering.

Seider, R. A., Gladstien, K. L., & Kidd, K. K. (1982). Language onset and concomitant speech and language problems in subgroups of stutterers and their siblings. *Journal of Speech and Hearing Research, 25,* 482–486.

Seider, R. A., Gladstien, K. L., & Kidd, K. K. (1983). Recovery and persistence of stuttering among relatives of stutterers. *Journal of Speech and Hearing Disorders, 48,* 402–409.

Shames, G. H., & Sherrick, C. E. (1963). A discussion of nonfluency and stuttering as operant behavior. *Journal of Speech and Hearing Disorders, 28,* 3–18.

Sheehan, J. G. (1958). Conflict theory of stuttering. In J. Eisenson (Ed.), *Stuttering: A symposium* (pp. 121–166). New York: Harper & Row.

Sheehan, J. G. (1970). *Stuttering: Research and theory.* New York: Harper & Row.

Sheehan, J., & Martyn, M. (1966). Spontaneous recovery from stuttering. *Journal of Speech and Hearing Research, 9,* 121–135.

Shine, R. (1980). Direct management of the beginning stutterer. In W. Perkins (Ed.), *Strategies in stuttering therapy* (pp. 339–350). An issue of *Seminars in Speech, Language, and Hearing.* New York: Thieme.

Shugart, Y., Mundorff, J., Kilshaw, J., Doheny, K., Doan, B., Wanyee, J., Green, E., & Drayna, D. (2003). Results of a genome-wide linkage scan for stuttering. *American Journal of Medical Genetics, 124A*, 133–135.

Siegel, G. (1998). Stuttering: Theory, research, and therapy. In A. Cordes & R. J. Ingham (Eds.), *Treatment efficacy for stuttering: A search for empirical bases* (pp. 103–114). San Diego, CA: Singular.

Silverman, E. M. (1972). Generality of disfluency data collected from preschoolers. *Journal of Speech and Hearing Research, 15*, 84–92.

Silverman, E. M. (1973). Clustering: A characteristic of preschoolers' speech disfluency. *Journal of Speech and Hearing Research, 16*, 578–583.

Sim, H. S. (1996). Kinematic analysis of the sound/syllable repetitions, sound prolongations and fluent speech of children who stutter. Unpublished doctoral dissertation, University of Iowa.

Sim, H. S., & Zebrowski, P. M. (1995, August). The ability of young children to imitate different speaking rates. In C. W. Starkweather & H. F. M. Peters (Eds.), *Stuttering: Proceedings of the First World Congress on Fluency Disorders* (pp. 206–209). Munich, Germany.

Smit, A. B., & Hand, L. (1997). *Smit–Hand Articulation and Phonology Evaluation manual.* Los Angeles: Webster Psychological Services.

Smith, A., & Kelly, E. M. (1995, August). Application of an integrated multifactorial theory to the development of stuttering. In C. W. Starkweather & H. F. M. Peters (Eds.), *Stuttering: Proceedings of the First World Congress on Fluency Disorders* (pp. 210–212). Munich, Germany.

Smith, A., & Kelly, E. M. (1997). Stuttering: A dynamic, multifactorial model. In R. F. Curlee & G. M. Siegel (Eds.), *Nature and treatment of stuttering: New directions* (2nd ed., pp. 204–217). Boston: Allyn & Bacon.

Smith, M. (1926). An investigation of the development of the sentences and the extent of vocabulary in young children. *University of Iowa studies: Studies in child welfare, 3*, No. 5.

Soderberg, G. A. (1962). What is "average" stuttering? *Journal of Speech and Hearing Disorders, 27*, 85–86.

St. Louis, K. O., Clausell, P. L., Thompson, J. N., & Rife, C. C. (1982). Preliminary investigation of EMG biofeedback induced relaxation with a preschool aged stutterer. *Perceptual and Motor Skills, 55*, 195–199.

St. Louis, K. O., & Hinzman, A. R. (1988). A descriptive study of speech, language, and hearing characteristics of school-aged stutterers. *Journal of Fluency Disorders, 13*, 331–355.

St. Louis, K. O., Murray, C. D., & Ashworth, M. S. (1991). Coexisting communication disorders in a random sample of school-aged stutterers. *Journal of Fluency Disorders, 16*, 13–23.

St. Onge, K. R. (1963). The stuttering syndrome. *Journal of Speech and Hearing Research, 6*, 195–197.

Stampe, D. (1973). *A dissertation on natural phonology.* Unpublished doctoral dissertation, University of Chicago, Chicago, IL.

Starkweather, C. W. (1982). The development of fluency in normal children. In J. Fraser (Ed.), *Stuttering therapy: Prevention and intervention with children* (pp. 9–49). Memphis, TN: Speech Foundation of America.

Starkweather, C. W. (1987). *Fluency and stuttering.* Englewood Cliffs, NJ: Prentice Hall.

Starkweather, C. W. (1990). Current trends in therapy for stuttering children and suggestions for future research. *ASHA Reports, 18,* 82–90.

Starkweather, C. W. (1997). Therapy for younger children. In R. F. Curlee & G. M. Siegel (Eds.), *Nature and treatment of stuttering: New directions* (2nd ed., pp. 257–279). Boston: Allyn & Bacon.

Starkweather, C. W., & Gottwald, S. (1984, November). *Children's stuttering and parents' speech rate.* Presented at the convention of the American Speech-Language-Hearing Association, San Francisco.

Starkweather, C. W., Gottwald, S., & Halfond, M. (1990). *Stuttering prevention.* Englewood Cliffs, NJ: Prentice Hall.

Stephanson-Opsal, D., & Bernstein Ratner, N. (1988). Maternal speech rate modification and childhood stuttering. *Journal of Fluency Disorders, 13,* 49–56.

Stevenson, R. L. (1886). *The strange case of Dr. Jekyll and Mr. Hyde.* London: Longmans, Green.

Still, A. W., & Griggs, S. (1979). Changes in the probability of stuttering following a stutter: A test of some recent models. *Journal of Speech and Hearing Research, 22,* 565–571.

Still, A. W., & Sherrard, C. (1976). Formalizing theories of stuttering. *The British Journal of Mathematical and Statistical Psychology, 29,* 129–138.

Stocker, B. (1976). *The Stocker Probe technique for diagnosis and treatment of stuttering in young children.* Tulsa, OK: Modern Education Corp.

Stocker, B., & Gerstman, L. J. (1983). A comparison of the Probe technique and conventional therapy for young stutterers. *Journal of Fluency Disorders, 8,* 331–339.

Stocker, B., & Goldfarb, R. (1995). *The Stocker Probe for fluency and language* (3rd ed.). Vero Beach, FL: The Speech Bin.

Stromsta, C. (1965). A spectrographic study of disfluencies labeled as stuttering by parents. *De Therapia Vocis et Loquelae, 1,* 317–318.

Stroop, J. R. (1935). Studies of interference in serial verbal reactions. *Journal of Experimental Psychology, 18,* 643–662.

Subramanian, A. (2001). *Identification of traits transmitted associated with stuttering.* Unpublished doctoral dissertation, University of Illinois, Urbana-Champaign.

Subramanian, A., Yairi, E., & Amir, O. (2003). Second formant transitions in fluent speech of persistent and recovered preschool children who stutter. *Journal of Communication Disorders, 36,* 59–75.

Tallal, P., Hirsch, L. S., Realpe-Bonilla, T., Miller, S., & Brzustowicz, L. M. (2001). Familial aggregation in specific language impairment. *Journal of Speech, Language, and Hearing Research, 44,* 1172–1182.

Taylor, G. (1937). *An observational study of the nature of stuttering at its onset.* Unpublished master's thesis, State University of Iowa, Iowa City.

Taylor, I., & Taylor, M. (1967). Test of predictions from the conflict hypothesis of stuttering. *Journal of Abnormal Psychology, 72,* 431–433.

Templin, M. C., & Darley, F. L. (1969). *The Templin–Darley Tests of Articulation: A manual and discussion of articulation testing* (2nd ed.). Iowa City: University of Iowa.

Thompson, J. (1983). *Assessment of fluency in school-age children: Resource guide.* Danville, IL: Interstate Printers and Publishers.

Throneburg, N. R. (1997). *Characteristics of disfluencies of preschool children who stutter: A longitudinal study regarding persistence and recovery.* Unpublished doctoral dissertation, University of Illinois, Urbana-Champaign.

Throneburg, R., Ambrose, N., & Yairi, E. (2003). *Secondary characteristics of children whose stuttering persisted or recovered.* Manuscript submitted for publication.

Throneburg, R. N., & Yairi, E. (1994). Temporal dynamics of repetitions during the early stage of childhood stuttering: An acoustic study. *Journal of Speech and Hearing Research, 37,* 1067–1075.

Throneburg, R. N., & Yairi, E. (2001). Durational, proportionate, and absolute frequency characteristics of disfluencies: A longitudinal study regarding persistence and recovery. *Journal of Speech, Language, and Hearing Research, 44,* 38–51.

Throneburg, R. N., Yairi, E., & Paden, E. P. (1994). Relation between phonologic difficulty and the occurrence of disfluencies in the early stage of stuttering. *Journal of Speech and Hearing Research, 37,* 504–509.

Tomaiuoli, D., Del Gado, A., Lucchini, E., Lattuca, S., & Spinetti, M. (2001). *The fantastic world of the tales.* Presented at the Second International Symposium on Stuttering, Rome, Italy.

Tomblin, J., & Buckwalter, P. (1994). Studies of genetics of specific language impairment. In R. Watkins & M. Rice (Eds.), *Specific language impairments in children* (pp. 17–34). Baltimore: Brooks.

Travis, L. (1931). *Speech pathology.* New York: Appleton-Century.

Tudor, M. (1939). *An experimental study of the effect of evaluative labeling on speech fluency.* Unpublished master's thesis, University of Iowa, Iowa City.

Van Lieshout, P. (1995). *Motor planning and articulation in fluent speech of stutterers and nonstutterers.* Nijmegen, The Netherlands: Nijmegen University Press.

Van Lieshout, P., Hulstijn, W., & Peters, H. (1996). Speech production in people who stutter: Testing the motor plan assembly hypothesis. *Journal of Speech, Language, and Hearing Research, 39,* 76–92.

Van Riper, C. (1939). *Speech correction: Principles and methods.* Englewood Cliffs, NJ: Prentice Hall.

Van Riper, C. (1948). *Stuttering.* Chicago: The National Society for Crippled Children and Adults.

Van Riper, C. (1954). *Speech correction: Principles and methods* (3rd ed.). New York: Prentice Hall.

Van Riper, C. (1958). Experiments in stuttering therapy. In J. Eisenson (Ed.), *Stuttering: A symposium* (pp. 273–390). New York: Harper & Row.

Van Riper, C. (1971). *The nature of stuttering.* Englewood Cliffs, NJ: Prentice Hall.

Van Riper, C. (1972). *Speech correction: Principles and methods* (5th ed.). Englewood Cliffs, NJ: Prentice Hall.

Van Riper, C. (1973). *The treatment of stuttering.* Englewood Cliffs, NJ: Prentice Hall.

Van Riper, C. (1982). *The nature of stuttering* (2nd ed.). Englewood Cliffs, NJ: Prentice Hall.

Vanryckeghem, M., & Brutten, G. J. (1997). The speech-associated attitudes of children who do and do not stutter and the differential effect of age. *American Journal of Speech-Language Pathology, 6*(4), 67–73.

Vanryckeghem, M., & Brutten, G. J. (2002, November). *Kiddy CAT: A measure of stuttering and nonstuttering preschoolers' attitude.* Poster presented at the convention of the American Speech-Language-Hearing Association, Atlanta, GA.

Vanryckeghem, M., Hylebos, C., Brutten, G. J., & Peleman, M. (2001). The relationship between communication attitude and emotion of children who stutter. *Journal of Fluency Disorders, 26,* 1–15.

Vlasova, N. A. (1962). Prevention and treatment of children's stuttering in U.S.S.R. *Ceskoslovenska Otolaryngologie, 11,* 30–32.

Wakaba, Y. (1983). Group play therapy for Japanese children who stutter. *Journal of Fluency Disorders, 8,* 93–118.

Wakaba, Y. (1992). Process of recovery from stuttering of a three-year-old stuttering child. *Tokyo Gakugei University Research Institute for the Education of Exceptional Children, 41,* 35–46.

Wakaba, Y. (1998). Research on temperament of stuttering children with early onset. In E. C. Healey & H. Peters (Eds.), *Proceedings of the Second World Congress on Fluency Disorders* (pp. 84–87). Nijmegen, The Netherlands: Nijmegen University.

Wakaba, Y. (1999). *Research on remedial process of stuttering with early onset.* Unpublished doctoral dissertation, Nagoya University, Nagoya, Japan.

Walker, H. (1983). *Walker Problem Behavior Identification Checklist.* Los Angeles: Western Psychological Services.

Watkins, K., Gadian, D., & Vargha-Khadem, F. (1999). Human genetics '99: Functional and structural brain abnormalities with a genetic disorder of speech and language. *American Journal of Human Genetics, 65,* 1215–1221.

Watkins, R. V., & Yairi, E. (1997). Language production abilities of children whose stuttering persisted or recovered. *Journal of Speech, Language, and Hearing Research, 40,* 385–399.

Watkins, R. V., Yairi, E., & Ambrose, N. G. (1999). Early childhood stuttering III: Initial status of expressive language abilities. *Journal of Speech, Language, and Hearing Research, 42,* 1125–1135.

Watkins, R. V., Yairi, E., Ambrose, N., Evans, K., DeThorne, L., & Mullen, C. (2000, November). *Grammatical influences on stuttering in young children.* Paper presented at the convention of the American Speech-Language-Hearing Association, Washington, DC.

Webb, S., Monk, C., & Nelson, C. (2001). Mechanisms of postnatal neurobiological development: Implications for human development. *Developmental Neuropsychology, 19,* 147–171.

Webster, R. L. (1980). Evolution of a target-based behavioral therapy for stuttering. *Journal of Fluency Disorders, 5*, 303–320.

Weiss, A. (1995). Conversational demands and their effect on fluency and stuttering. In *Topics in Language Disorders, 15*(3), 18–31.

Weiss, A. L. (2002). Recasts in parents' language to their school-age children who stutter: A preliminary study. *Journal of Fluency Disorders, 27*, 243–266.

West, R., Kennedy, L., & Carr, A. (1947). *The rehabilitation of speech* (rev. ed.). New York: Harper & Bros.

West, R., Nelson, S., & Berry, M. (1939). The heredity of stuttering. *Quarterly Journal of Speech, 25*, 23–30.

Wexler, K. B. (1982). Developmental disfluency in 2-, 4-, and 6-year old boys in neutral and stress situations. *Journal of Speech and Hearing Research, 25*, 229–234.

Williams, D. E., & Kent, L. R. (1958). Listener evaluations of speech interruptions. *Journal of Speech and Hearing Research, 1*, 124–131.

Williams, D. E., & Silverman, F. H. (1968). Note concerning articulation of school-age stutterers. *Perceptual and Motor Skills, 27*, 713–714.

Williams, D. E., Silverman, F. H., & Kools, J. A. (1968). Disfluency behavior of elementary school stutterers and nonstutterers: The adaptation effect. *Journal of Speech and Hearing Research, 11*, 622–630.

Wingate, M. E. (1962). Evaluation of stuttering: III. Identification of stuttering and the use of a label. *Journal of Speech and Hearing Disorders, 27*, 368–377.

Wingate, M. E. (1964). Recovery from stuttering. *Journal of Speech and Hearing Disorders, 29*, 312–321.

Wingate, M. E. (1976). *Stuttering: Theory and treatment.* New York: Irvington.

Wingate, M. E. (1988). *The structure of stuttering: A psycholinguistic analysis.* New York: Springer-Verlag.

Wingate, M. E. (2001). SLD is not stuttering. *Journal of Speech, Language, and Hearing Research, 44*, 381–383.

Wischner, G. J. (1950). Stuttering behavior and learning: A preliminary theoretical formulation. *Journal of Speech and Hearing Disorders, 15*, 324–335.

Wittgenstein, L. (1922). *Tractatus logico-philosophicus.* London: Routledge & Kegan Paul.

Wohl, M. T. (1968). The electric metronome—An evaluative study. *British Journal of Disorders of Communication, 3*, 89–98.

Wolk, L., Blomgren, M., & Smith, A. B. (2000). The frequency of simultaneous disfluency and phonological errors in children: A preliminary investigation. *Journal of Fluency Disorders, 25*, 269–281.

Wolk, L., Edwards, M. L., & Conture, E. G. (1993). Coexistence of stuttering and disordered phonology in young children. *Journal of Speech and Hearing Research, 36*, 906–917.

Wood, K. (1948). The parent's role in the clinical program. *Journal of Speech and Hearing Disorders, 13*, 209–210.

World Health Organization. (1977). *Manual of international statistical classification of diseases, injuries, and causes of death* (Vol. 1). Geneva, Switzerland: World Health Organization.

World Health Organization. (2001). *International classification of functioning, disability, and health.* Geneva, Switzerland: World Health Organization.

Wyatt, G. L., & Herzan, H. M. (1962). Therapy with stuttering children and their mothers. *American Journal of Orthopsychiatry, 23,* 645–659.

Yairi, E. (1972). Disfluency rates and patterns of stutterers and nonstutterers. *Journal of Communication Disorders, 5,* 225–231.

Yairi, E. (1974). *Personal observations of the onset of stuttering and its early stage: A case report.* Unpublished manuscript.

Yairi, E. (1976). Effects of binaural and monaural noise on stuttering. *Journal of Auditory Research, 16,* 114–119.

Yairi, E. (1981). Disfluencies of normally speaking two-year-old children. *Journal of Speech and Hearing Research, 24,* 490–495.

Yairi, E. (1982a). Longitudinal studies of disfluencies in two-year-old children. *Journal of Speech and Hearing Research, 25,* 155–160.

Yairi, E. (1982b). *An outline for counseling of parents of pre-school aged beginning stutterers.* Unpublished manuscript.

Yairi, E. (1983). The onset of stuttering in two- and three-year-old children: A preliminary report. *Journal of Speech and Hearing Disorders, 48,* 171–177.

Yairi, E. (1985). *Speech rate modification program for preschool-age children who stutter.* Unpublished manuscript.

Yairi, E. (1990). Subtyping child stutterers for research purposes. *ASHA Reports, 18,* 50–57.

Yairi, E. (1993). Epidemiology and other considerations in treatment efficacy research with preschool age children who stutter. *Journal of Fluency Disorders, 18,* 197–219.

Yairi, E. (1996). Applications of disfluencies in measurements of stuttering. *Journal of Speech and Hearing Research, 39,* 402–403.

Yairi, E. (1997a). Disfluency characteristics of early childhood stuttering. In R. F. Curlee & G. M. Siegel (Eds.), *Nature and treatment of stuttering: New directions* (2nd ed., pp. 49–78). Boston: Allyn & Bacon.

Yairi, E. (1997b). Home environments of stuttering children. In R. F. Curlee & G. M. Siegel (Eds.), *Nature and treatment of stuttering: New directions* (2nd ed., pp. 49–78). Boston: Allyn & Bacon.

Yairi, E. (1998, November). *Is the basis of stuttering genetic?* Paper presented at the convention of the American Speech-Language-Hearing Association, San Antonio, TX.

Yairi, E. (1999). Epidemiologic factors and stuttering research. In N. Bernstein Ratner & C. Healey (Eds.), *Stuttering research and practice: Bridging the gap* (pp. 45–53). Mahwa, NJ: Erlbaum.

Yairi, E. (2001). The state of art of research in stuttering. Keynote presentation, Symposium on stuttering, Rome, Italy.

Yairi, E., & Ambrose, N. (1992a). A longitudinal study of stuttering in children: A preliminary report. *Journal of Speech and Hearing Research, 35*, 755–760.

Yairi, E., & Ambrose, N. (1992b). Onset of stuttering in preschool children: Selected factors. *Journal of Speech and Hearing Research, 35*, 782–788.

Yairi, E., & Ambrose, N. G. (1999a). Early childhood stuttering I: Persistency and recovery rates. *Journal of Speech, Language, and Hearing Research, 42*, 1097–1112.

Yairi, E., & Ambrose, N. (1999b). Spontaneous recovery and clinical trials research in early childhood stuttering: A response to Onslow and Packman (1999). *Journal of Speech, Language, and Hearing Research, 42*, 402–410.

Yairi, E., & Ambrose, N. G. (2001). Longitudinal studies of childhood stuttering: Evaluation of critiques. *Journal of Speech, Language, and Hearing Research, 44*, 867–872.

Yairi, E., & Ambrose, N. G. (2002). Evidence for genetic etiology in stuttering. *Perspectives, 12*(2), 10–15.

Yairi, E., Ambrose, N., & Cox, N. (1996). Genetics of stuttering: A critical review. *Journal of Speech and Hearing Research, 39*, 771–784.

Yairi, E., Ambrose, N. G., & Niermann, R. (1993). The early months of stuttering: A developmental study. *Journal of Speech and Hearing Research, 36*, 521–528.

Yairi, E., Ambrose, N. G., Paden, E. P., & Throneburg, R. N. (1996). Predictive factors of persistence and recovery: Pathways of childhood stuttering. *Journal of Communication Disorders, 29*, 51–77.

Yairi, E., & Carrico, D. M. (1992). Early childhood: Pediatricians' attitudes and practices. *American Journal of Speech–Language Pathology, 1*(3), 54–62.

Yairi, E., & Clifton, N. F. (1972). Disfluent speech behavior of preschool children, high school seniors, and geriatric persons. *Journal of Speech and Hearing Research, 15*, 714–719.

Yairi, E., & Curlee, R. (1997). The clinical–research connection in early childhood stuttering. *American Journal of Speech–Language Pathology, 6*(4), 85–86.

Yairi, E., Gintautas, J., & Avent, J. (1981). Disfluent speech associated with brain damage. *Brain and Language, 14*, 49–56.

Yairi, E., & Hall, K. D. (1993). Temporal relations within repetitions of preschool children near the onset of stuttering: A preliminary report. *Journal of Communication Disorders, 26*, 231–244.

Yairi, E., & Jennings, S. M. (1974). Relationship between the disfluent speech behavior of normal-speaking preschool boys and their parents. *Journal of Speech and Hearing Research, 17*, 94–98.

Yairi, E., & Lewis, B. (1984). Disfluencies at the onset of stuttering. *Journal of Speech and Hearing Research, 27*, 154–159.

Yairi, E., Watkins, R., Ambrose, N., & Paden, E. (2001). What is stuttering? *Journal of Speech, Language, and Hearing Research, 44*, 585–592.

Yairi, E., & Williams, D. E. (1970). Speech clinicians' stereotypes of elementary school boys who stutter. *Journal of Communication Disorders, 3*, 161–170.

Yairi, E., & Williams, D. E. (1971). Reports of parental attitudes by stuttering and by nonstuttering children. *Journal of Speech and Hearing Research, 14*, 596–604.

Yaruss, J. S. (1997). Clinical implications of situational variability in preschool children who stutter. *Journal of Fluency Disorders, 22,* 187–203.

Yaruss, J. S. (1999). Utterance length, syntactic complexity, and childhood stuttering. *Journal of Speech, Language and Hearing Research, 42,* 329–344.

Yaruss, J. S., & Conture, E. G. (1993). F2 transitions during sound/syllable repetitions of children who stutter and predictions of stuttering chronicity. *Journal of Speech and Hearing Research, 36,* 883–896.

Yaruss, J. S., & Conture, E. G. (1996). Stuttering and phonological disorders in children: Examination of the covert repair hypothesis. *Journal of Speech and Hearing Research, 39,* 349–364.

Yaruss, J. S., LaSalle, L. R., & Conture, E. G. (1998). Evaluating stuttering in young children: Diagnosing data. *American Journal of Speech–Language Pathology, 7*(4), 62–76.

Yaruss, J. S., & Quesal, R. (2004). Stuttering and the International Classification of Functioning, Disability, and Health (ICF): An update. *Journal of Communication Disorders, 37*(1), 35–52.

Young, E., & Hawk, S. (1955). *Moto-kinesthetic speech training.* Stanford, CA: Stanford University.

Young, M. A. (1975). Onset, prevalence, and recovery from stuttering. *Journal of Speech and Hearing Disorders, 40,* 49–58.

Young, M. A. (1984). Identification of stuttering and stutterers. In R. F. Curlee & W. H. Perkins (Eds.), *Nature and treatment of stuttering: New directions* (pp. 13–30). San Diego, CA: College-Hill.

Zebrowski, P. M. (1991). Duration of speech disfluencies of beginning stutterers. *Journal of Speech and Hearing Research, 34,* 483–491.

Zebrowski, P. M. (1994). Duration of sound prolongation and sound/syllable repetition in children who stutter: Preliminary observations. *Journal of Speech and Hearing Research, 37,* 254–263.

Zebrowski, P. M. (1997). Assisting young children who stutter and their families: Defining the role of the speech–language pathologist. *American Journal of Speech–Language Pathology, 6*(2), 19–28.

Zebrowski, P. M., & Conture, E. G. (1989). Judgment of disfluency by mothers of stuttering and normally fluent children. *Journal of Speech and Hearing Research, 32,* 625–634.

Zebrowski, P. M., Conture, E. G., & Cudahy, E. A. (1985). Acoustic analysis of young stutterers' fluency: Preliminary observations. *Journal of Fluency Disorders, 10,* 173–192.

Zebrowski, P. M., Moon, J., & Robin, D. (1997). Visuomotor tracking abilities of stuttering and nonstuttering children. In H. W. Hulstijn, H. F. M. Peters, & P. H. H. M. Van Lieshout (Eds.), *Speech production: Motor control, brain research, and fluency disorders—Proceedings of the 3rd International Conference on Speech Motor Production and Fluency Disorders* (pp. 579–584). Amsterdam, The Netherlands: Elsevier.

Zebrowski, P. M., & Schum, R. (1993). Counseling parents of children who stutter. *American Journal of Speech–Language Pathology, 2*(2), 65–73.

Zebrowski, P. M., Weiss, A., Savelkoul, E., & Hammer, C. (1996). The effect of maternal rate reduction on the speech rates and linguistic productions of children who stutter: Evidence from individual dyads. *Clinical Linguistics and Phonetics, 10,* 189–206.

Zimmermann, G. (1980a). Articulatory behaviors associated with stuttering: A cinefluorographic analysis. *Journal of Speech and Hearing Research, 23,* 108–121.

Zimmermann, G. (1980b). Stuttering: A disorder of movement. *Journal of Speech and Hearing Research, 23,* 122–126.

Zimmerman, I., Steiner, V., & Pond, R. (1979). *Preschool Language Scale.* San Antonio, TX: Psychological Corp.

Zwitman, D. (1978). *The disfluent child.* Baltimore: University Park.

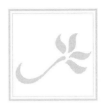

Index

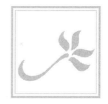

About the Authors

Ehud Yairi, PhD, CCC-SLP, received his BA from Tel Aviv University, Israel, in psychology and African studies, and his MA and PhD in speech–language pathology and audiology from the University of Iowa. Professor Yairi has been with the Department of Speech and Hearing Science at the University of Illinois at Urbana-Champaign since 1977. Currently his research centers on the onset and development of early childhood stuttering, including speech and nonspeech characteristics, and genetic aspects. Yairi is a recipient of the King James McCristal Distinguished Scholar Award from the University of Illinois, the Distinguished Alumnus Award from the University of Iowa Department of Speech Pathology and Audiology, the Researcher Award of Distinction from the International Fluency Association, and the Honors of the Association from the American Speech-Language-Hearing Association.

Nicoline Grinager Ambrose, PhD, CCC-SLP, received her BA in anthropology from the University of Massachusetts, an MA in linguistics from the University of California at Berkeley, and an MA and PhD in speech and hearing science from the University of Illinois at Urbana-Champaign. Professor Ambrose has been with the Department of Speech and Hearing Science at the University of Illinois since 1989. Her primary scientific interests include early childhood stuttering, genetics, and the evolution of human communication.